Handbook of Ocular Drug Therapy and Ocular Side Effects of Systemic Drugs

WILLIAM M. DELL, O.D., M.P.H.

Handbook of Ocular Drug Therapy and Ocular Side Effects of Systemic Drugs

Deborah Pavan-Langston, M.D., F.A.C.S.

Associate Professor of Ophthalmology, Harvard Medical School; Senior Scientist, Eye Research Institute; Surgeon, Massachusetts Eye and Ear Infirmary, Boston

and

Edmund C. Dunkel, Ph.D.

Assistant Professor of Ophthalmology, Harvard Medical School; Associate Scientist, Eye Research Institute, Boston

Little, Brown and Company
Boston/Toronto/London

Library of Congress Catalog Card No. 90-61769

ISBN 0-316-69545-9

Printed in the United States of America

RRD-VA

To Tao, Wyndy, Johanna, Sam, and Willie

Contents

Preface

With the rapid proliferation of varied pharmacologic approaches both to ocular and systemic disease in the last decade, it has become increasingly difficult for the practicing health professional to stay abreast of the plethora of new information. In response to the need for a concise and practical guide for well-informed, often daily decisions involving the visual system, we have put together two books in one.

Part I, Ocular Drug Therapy, presents succinct synopses of the pharmacologic agents used in a wide variety of ocular procedures or in afflictions such as bacterial, viral, fungal, and parasitic infections, immune and inflammatory diseases, allergic states, and the glaucomas. Discussions include clinical indications, mechanisms of drug action, local and systemic side effects, contraindications, and dosages (topical, systemic, intravitreal, subconjunctival), as well as a succinct presentation of the clinical management of the individual disease states themselves. The FDA status of drug use in the various situations is so indicated.

Information is presented both in tabular and text outline format for rapid retrieval of data on an extensive list of drugs. Included are not only current uses of older drugs such as carbachol or corticosteroids, but the latest developments in use of new ocular therapeutic agents such as third-generation cephalosporins, fifth-generation penicillins, ganciclovir and AZT, apraclonidine, propamidine, cyclophosphamide and other immunosuppressives, nonsteroidal anti-inflammatory drugs, cromolyn, natamycin, and flucytosine. The advantages and limitations of each are reviewed in detail, and recommended doses for adults and, where indicated, children and infants are clearly delineated. At the end of each chapter is the list of references from which information in the text was taken, as well as additional selected resources indicating material covered in each. Extensive indexes further assist the reader in rapid information retrieval, whether by drug or disease.

Part II, Ocular Side Effects of Systemic Drugs, is the tabular presentation of an area of rapidly expanding information crucial to the safe and informed use of the older and the newest drugs alike. The tables are organized alphabetically by therapeutic use (e.g., "Cardiovascular Agents—Vasodilators"), the drugs listed generically and alphabetically within, and under chemical family, if pertinent. For most convenient information access, the side effects are organized under ocular anatomic location or by visual symptoms. In those instances where only the commercial but not the generic drug name is known to the practitioner, the reader may refer to the extensive Part II Index of drug proprietary names following the tables. These names are listed in alphabetical order; proprietary names are followed by their generic names, so that they can be located in the tables. This system is, in turn, backed up by the Part I Index.

The information included in this book is based not only on the most current literature but on two decades of experience in patient care and in teaching medical students, residents, fellows, other physicians, and a wide variety of health care practitioners. It is a practical approach to knowledge needed by the practitioner for the most efficacious and safest care of the patient.

D.P.-L.
E.C.D.

Acknowledgments

The authors are forever grateful to the hard-driving, highly accurate, and always good-humored Leona Greenhill, Chief of Editorial Services at the Eye Research Institute. She and her skilled assistants, Ava Bell and Margie Leak, kept us on the move and on schedule. We are also indebted to the expert and kindly editorial guidance of Susan Pioli, Senior Medical Editor at Little, Brown and Company. Last, but not least, we thank Mary Lou Moar, Administrative Assistant at the Massachusetts Eye and Ear Infirmary, and Patricia Geary, Research Associate at the Eye Research Institute, for their gentle prodding and inestimable patience as we worked to bring this project to fruition.

Ocular Drug Therapy

Notice

The indications and dosages of all drugs in this book have been recommended in the medical literature and conform to the practices of the general medical community. The medications described do not necessarily have specific approval by the Food and Drug Administration for use in the diseases and dosages for which they are recommended. The package insert for each drug should be consulted for use and dosage as approved by the FDA. Because standards for usage change, it is advisable to keep abreast of revised recommendations, particularly those concerning new drugs.

Pharmacokinetics of Ophthalmic Drug Administration

Effective therapy of ocular disease relies in large part on a correct diagnosis based on an understanding of the pathophysiology of a given disorder. Of equal importance, however, is sufficient knowledge of the available therapeutic agents to make a rational and judicious decision in determining appropriate treatment. This knowledge includes not only drug actions and dosages, but also adverse reactions, precautions, and contraindications.

The vast majority of medications prescribed today are potent chemicals with as much capability for harm as for relief of disease. A brief review of the pharmacokinetics of ophthalmic drugs and reasons for therapeutic failure may avoid many of the negative aspects of therapy.

I. Factors in Pharmacokinetics

The pharmacokinetics of ocular therapy depend on drug concentration, frequency of administration, and route of administration.

A. **Eye drops** should be no larger than 20 μl (the usual drop size from a dropper bottle or standard eye dropper). Given the anatomic considerations of drug flow from the tear meniscus down the lacrimal puncta to the nasopharynx, two rapid-succession drops, or a drop larger than standard, will stimulate excess tearing through irritation, and thus dilute dosage. By sheer volume, the drug–tear mix will either spill over the lid margin or be washed down the puncta as a function of increased lacrimation. Reflex stimulation from a single drop requires 5 minutes to subside, and the maximum volume accommodated by the lids and tear film is 30 μl. Therefore, to achieve maximum therapeutic effect, a second drop of the same or a different medication should not be given sooner than 5 minutes after the first drop. The penetration of any drug is enhanced in the presence of unhealthy, irregular, or ulcerated epithelium.

B. **Antibiotic ointments** have a longer duration of action than drops, but usually do not provide full therapeutic coverage overnight unless reinstilled every few hours. Like eye drops, ointments are cleared from the eye via the lacrimal drainage system. The physiologic turnover rate of tears is approximately 16% per minute, but drugs in ointment form turn over at a rate of approximately 0.5% per minute. Although ointments have the advantage of less-frequent administration than drops, they cannot achieve as high tissue-drug concentrations as frequent eye drops (every 30 minutes to 1 hour when such intensive therapy is required). In addition, fortified (extremely high concentration) antibiotics are not available in ointment form unless made up by special request in hospital pharmacies. Fortified drops can be formulated easily and can achieve even better results. Corneal and intraocular penetration of tetracycline, fluorescein, and pilocarpine is significantly higher as an ointment than as an eye drop, but these are exceptions to the rule, and eye drops should be the form of choice when intensive therapy is required. In routine therapy, however, there is no question that an antibiotic ointment maintains the desired therapeutic levels in the tears and in some cases in the aqueous humor for 2–4 hours; in drop form the duration of therapeutic levels may be only 20–30 minutes, thereby requiring more frequent application.

C. **Topical drug vehicle selection.** Although ointments have the advantage of less frequent administration and of lubricating unhealthy epithelium, they also may act as a mechanical barrier to the instillation and penetration of concomitant eye drop therapy. Patients should be instructed to administer eye drops before instilling ointment, or they will effectively block the instillation of the drug solution form. Some patients will not tolerate an ointment because of the blurring of vision and deposition on the eyelids, with subsequent discomfort and undesirable cosmetic appearance. To assure better patient compliance, the physician may select the drug form based on the patient's visual requirements and preference for a more frequent drop over a less frequent ointment.

D. **Subconjunctival injection** of drug has the advantage of extremely rapid delivery of high levels of drug to the anterior segment of the eye. Therapeutic drug levels of non-depot forms persist 3–6 hours after injection, and then taper over the ensuing 24 hours. The use of subconjunctival administration is **decreasing** for several reasons: (1) studies have shown that similar therapeutic drug levels may be maintained in the cornea and anterior chamber with frequent topical fortified drops; (2) subconjunctival injection often is painful, even when used with local anesthetic; and (3) repeating the injection is often difficult and inconvenient for both patient and physician. Subconjunctival injection is largely reserved for use in a deeply infiltrating corneal infection, when high drug levels are desired quickly, when fortified topical antibiotic drops are not available, or where patient compliance is poor. Many cataract surgeons routinely give subconjunctival antibiotic and steroid at the end of the surgical procedure. There appears to be no difference between the incidence of endophthalmitis in patients receiving such injections and those who do not. The therapy of endophthalmitis itself, however, usually involves subconjunctival injection at the time of vitrectomy accompanied by intravitreal injection of antibiotic and steroid. Even in these cases, subsequent subconjunctival injection is rarely used, the routes of choice being intravenous and topical administration of drug.

E. The **systemic administration** of drugs, either orally or intravenously, delivers fairly low corneal concentrations, but often therapeutically useful intraocular drug levels. As a result, intravenous antibiotic therapy is used frequently in the management of a perforated, infected corneal ulcer, extension of corneal disease to sclera, or a traumatic perforation of the eye, as well as in globe-threatening infections such as those caused by *Neisseria* or *Hemophilus* endophthalmitis and, of course, in the life-threatening situation of orbital cellulitis. Systemic steroids are also administered orally or intravenously in selected patients to combat damage secondary to intraocular inflammation.

II. When the Patient Fails to Respond to Treatment

Unfortunately, despite the most judicious and well-informed therapeutic regimen, a few patients fail to respond adequately to therapy. Should this be the case, the physician should reassess the situation and review the following possible causes of therapeutic failure.

A. Drug factors

1. **Timing.** Therapy may not have been initiated in sufficient time to reverse the effects of rampant infection or inflammation.
2. **Dosage.** Despite the best-recommended drug dosages for a given disease, this dosage may be suboptimal.
3. **Wrong drug.** An infecting organism or inflammatory reaction may not be sensitive to the particular drug selected.
4. **Resistance.** The metabolic state of an infecting agent may change, and the microorganism may develop resistance to the drug in use.
5. **Tissue inaccessibility.** The chemical nature of the drug itself may interfere with appropriate delivery. For example, a relatively hydrophilic drug will penetrate the eye poorly, whereas a lipophilic or, better yet, a bipolar drug such as timolol will penetrate both epithelial and stromal layers much more effectively.
6. **Antagonism.** Interdrug antagonism may be operating, such as noted when chloramphenicol or tetracyclines are used concomitantly with any of the penicillins. Sulfonamides are inactivated by aminobenzoic acid in the presence of purulent material. Ocular variations in pH may alter drug activity.

B. Patient factors

1. **Poor compliance,** probably the most common cause of therapeutic failure.
2. **Impairment** of the patient's **immune** system.
3. **Environment.** Any adverse effects caused by environmental factors, e.g., chemical irritants or pollutants.
4. **Pre-existing disease.** Concomitant ocular disease such as dry eyes or chronic intermittent obstruction of the nasolacrimal drain may contribute to poor therapeutic response.

   Having reassessed all of these factors, the physician will frequently be able to pinpoint the source(s) of therapeutic failure and adjust the regimen accordingly.

Information Sources and Suggested Reading (*Pharmacokinetics*)

1. Benet, L., and Sheiner, L., Pharmacokinetics: The dynamics of drug absorption, distribution, and elimination. In Gilman, A.G., Goodman, L.S., Rall, T., and Murad, F. (Eds.), *The Pharmacological Basis of Therapeutics,* 7th ed. New York: Macmillan, 1985, pp. 3–34.
2. Gilman A.G., Goodman, L.S., Rall, T., and Murad, F. (Eds.), *The Pharmacological Basis of Therapeutics,* 7th ed. New York: Macmillan, 1985, pp. 3–35 (pharmaco-kinetics and dynamics).
3. Maurice, D.M., and Mishima, S., Ocular pharmacokinetics. In Sears, M.L. (Ed.), *Pharmacology of the Eye,* vol. 69, Handbook of Experimental Pharmacology. New York: Springer-Verlag, 1984, pp. 19–116.
4. Palmer, E., How safe are ocular drugs in pediatrics? Ophthalmology 93:1038–1040, 1986.
5. Ross, E., and Gilman, A.G., Pharmacodynamics: mechanisms of drug action and the relationship between drug concentration and effect. In Gilman, A.G., Goodman, L.S., Rall, T., and Murad, F. (Eds.), *The Pharmacological Basis of Therapeutics,* 7th ed. New York: Macmillan, 1985, pp. 35–48.
6. Shichi, H., Biotransformation and drug metabolism. In Sears, M.L. (Ed.), *Pharmacology of the Eye,* vol. 69. Heidelberg: Springer-Verlag, 1984, pp. 117–148.

2

Anti-Allergy Agents and Ocular Decongestants

I. Ocular Allergy

A. Predisposing factors and general clinical manifestations.

Because nearly 20% of the American population has at least one allergic condition, ocular allergy is a problem frequently seen in the ophthalmologist's office. It is commonly familial, with early onset being associated with more severe and long-lasting disease. Approximately 75% of asthmatic and hay fever patients have positive family histories for the same or some other atopy.

Although the immunologic basis for many diseases classified as ocular allergy is weak, three characteristics are common to all ocular allergic conditions: **chronicity, inflammation,** and **fluctuating recurrences.** The hallmarks of hyperemia, pain, itching, swelling, and warmth characterize the inflammatory component of these diseases. They tend to last for several weeks to months, and follow a waxing and waning course regardless of whether therapy is given. Hay fever conjunctivitis is the only condition proven to be a true allergic state. This extremely common ocular atopy is manifested by itching, redness, and swelling of the lids and conjunctiva, and is most often precipitated on a seasonal basis by exposure to airborne substances such as pollen, grasses, weeds, molds, dust, and animal dander. Hay fever conjunctivitis may or may not be associated with the major atopies of seasonal rhinitis (hay fever), chronic rhinitis with or without nasal polyps, bronchial asthma, and eczema. The minor atopies that may also be associated with the ocular reaction are food allergies, urticaria, nonhereditary angioedema, and some forms of chronic allergic bronchitis.

B. Mechanisms of disease

1. **Mast cell degranulation** is probably the most important event in the ocular allergic reaction. Mast cells, which have up to 500,000 gamma E immunoglobulin (IgE) receptors on their surface membranes, are located in the skin and mucous membranes and around venules. The specific binding of an antigen to two IgE antibodies on the mast cell receptors induces two events leading to degranulation: a rapid rise in cyclic adenosine monophosphate (cAMP), and Ca^{2+} influx into the mast cell. Both events contribute to the subsequent granule swelling, migration to and fusion with the mast cell membrane, and release of the chemical mediators of allergic reaction—histamine, leukotrienes, eosinophil chemotactic factor, prostaglandins, serotonin, and heparin. High cAMP levels appear to yield a negative feedback, resulting in inhibition of additional mediator release. Non-IgE inducers of degranulation include IgG, the cationic compounds polymyxin F and morphine, and ionophores that induce elevated intraocular Ca^{2+} levels.

2. **Anatomic distribution of mast cells.** The eye has a wealth of mast cells, with the greatest number being in the lid, followed by tarsal conjunctiva, orbit, bulbar conjunctiva, and, in lower but significant numbers, episclera, limbal tissues, orbital nerves, choroid, and ciliary body. There are no mast cells in the iris, despite their presence in other uveal structures, and none in the cornea, retina, or optic nerve. Because of the vastly greater number of mast cells in the lids and conjunctiva, ocular allergic reaction is manifested primarily in these structures, with the most adverse symptoms induced by histamine (itching, conjunctival vasodilation), the leukotriene slow-reacting substance of anaphylaxis (SRS-A, increased vascular permeability), and various prostaglandins (stimulation of mucus secretion, neutrophil chemotaxis, and increased capillary permeability). Increased levels of all three mediator groups have been documented in the tear film of patients with vernal conjunctivitis, contact lens-associated giant papillary conjunctivitis, hay fever conjunctivitis, and other ocular inflammatory conditions.

C. **General therapeutic considerations.** Therapy of ocular allergic disease includes minimizing exposure to the offending allergen, inhibition of the chemical mediators released, and mast cell stabilization. The first factor is achieved by repeated careful history-taking; the second and third, by topical antihistamine-decongestants and mast cell stabilizers, respectively, either treatment being given with or without the other or with adjunctive topical or systemic steroidal or nonsteroidal agents as needed.

1. **Initial pharmacologic measures** include local symptomatic relief by the use of vasoconstrictive drops, such as naphazoline or phenylephrine with topical antihistamines. In the presence of conjunctival swelling, frequent use of artificial tears will enhance stabilization of the tear film and corneal wetting with washout of the offending antigen. In milder cases and especially in hay fever conjunctivitis, topical corticosteroids should be avoided, as the risks often outweigh the benefits. However, if the cornea becomes involved in a true atopic keratoconjunctivitis, 0.1% dexamethasone or 1% prednisolone 2–4 times daily should be started, rapidly tapered toward ⅛% prednisolone, and then, if possible, discontinued as the therapeutic effect is achieved. The mast cell stabilizers, cromolyn and ketotifen, are relatively new drugs that may offer sufficient symptomatic control so that steroids may be avoided or used in significantly lower doses. Ketotifen is not yet available in the United States.

2. **Supportive measures.** In addition to topical therapy, patients often require supportive treatment: cold compresses 4–5 times daily to decrease itching, and oral antihistamines. The latter's action may be enhanced by the addition of 600 mg of aspirin daily for patients with severe itching.

II. Specific Pharmacologic Agents

Cromolyn, antihistamine-decongestants, single decongestants, steroidal and nonsteroidal anti-inflammatory drugs (NSAIDs), and systemic antihistamines will be discussed before review of the diagnosis and management of specific ocular allergic conditions.

A. Mast cell stabilizers

1. Cromolyn sodium

a. **Pharmacology and mechanism of action.** Cromolyn sodium, or disodium cromoglycate (DSCG), is made up of two chromone rings joined by a flexible carbon chain, each ring possessing a polar carboxyl group. The precise mechanism of action is unclear, but it is known that DSCG inhibits the enzyme phosphodiesterase, resulting in increased intracellular cAMP. This, in turn, reduces Ca^{2+} transport across the mast cell membrane, thus stabilizing the cell and preventing the intracellular calcium rise necessary for degranulation. Cromolyn sodium has no intrinsic vasoconstrictor, antihistaminic, or anti-inflammatory action, but its effective use may obviate the need for such adjunctive drug therapy. In humans, the drug acts only on the ocular, nasal, and bronchial mucosa. As it is poorly absorbed from the gastrointestinal tract, it must be administered topically to the eye or as an inhalant for nasal congestion or bronchial asthma. It is not metabolized, but excreted intact in bile and urine.

b. **Ocular indications and use.** Cromolyn sodium is indicated for therapy of certain ocular allergies included in the terms vernal keratoconjunctivitis, vernal conjunctivitis, giant papillary conjunctivitis (GPC), contact lens GPC, vernal keratitis, allergic keratoconjunctivitis, and possibly ligneous conjunctivitis. Patients with atopy and elevated IgE levels are more responsive than those with ocular findings alone. The usual dosage is 4% cromolyn sodium 4–6 times daily. The anticipated symptomatic response to therapy—reduced itching, tearing, redness, and discharge—usually occurs within a few days, but occasionally may take up to 6 weeks. Therapy should be continuous, not intermittent, and maintained after symptomatic improvement for as long as necessary to sustain that improvement. It is often advisable to initiate therapy well before the onset of allergic disease, as patients head into an adverse season, thereby achieving early control over the reaction. Soft contact lens wearers should not use their lenses while under treatment, but may reinstitute their use several hours after discontinuation of the drug. The drug is commercially available in the United States as Opticrom.

c. **Precautions and adverse side effects.** Carcinogenesis, mutagenesis, and impairment of fertility have not been demonstrated in laboratory studies investigating these parameters. There is no known effect on pregnancy in laboratory animals, but no adequately controlled human studies have been done. It is also not known whether the drug is excreted in human milk. Safety and efficacy of this drug have not been conclusively established in children below the age of 4 years. The drug should not be used in any patient with known cromolyn hypersensitivity.

Transient ocular stinging or burning on instillation may occur, and bulbar conjunctival hyperemia and chemosis may develop in up to ⅓ of patients. Less well-established adverse reactions—conjunctival injection, watery eyes, itchy eyes, periocular dryness, puffy eyes, eye irritation, and styes—have been reported, but are not known to be directly attributable to the drug.

2. **Ketotifen** (Zaditen) is a mast cell stabilizer that works by calcium antagonism, thus blocking the rise in intracellular Ca^{2+} necessary for granule swelling. It is in clinical use outside the United States for prophylaxis of atopic disease and asthma. Ketotifen is currently under investigation in the United States for ocular use, and is of particular interest because of its excellent systemic absorption after oral administration.

B. **Antihistamine-decongestant combinations**
1. **Histamine action.** Histamine is released during acute allergic or inflammatory reactions from mast cells, basophils, and platelets. It exerts its action by binding to histamine receptor sites, classified as H_1 or H_2, found on cell membranes in organ systems throughout the body. In the eye and periocular tissues, H_1 receptor stimulation results in itching and mild conjunctival hyperemia, and H_2 receptor stimulation results in diffuse, more intense conjunctival and lid vasodilation and edema.

2. **Antihistamines.** Histamine blockers, or antihistamines, are also classified by the receptor sites H_1 and H_2. Currently only three H_1 blockers are commercially available for topical use in the eye: pheniramine maleate, antazoline phosphate, and pyrilamine maleate. No topical H_2 blockers are FDA approved for ocular use, although oral **cimetidine,** an H_2 blocker used to treat gastric ulcers, is useful as adjuvant therapy in the acute inflammatory stages of herpes zoster ophthalmicus (see Chap. 7, Antiviral Drugs).

a. **Pharmacology and mechanism of action.** The ocular preparations are in two of the five classes of H_1 antihistamines: the alkylamine **pheniramine maleate,** and the ethylenediamines **antazoline phosphate** and **pyrilamine maleate.** The mechanism of action is a reversible blocking of the histamine receptor sites on susceptible tissues. Antihistamines do not prevent the release of histamine from inflammatory cells, only its action on target sites after it has been released.

b. **Indications and dosage.** Topical antihistamines are most useful in controlling the manifestations of mild to moderate ocular allergy such as hay fever or mild vernal conjunctivitis. By blocking histamine-induced, increased capillary permeability, they inhibit tissue edema, flare, and itch. Many H_1 blockers have a local anesthetic effect by blocking histamine receptors on nerve endings. This occurs, however, only at doses much higher than needed for therapeutic efficacy in allergic conditions. In more severe allergic disease, such as vernal or contact lens-associated GPC, topical antihistamines are useful adjuncts to mast cell stabilizers, corticosteroids, NSAIDs, and oral antihistamines. As histamine is not a component of microbial or contact hypersensitivity reactions, antihistamines are not indicated in their treatment.

(1) **Topical** ocular **antihistamines** are currently available only in combination with the **decongestants** 0.05% or 0.025% **naphazoline HCl**, 0.05% or 0.025% **tetrahydrozoline HCl**, or 0.12%–0.125% **phenylephrine HCl.** These latter drugs are sympathomimetics that induce vasoconstriction, thus whitening the eye and enhancing comfort. The decongestants are available also as single agents (see below). Table 2-1 lists the available antihistamine-decongestant combinations. Dosage is commonly 1–2 drops 2–4 times daily.

(2) **Oral antihistamines** of particular use in ocular allergic conditions include the ethanolamine **diphenhydramine** 25–50 mg po tid to qid, the ethylenediamine **tripelennamine** 25–50 mg po q4–6h, and the piperazine **hydroxy-**

Table 2-1. Antihistamine-decongestant combinations

Generic name	Commercial preparations*	Recommended dosage
Antazoline PO$_4$ (0.5%) Naphazoline HCl (0.05%)	Albalon A Vasocon A	1–2 drops/eye q3–4h or less to relieve symptoms
Pheniramine maleate (0.3%) Naphazoline HCl (0.025%)	AK-Con A Opcon A Naphcon A	1–2 drops/eye q3–4h or less to relieve symptoms
Pyrilamine maleate (0.1%) Phenylephrine (0.12%)	Prefrin-A	1–2 drops/eye q3–4h or less to relieve symptoms

* Prescription required for all preparations listed.

zine HCl, 25 mg po tid. Sustained-release **chlorpheniramine** 8–10 mg q12h or **triprolidine** 2.5 mg (with pseudoephedrine) q8h also may offer relief. If sedation is excessive with use of these drugs, alternatives include slow-release **brompheniramine** 12 mg q8h, **terfenadine** 60 mg bid to tid, or **phenindamine** 25 mg q4h. All oral antihistamines are available as single agents or in combination with decongestants.

c. **Precautions and adverse side effects**

(1) **Topical antihistamines.** Although undesirable side effects of topical antihistamines are rare, these drugs are available only in combination with sympathomimetic decongestants, thus necessitating the following warnings concerning use of these drug combinations. Contraindications include hypersensitivity to any component of the combination drug. Because of potential induced mydriasis by either the antihistamine or decongestant, these drugs should not be used in the presence of untreated narrow-angle glaucoma. Patients using monoaminoxidase inhibitors may suffer severe hypertensive crisis if given sympathomimetic drugs such as naphazoline. Use in young children may cause CNS depression, leading to coma and hypothermia.

Because of potential systemic vasoconstriction, topical antihistamines should be used with caution in older patients with severe cardiovascular disease including arrhythmia, poorly controlled hypertension, or brittle diabetes. Carcinogenesis, mutagenesis, impairment of fertility and pregnancy, and effect on pregnancy and nursing mothers have not been evaluated with respect to safety and efficacy of all combination drugs, but systemic piperazines have induced experimental teratogenesis.

Pupillary dilation, increase or decrease in intraocular pressure, and mild transient stinging, burning, tearing, or diffuse epithelial haze may be noted. Systemic effects are very rare; they include lightheadedness, hyperglycemia, hypothermia, weakness, nausea, nervousness, anaphylaxis, and drowsiness.

(2) **Oral antihistamines** commonly cause variable levels of sedation that may be sufficiently severe to necessitate cessation of the drug. They also have an atropinic effect in inducing dry eyes, which may cause contact lens intolerance or keratoconjunctivitis sicca as well as pupillary mydriasis. In untreated, predisposed individuals, the mydriasis potentially may precipitate acute angle-closure glaucoma. This latter reaction is very rarely if ever seen, and a major

study on the use of oral nasal decongestants in the presence of narrow angles was unable to prove that these drugs actually induce angle narrowing, mydriasis, or elevated intraocular pressure. Other ocular or visual system side effects include blurred vision secondary to ciliary muscle paresis and decreased accommodation and, in overdosage, visual hallucinations, pupillary paralysis, and temporary blindness.

Other systemic side effects related to the gastrointestinal tract may be minimized by ingestion of the pills with meals. The symptoms include anorexia, nausea, vomiting, and constipation or diarrhea. Central nervous system effects include dizziness, fatigue, tinnitus, loss of coordination, euphoria, insomnia, and tremulousness.

As noted under topical combinations, the piperazines may induce teratogenesis. Safety in pregnancy has not been established for the systemic antihistamines.

C. Single-agent decongestants. These sympathomimetic vasoconstrictors may be therapeutically effective when used alone for mild, nonspecific ocular irritation or allergy. Available agents are listed in Table 2-2. Because these agents are sympathomimetics, precautions and adverse side effects are similar to those noted under antihistamine-decongestant combinations.

D. Corticosteroids. These drugs include, in increasing order of potency, the ocular topical agents **fluoromethalone** (0.1–1.0% FML), **prednisolone** (⅛ or 1%), and **dexamethasone** (0.1%). They induce the formation of the cell surface proteins lipomodulin or macrocortin, thereby inhibiting transmembrane phospholipase A_2 necessary for formation of leukotriene SRS-A and prostaglandins. Topical corticosteroids, like the systemic nonsteroidals and antihistamines, are used in the more recalcitrant cases of ocular allergy and particularly if the cornea is involved. Dose frequencies are 2–6 times daily in a potency warranted by the extent of ocular disease and slowly tapered to maintenance levels over several weeks. Systemic steroids are of little or no use in ocular allergy, but ointments such as 0.05% dexamethasone or 0.1% fluoromethalone ocular preparation 2–3 times daily may reduce disease manifestations more rapidly than drops alone. However, these drugs interfere with wound healing, and their use in breaking the itch–scratch reaction may ultimately be limited if the lids macerate in an atopic patient.

Corticosteroids are discussed in greater detail in Chap. 8 on intraocular inflammation and immune disease of the eye.

E. Nonsteroidal anti-inflammatory agents (NSAIDs). **Aspirin, diflunisal** (Dolobid) 500 mg po q12h, **naproxen** (Naprosyn) 250-500 mg po q12h, and **indomethacin** (Indocin) 25 mg po tid are the most effective adjunctive drugs of this class in ocular inflammation and allergy. They

Table 2-2. Ocular decongestants, decongestant-astringents,* decongestant-antibacterials

Generic name	Commercial preparations (drops)	Usual recommended dosage (7–14 days)
Decongestants		
Naphazoline (0.12% [Rx]; 0.012% [OTC])	Albalon (Rx) Clear Eyes (OTC) Degest-2 (OTC) Opcon (Rx) Naphcon (OTC) Naphcon Forte (Rx) Vasoclear (OTC) Vasocon Regular (Rx)	1 drop/eye q3–4h or less to relieve symptoms
Phenylephrine (0.12%)	AK-nephrine (OTC) Prefrin (OTC) Relief (OTC)	1 drop/eye q3–4h or less to relieve symptoms
Tetrahydrozoline HCl (0.05%)	Collyrium (OTC) Murine PLUS (OTC) Visine (OTC)	1 drop/eye q3–4h or less to relieve symptoms
Decongestant-astringents		
Naphazoline (0.02%) Zinc SO$_4$ (0.25%)	Vasoclear A (OTC)	1–2 drops/eye up to 4 times daily
Phenylephrine HCl (0.12%) Zinc SO$_4$ (0.25%)	Visine AC (Rx)	1–2 drops/eye up to 4 times daily
Tetrahydrozoline HCl (0.05%) Zinc SO$_4$ (0.25%)	Zincfrin (Rx)	1–2 drops/eye up to 4 times daily
Decongestant-antibacterials		
Phenylephrine HCl (0.12%) Sulfacetamide Na (15%)	Vasosulf (Rx)	1–2 drops/eye q2–4h

OTC = over the counter; Rx = prescription required.
* Astringents (eg, ZnSO$_4$) precipitate protein, helping to clear mucus from the ocular surface.

inhibit conversion of arachidonic acid to prostaglandins by blocking the cyclo-oxygenase pathway. Of the listed drugs, aspirin 600 mg po qid has been the most useful in ocular allergic disease as adjunctive therapy in conditions resistant to combined topical therapies and systemic antihistamines. All NSAIDs should be taken with a meal or milk. The other nonsteroidal agents are discussed in greater detail in Chap. 8 with reference to intraocular inflammation and macular edema, as their role in ocular allergy has not been conclusively demonstrated.

III. **Specific Ocular Allergies** affect the conjunctiva so frequently as to make allergic conjunctivitis synonymous with ocular allergy. These allergies are classified into six clinical entities: **seasonal allergic conjunctivitis, perennial allergic conjunctivitis, vernal conjunctivitis, giant papillary conjunctivitis,** and **conjunctival contact allergy.**

A. **Seasonal and perennial allergic conjunctivitis (SAC and PAC),** otherwise known as hay fever, account for more than 50% of all cases of allergic conjunctivitis. The most common inciting antigens are grass pollens in the spring and ragweed pollen in late summer and fall, thus lending the seasonal quality to SAC.

1. **Clinical findings of SAC** include the symptoms of mildly hyperemic, itchy, watery eyes often associated with rhinitis or allergic pharyngitis. Ocular signs are often minimal, with mild lid edema, fine papillary hypertrophy on the conjunctival side of the lid, bulbar conjunctival vascular dilation, especially near the corneal limbus, and, in more severe cases, milky edema of the bulbar conjunctiva. Corneal involvement is rare.

2. Clinically, **PAC** is a less common and less severe form of SAC but tends to occur on a year-round basis because of the nonseasonal nature of the antigens, eg, dust, animal dander, molds, house mite feces, and certain foods. When PAC is exacerbated seasonally, it is often difficult to distinguish from SAC. The chronic symptoms of ocular itchiness and tearing in normal-appearing eyes often indicate a diagnosis of PAC as opposed to SAC, which has more obvious clinical findings.

3. **Conjunctival scrapings** reveal eosinophils in about ½ to ¾ of both SAC and PAC patients.

4. **Differential diagnosis** of SAC and PAC includes seborrheic or chronic blepharitis, contact allergies (eg, cosmetics), and conjunctivitis sicca. Allergy conjunctivitis may be differentiated from blepharitis or dry eyes by the frequent history of systemic allergies such as hay fever, eczema, and food allergies, ocular itching, fine papillary hypertrophy of the tarsal conjunctiva, and frequently eosinophils in conjunctival scrapings and elevated tear IgE levels. Contact allergies resolve with removal of the offending antigen.

5. **Treatment** of SAC and PAC are similar except for the seasonal component.

   a. **Remove offending antigen.** This approach is usually successful for dust, dander, house mites, and wool, but not for pollen allergy. Densensitization may be tried but is less successful for ocular allergy than for rhinitis. Because of the self-limited and usually annoying but benign nature of the disease, therapy is oriented primarily toward alleviating symptoms rather than attempted cure.

   b. **Cold compresses** applied as a clean, wet facecloth 5–10 minutes 3 times daily alleviate itching, burning, and some hyperemia via vasoconstriction and inhibition of the inflammatory response.

      c. Vasoconstrictors and antihistamines (see Tables 2-1 and 2-2) applied **topically** 3–5 times daily will alleviate many of the symptoms. Patient comfort may be further enhanced by use of **systemic antihistamines** such as chlorpheniramine 4 mg po bid to tid (Histamic), diphenhydramine HCl 25–50 mg po every day to bid (Benadryl), and terfenadine (Seldane) 60 mg po bid or tid, especially during acute exacerbation of disease. See Sec. **II.B.2.** for other systemic antihistamines. Systemic **side effects** include anticholinergic action such as sedation and dry mouth and eyes. Terfenadine appears to be the least offensive in terms of side effects.

      d. Cromolyn eye drops stabilize the ocular mast cells and frequently relieve ocular itching and burning. Clinical therapeutic effect may not be noted for 1–2 weeks after starting treatment. Patients are then often able to reduce or stop systemic antihistamines without exacerbation of symptoms. Cromolyn dosage is 4% drops 4–6 times daily **without omission** and is particularly effective during pollen and ragweed season when coupled with cromolyn nasal spray for allergic rhinitis.

      e. Corticosteroids are a last but not infrequent resort. They are extremely effective in relieving both signs and symptoms of ocular allergy. Because of potential adverse side effects such as glaucoma, cataract, and infection, however, corticosteroid use should be limited to short-term therapy to bring acute disease under control. Prednisolone 0.125% one drop 1–3 times daily with tapering off over 2 weeks should be sufficient in most cases.

      f. Oral immunotherapy is still a controversial approach despite reports that administration of enterosoluble birch-pollen capsules decreased ocular signs and symptoms of birch pollenosis.

B. Atopic keratoconjunctivitis (AKC) is a component of atopic dermatitis and frequently associated with other atopic illness such as eczema and asthma in either the patient or other family members. Unlike the dermatitis that is usually seen in the early years of life and largely resolves before the teen years, AKC appears in the late teens and early 20s, more often in men than women, peaks in incidence between the ages of 30 and 50 years, and then gradually recedes.

1. Clinical symptoms and signs include bilateral tearing, itching, and burning. The lids are red, swollen, and often macerated from chronic tearing and rubbing or from a superimposed staphylococcal infection. The bulbar conjunctiva is red and chemotic, and the palpebral conjunctiva manifests a papillary hypertrophy, worse on the lower lids than the upper (unlike vernal conjunctivitis). Corneal signs may be present in the form of punctate keratitis of the lower third of the cornea, neovascularization, ulcers, superficial nebulous scarring, and, rarely, Trantas' dots (limbal follicles).

2. **Differential diagosis** of AKC includes blepharitis and vernal keratoconjunctivitis. The association of other atopic disease such as asthma and the findings of intense itching, swelling, and lid maceration with or without corneal changes strongly suggest AKC over a chronic or acute seborrheic-staphylococcal blepharitis. The two diseases may coexist, however, and each requires its own appropriate therapy. Differentiation of AKC from vernal KC is aided by the fact that vernal occurs in younger patients, is seasonal, and is rarely associated with lid dermatitis, and the papillary hypertrophy predominates in the upper lid, as opposed to the lower lid in AKC.

3. **Associated conditions** include keratoconus, anterior and posterior subcapsular cataract, secondary lid inversion and punctal stenosis, and chronic recurrent herpes simplex keratitis, often bilateral and tending to persistent sterile epithelial defects after appropriate antiviral therapy.

4. **Treatment** of AKC, like SAC and PAC, involves the use of multiple drugs for optimal effect.

   a. **Lid hygiene** is extremely important both to treat and prevent secondary staphylococcal blepharitis and enhance drug delivery to the affected tissues. Patients should perform lid scrubs once or twice daily using baby shampoo diluted 50:50 in tepid water or a commercial lid scrub such as Ocu-soft or I-Scrub. Lathering the fingertips and then gently massaging the lid margins of the closed (not squeezed shut!) lids for 2 minutes before rinsing clean may be easier and more effective than the use of cotton balls or cotton-tip applicators. This should be followed by a 10-minute **cold wet compress** to alleviate itching, which may be intensified by the warm water used in the lid hygiene.

   b. **Topical corticosteroids** given over 1–3 weeks will alleviate both lid and conjunctival symptoms and signs. Common dosage is 0.125% prednisolone 2–4 times daily, with gradual taper and discontinuation. In the interim, other, more benign drugs, as noted below, may be instituted for long-term therapy. Short-term courses of steroids may have to be repeated periodically, however, for acute exacerbations despite use of other drugs. Use of the minimum steroid necessary to relieve the more severe aspects of the allergy should be the guiding rule. It is usually more effective to use low-dose steroid such as 0.125% prednisolone 4 times daily than 0.1% dexamethasone once daily, yet the total effective drug dosage is lower using the former regimen. Application of 0.05% dexamethasone or 0.1% fluoromethalone ophthalmic **ointment** to the lids once or twice daily for 2–6 weeks may reduce the need for drops to a lower frequency. Steroid ointment will ultimately thin the skin of the lids if usage is prolonged, thus worsening any maceration.

c. **Topical antihistamines** as listed in Table 2-1 will further alleviate itching and chemosis and, when coupled with a **vasoconstrictor,** relieve hyperemia as well. Dosage ranges from 2–4 times daily. Systemic antihistamines may have some beneficial effect, but side effects may outweigh the added benefit.

d. **Cromolyn** 4% eye drops 4–6 times daily will begin to alleviate both symptoms and signs of AKC after 10 days of treatment in about two thirds of patients so treated. Long-term maintenance therapy with qid drops reduces or eliminates the need for topical steroids and should be coupled with lid hygiene, cold compresses, and topical antihistamine-vasoconstrictors for maximum relief.

C. **Vernal keratoconjunctivitis (VKC)** is a seasonally recurrent (spring and fall), bilateral, ocular allergic condition appearing in the preteen years, affecting males more than females, and usually disappearing spontaneously by the third decade of life. In a few unfortunate individuals the disease is active throughout the year, with fluctuations from bad to worse.

1. **Clinical symptoms and signs** include intense itching, tearing, photophobia, and a thick, elastoid discharge. The skin of the lids is normal, but the palpebral conjunctiva displays firm, elevated, discrete, cobblestone giant papillae much more severe on the upper than the lower lid. There may be limbal conjunctival edema and folliculosis and limbal Trantas' dots. Corneal signs range from punctate staining to shield ulcers from the rubbing of the cobblestones.

2. **Differential diagnosis** of VKC, discussed earlier in the chapter, includes seasonal allergic conjunctivitis and allergic keratoconjunctivitis.

3. **Pathophysiologic changes** associated with the above physical findings include elevated levels of locally produced immunoglobulins IgE, IgG, and IgM. The IgE and IgG antibodies are not always elevated together in the same patient, but do appear to be pollen specific to rye grass and ragweed antigen. Gamma G immunoglobulin activates the complement cascade of immune events, and IgE mediates mast cell stimulation. Patients with VKC have decreased tear lactoferrin, an inhibitor of the complement system. This enhances the activity of the complement cascade, further promoting disease.

4. **Treatment** of VKC involves the multiple-factor approach seen with the ocular allergies.

a. **Cold wet compresses** 10 minutes 2–4 times daily, and **removal of the ropy discharge** with cotton-tip applicators will alleviate much of the itching and ocular irritation.

b. **Cromolyn** 4% drops used 6 times daily is effective

in controlling the mast cell-mediated (IgE-activated) component of the acute disease. Therapeutic efficacy begins after the first 10–14 days of treatment, with marked improvement in conjunctival and limbal hyperemia and edema, tearing, and itching, and decreased discharge. Atopic patients (hay fever, asthma, eczema) are, as a rule, more responsive to cromolyn than those with VC but no other allergic disease. Therapy should be maintained at 6 times daily levels throughout the seasons of exacerbation and at 2–4 times daily the remainder of the year.

   c. **Topical antihistamine-vasoconstrictors** 2–4 times daily may relieve some of the mast cell histamine itch-and-dilate effect. Systemic antihistamines have little or no efficacy.

   d. **Aspirin,** a prostaglandin inhibitor, is effective in a large majority of patients with VKC. Dosages of 0.5–1.5 g/day, depending on age, for 6 weeks followed by gradual weaning may result in improvement in corneal punctate keratopathy and reduced limbal infiltration, itching, and irritation. The lid cobblestones persist but become less inflamed. It should be remembered, however, that VKC occurs in the same age group as those susceptible to **Reye's syndrome.** Other potential adverse side effects are gastritis and aggravation of asthma.

   e. **Topical steroids** are reserved for patients who are severely affected or who have corneal involvement. Attempts should be made to keep the patient on short-term, low-dose steroid, although some will require initial hourly treatment for 48 hours and taper to 1 or 2 drops of 0.125% prednisolone daily for many weeks. These patients may still be somewhat symptomatic despite addition of the other therapeutic modalities discussed in this section. Most patients, however, will be able to stop topical steroid after the acute phase has passed and require only occasional pulsed treatment during seasonal reactivation of disease.

   f. **Shield ulcers or erosions of the cornea** should be managed with therapeutic contact lenses to protect the ocular surface from further mechanical damage from the lids, enhance healing, and allow the disease to be brought under better control with medical therapy. Topical antibiotic drops should be used bid as long as an epithelial ulcer persists.

D. **Giant papillary conjunctivitis (GPC)** is a local ocular allergy associated with hard and soft contact lenses, sutures, and ocular prosthetic devices.

   1. **Clinical symptoms and signs** include itching, photophobia, increased mucus production, diffuse conjunctival erythema, punctate staining at the upper limbus, and, above all, giant papillae greater than 0.3 mm in diameter on the upper tarsal conjunctiva. There is also a decreased tolerance of contact lens wear and in-

creased awareness of contact lenses while they are worn.

2. **Differential diagnosis** of GPC is VKC. As the clinical and histologic findings are similar in the two diseases, they are differentiated primarily by the presence or absence of the associated factors of contact lenses, sutures, or prostheses. In the case of GPC, the **stimulating factor** is thought to be a coating of the contact lens with an antigen, which then stimulates local production of elevated tear levels of IgE, IgG, and IgM. This, as in VKC, leads to activation of the complement cascade and mast-cell system.

3. **Treatment** of GPC differs somewhat from that of other ocular allergic conditions because of the rather specific nature of the allergen.

    a. **Eliminate contact lens** wear (or remove offending sutures or prostheses) for at least 4 weeks and until the eyes are totally uninflamed and all punctate staining has cleared. The appearance of the upper tarsal plate will remain unchanged for many weeks, however.

    b. **Contact lens management.** Once the eye is quiet and nonstaining, the patient should be carefully instructed in fastidious lens care and cleaning on a daily basis with nonpreserved saline. He or she should also use enzymatic lens treatment 1–2 times weekly and hydrogen peroxide or other cold disinfection daily (heat may bake antigen on the lens surface). The patient then is fitted with a pair of new contact lenses, preferably of a material different from the original offending set and even of a different design. At the first sign of return of increased mucus production, the patient should obtain a new set of lenses.

    c. **Recurrent GPC.** If the disease itself returns despite the proper contact lens management, 4% cromolyn 4–6 times daily should be added to the regimen. If all of the above are carried out, the success rate of GPC patients being able to continue contact lens (or prosthesis) wear approaches 90%.

E. **Contact allergies** of the lids or conjunctiva are frequently the result of sensitization to topical medications or contact lens solutions or their preservatives.

1. **Offending drugs** include most commonly neomycin (18%), bacitracin (7%), polymyxin B (<4%), and atropine (4%); sensitizing preservatives include thimerosol (4%) and benzalkonium chloride (4%). Antivirals such as idoxuridine are also sensitizing, but to a lesser extent.

2. **Clinical symptoms and signs** are itching, burning, tearing, lid edema, and hyperemia with leathery, scaling dermatitis and papillary hypertrophy of the conjunctiva. Corneal manifestations are gray anterior stromal infiltrates, diffuse punctate keratopathy, and epithelial opacities.

3. **Treatment**

a. Identification and discontinuation of offending agent. For patients on several eye medications, those most suspect should be stopped first. In a few cases, however, all drugs may have to be temporarily discontinued, if possible, and then only those necessary reinstituted one at a time.

b. Topical corticosteroid ointments such as 0.05% dexamethasone will relieve acute lid reaction, and a short course of topical 0.125% prednisolone 2–3 times daily may be necessary for a few days in those severely affected. Most patients will not require steroids, however, but will recover just by discontinuing the sensitizing medication and using cold compresses for symptomatic relief for a few days.

Information Sources and Suggested Reading (*Antiallergy*)

1. Abelson, M., and Allansmith, M., Ocular allergies. In Smolin, G., and Thoft, R.A. (Eds.), *The Cornea,* 2nd ed. Boston: Little, Brown, 1987, pp. 307–320.

2. Abelson, M.B., and Weston, J., Antihistamines. In Lamberts, D.W., and Potter, D.E. (Eds.), *Clinical Ophthalmic Pharmacology.* Boston: Little, Brown, 1987, pp. 417–424.

3. Butrus, S., Weston, J., and Abelson, M.B., Ocular mast cell stabilizing agents. In Lamberts, D.W., and Potter, D.E. (Eds.), *Clinical Ophthalmic Pharmacology.* Boston: Little, Brown, 1988, pp. 483–496.

4. Douglas, W., Histamine and serotonin and their antagonists. In Goodman, L., Gilman, A., Rall, T., and Murad, F., (Eds.), *The Pharmacologic Basis of Therapeutics,* 7th ed. New York: Macmillan, 1985, pp. 605–638.

5. Ellis, P., *Ocular Therapeutics and Pharmacology,* 7th ed. St. Louis: C.V. Mosby, 1985, pp. 278–282 (antihistamines).

6. Fraunfelder, F., and Roy, F.H. (Eds.), *Current Ocular Therapy 3,* 3rd ed. Philadelphia: W.B. Saunders, multiple contributing authors, 1990, pp. 400, 411, 420 (allergic conjunctivitis).

7. Smolin, G., and Friedlaender, M. (Eds.), *Ocular Allergy.* Int. Ophthalmol. Clin., 28 (4), 1988. Boston: Little, Brown, 1989, pp. 262–266 (immunological mechanisms, Stock, E.), pp. 267–274 (mast cells and eosinophils, Rothenberg, M., Owen, W. Jr., Stevens, R.), pp. 275–281 (differential diagnosis, Udell, I.), pp. 282–293 (evaluation and treatment, Christiansen, S.), pp. 294–302 (conjunctivitis, Donshik, P.), p. 308 (vernal, Buckley, R.), pp. 309–316 (giant papillary conjunctivitis, Allansmith, M., Ross, R.), pp. 317–320 (contact allergy and toxicity, Friedlaender, M.).

8. Smolin, G., and O'Connor, G.R., *Ocular Immunology,* 2nd ed. Boston: Little, Brown, 1986, pp. 135–192 (atopic diseases affecting the eye).

9. Stjernschantz, J., Autacoids and neuropeptides (histamine, hydroxytryptamine, kinins). In Sears, M.L. (Ed.), *Pharmacology of the Eye.* Handbook of Experimental Pharmacology, Vol. 69. New York: Springer–Verlag, 1984, pp. 311–336.

3

Antibiotics

I. **Bacterial Structure and Function**
   A. **The bacterial cell wall** structure affects reaction to the gram stain and as such determines the classification of bacteria into two groups, gram-positive and gram-negative. Gram-positive organisms such as *Staphylococcus* and *Streptococcus* possess a very thick wall made largely of layered peptidoglycan. This cellular "armor" determines the sensitivity of organisms to certain antibiotics and lends mechanical strength to the organism, making it more resistant to damage from physical forces. Gram-negative organisms such as *Pseudomonas* and *Neisseria* possess a very thin peptidoglycan wall. This wall lies, however, within an outer membrane composed of liposaccharide and lipoprotein, substances that make the organisms resistant to rupture by the enzyme lysozyme, a key defense mechanism of the tear film.
   B. **The cytoplasmic membrane** lines the cell wall and is a semipermeable structure delineating the anatomic limits of the living organism. The bacterial DNA lies as a single strand free within the cytoplasm rather than bound within a nuclear membrane. This DNA strand is the source of the genetic information critical to cell growth and replication. The bacterial cytoplasm lacks true organelles but contains two ribosome types (subunits -[S]) of different weights, 30S and 50S. A messenger RNA (mRNA) is synthesized along the sequence of nucleotide bases on the DNA strand, thus transcribing the genetic message. The mRNA binds to a specific site on a 30S ribosome subunit and stimulates the binding of a transfer RNA (tRNA) to the 50S ribosomal subunit at its specific binding site. Ribosomes are the site of protein synthesis within the bacteria. They function by presenting sequential areas of DNA-programmed mRNA to tRNA molecules carrying the building blocks of protein amino acids. The tRNA inserts the amino acids in correct sequence within the polypeptide chain. The ribosomes and DNA, like the cell wall, are critical sites for antibiotic and antimicrobial drug action.

II. **Pharmacologic Overview of Drug Mechanisms and Microbial Resistance**
   A. **Mechanisms of action.** Drugs used against bacteria are either bactericidal or bacteriostatic. The former kill the organisms; the latter inhibit their growth. Bactericidal drugs include the penicillins, aminoglycosides, and cephalosporins. Bacteriostatic agents include erythromycin, tetracyclines, chloramphenicol, and sulfonamides, although in sufficiently high doses any of these may become bactericidal as well.

   The mechanisms of action of antibiotics and antimicrobials are discussed under specific drugs, but in general these agents work by inhibiting protein synthesis, cell wall function, or nucleic acid synthesis.

   1. **Inhibition of bacterial protein synthesis** is a com-

mon antibiotic function characteristic of both the bactericidal and bacteriostatic drugs: aminoglycosides, tetracyclines, erythromycin, clindamycin, and chloramphenicol. Inhibition of protein synthesis occurs after specific target effects on bacterial ribosomes. Host ribosomal functions are spared and toxicity to the host is minimized.

2. **Impairment of cell wall function,** effected by the bactericidal agents, the penicillins, bacitracin, the cephalosporins, and vancomycin, occurs through interference with peptidoglycan synthesis critical to protecting the organisms from mechanical damage and destructive action of autolytic enzymes. The bactericidal polymyxins and gramicidin also affect cell wall function, but function by a detergent-like action that allows transmembrane loss of essential ions and molecules.

3. **Inhibition of nucleic acid synthesis** is a mechanism common to bacteriostatic drugs such as the sulfonamides, trimethoprim, and pyrimethamine. These drugs compete with bacteria for para-aminobenzoic acid (PABA), thus depriving the organisms of their source of folic acid essential to production of new bacterial DNA. These drugs vary in the severity of their action against host cell PABA, eg, pyrimethamine is more host toxic than trimethoprim on this basis. Ciprofloxacin, like all 4-quinolone compounds, inhibits DNA gyrase, an enzyme involved in chromosomal supercoiling, and thus inhibits the replication of bacterial DNA. Rifampicin also inhibits bacterial replication pathways, but by direct binding to RNA polymerase. This action interferes with mRNA alignment along the bacterial DNA template, thus blocking transmission of genetic information to progeny bacteria.

B. **Drug resistance.** Bacterial resistance to antibiotics and antimicrobials is a problem of increasing concern. The mechanisms of bacterial resistance to drug action are not related to mechanisms of action of the drugs. They are, rather, developed totally independently by a variety of routes: enzymatic resistance, plasmid transfer of genetic information, and cell wall alterations.

1. **Enzymatic resistance** results from an organism developing the ability to produce enzymes destructive to the target drug. Beta lactamase hydrolyzes the beta lactam ring of certain but not all penicillins and cephalosporins, thereby inactivating the drugs. Beta lactamase is an enzyme produced by several strains of staphylococci, gram-negative bacilli, and certain *Hemophilus influenza* and *Neisseria* organisms. In addition to beta lactamase, gram-negative bacilli such as *Pseudomonas, Proteus,* and *Escherichia* are capable of producing a number of other enzymes that inactivate aminoglycosides, chloramphenicol, and a variety of other antibiotics by adenylation, phosphorylation, or acetylation. In response to increasing numbers and mecha-

nisms of drug resistance, the pharmaceutical industry has synthesized "designer drugs" aimed specifically at counteracting resistance to the drug-destructive action of bacterial enzymes. Semisynthetic and synthetic penicillins such as piperacillin, third-generation cephalosporins, and newer aminoglycosides (amikacin) are active against otherwise drug-resistant organisms. The bacteriostatic sulfur drugs are vulnerable to enzymatic resistance of a different sort. Excess enzymatic production by bacteria reduces the ability of antibacterial drugs to bind PABA. Thus, organisms are able to grow easily in the presence of otherwise therapeutic levels of drug.

2. **Plasmid transfer of resistance** is, in fact, an extension of enzymatic resistance. Plasmids are autoreplicating circular pieces of extrachromosomal DNA capable of incorporating foreign fragments of DNA, transposons, and transferring the information contained therein from one organism or cell to another. In the case of bacterial resistance, this involves the passage of the genetic code conferring biochemical capabilities responsible for drug degradation.

3. **Cell wall alterations** may affect resistance by a variety of mechanisms. Enhanced permeability of the cell wall prevents build-up of inhibitory drug concentrations within the bacterium by enhancing diffusion of drug out of the organism. This is a common mechanism in development of resistance to tetracycline, aminoglycosides, bacitracin, and vancomycin. Lack of autolytic enzymes normally present within the cell wall is a second mechanism of cell-wall–related resistance. Penicillin-induced cell wall lysis is dependent on these enzymes. The absence of the enzymes is responsible for organism inhibition (bacteriostatic) but not death in the face of treatment with members of the entire penicillin drug group. Methicillin, a semisynthetic penicillin, is also ineffective against *Staphylococcus* strains that have lost the ability to produce cell wall receptors for this drug. A lack of binding sites may occur also on the ribosomes, thus inducing resistance to erythromycin, clindamycin, and the aminoglycosides, all of which are ribosome activated.

III. **Management Considerations.** In ophthalmic practice, antimicrobials may be used empirically, specifically, or prophylactically, with the object being elimination or reduction of pathogenic organisms. For maximum therapeutic effect it is essential to know not only the organisms but also the appropriate antibiotics, their potential toxicity, absorption, and, in the case of systemic agents, mode of clearance from the body.

Rather than trying to master a vast list of agents, it is preferable for the physician to learn to use one or two drugs in each category well. Newer antibiotics should replace older ones only if clearly superior. It should be borne in mind that indiscriminate use of drugs broader in spectrum than warranted for a given disease state or their use for excessively long and unnecessary periods invites not only emergence of resistant organisms but also toxic reaction and excessive expense for the patient.

A. **Therapeutic approaches**

  1. **Empiric therapy.** Because of the need to preserve the integrity of the delicate ocular structures, initial treatment is begun immediately after the clinical history, physical exam, and gram-stained scrapings or aspirates are obtained. Common infections of the external eye such as blepharitis and conjunctivitis usually are treated with single drugs covering gram-positive organisms, the most common causative agent, or with solutions or ointments that cover both gram-positive and gram-negative organisms. For more serious infections, such as keratitis, orbital cellulitis, and endophthalmitis, where the nature of the organism is not immediately apparent, empiric therapy often involves a second- or third-generation cephalosporin or fifth-generation penicillin in combination with an aminoglycoside (Tables 3-1 and 3-2). Such drug group combinations are selected to cover a very wide range of gram-positive and gram-negative bacteria, including penicillin-resistant staphylococci. Despite suggestive organisms on scrapings, broad-spectrum coverage is advisable until culture and sensitivity data are available, because a more proliferative organism may mask the presence of a slower-growing one. Occasionally patients may have been partially treated with antibiotics before smears and cultures were taken, resulting in negative smears and "no growth" cultures. Such a situation is also an indication for empiric, very broad-spectrum therapy. Smears and scrapings are positive only about 50–70% of the time, but they may give some useful early indication of the nature of the organism and guide the physician's selection of drugs within the broad-spectrum, empiric coverage regimen.

  2. **Specific therapy.** Specific therapy may be instituted after identifying the causative agents by culture. Information on microbial drug sensitivity is usually available in 36–48 hours. For gram-negative bacilli such as *Pseudomonas aeruginosa,* this often means a change to such drugs as carbenicillin or ticarcillin in combination with an aminoglycoside such as tobramycin or amikacin. Multi-agent therapy is recommended in an attempt to prevent emergence of resistant organisms and to promote possible synergistic drug action. Penicillin G is still the drug of choice for **non–penicillinase-producing *Staphylococcus aureus,*** provided there is no history of penicillin allergy. This drug is less toxic, less expensive, and more effective than other penicillins or cephalosporins in treating this organism. **Penicillinase-producing *S. aureus,*** however, must be treated with a penicillinase-resistant penicillin such as oxacillin or nafcillin or with a first-generation cephalosporin such as cefazolin.

continued on page 36

Table 3-1. Antibacterial drugs of choice for ocular and periocular infections[a]

Microorganism	First-choice drugs	Effective alternative drugs
Gram-positive cocci		
Staphylococcus aureus or *S. epidermidis* Non–penicillinase-producing	Penicillin G or V	A cephalosporin, vancomycin, imipenem, clinda- mycin, ciprofloxacin
Penicillinase-producing	A penicillinase-resistant penicillin (cloxacillin, dicloxacillin, methicil- lin, nafcillin, oxacillin)	A cephalosporin, vancomycin, amoxicillin-clavu- lanic acid; ticarcillin-clavulanic acid, ampicillin- sulbactam; imipenem, clindamycin, ciprofloxacin
Methicillin-resistant[b]	Vancomycin and/or gentamicin or bacitracin	Trimethoprim-sulfamethoxazole, ciprofloxacin
Streptococcus pyogenes (Groups A, C, G)	Penicillin G or V	Erythromycin, a cephalosporin, vancomycin, baci- tracin
Streptococcus (Group B)	Penicillin G or ampicillin	A cephalosporin, vancomycin, erythromycin
Streptococcus viridans	Penicillin G with or without genta- micin	A cephalosporin, vancomycin
Streptococcus (enterococcus)	Ampicillin or amoxicillin	Norfloxacin, ciprofloxacin
Streptococcus (anaerobic) or Peptostrep- tococcus	Penicillin G	Clindamycin, a cephalosporin, vancomycin
Streptococcus pneumoniae (pneumococ- cus)	Penicillin G or V	Erythromycin, a cephalosporin, chloramphenicol, vancomycin

Gram-negative cocci		
Neisseria gonorrhoeae (gonococcus)	Penicillin G, ceftriaxone, ciprofloxacin, norfloxacin	Erythromycin, tetracycline, ampicillin, bacitracin, gentamicin, amoxicillin with probenecid, spectinomycin, chloramphenicol
Neisseria meningitidis (meningococcus)	Penicillin G, rifampin	As for *N. gonorrhoeae*
Gram-positive bacilli		
Bacillus anthracis (anthrax)	Penicillin G	Erythromycin,[c] tetracycline
Clostridium perfringens	Penicillin G	Chloramphenicol, metronidazole, clindamycin, a tetracycline
Clostridium tetani	Penicillin G	A tetracycline
Corynebacterium diphtheriae	Erythromycin	Penicillin G
Corynebacterium (Groups J, K)	Vancomycin	—
Listeria monocytogenes	Ampicillin[c] with or without gentamicin[c]	Trimethoprim-sulfamethoxazole,[c] erythromycin
Enteric gram-negative bacilli (Enterobacteriaceae)		
Bacteroides	Clindamycin	Penicillin G, a second- or third-generation cephalosporin, chloramphenicol, ticarcillin or piperacillin, imipenem, ampicillin-sulbactam, polymyxin B
Enterobacter	Ceftriaxone, gentamicin, tobramycin, amikacin	Cefotaxime, ceftizoxime, imipenem, carbenicillin, ticarcillin, mezlocillin, piperacillin, ceftazidime, ciprofloxacin, norfloxacin, chloramphenicol, polymyxin B

Table 3-1. (continued)

Microorganism	First-choice drugs	Effective alternative drugs
Escherichia coli	Gentamicin, tobramycin, or amikacin with or without ampicillin	As under *Enterobacter*, amoxicillin-clavulanic acid, ticarcillin-clavulanic acid, ampicillin-sulbactam, a tetracycline, polymyxin B
Klebsiella pneumoniae	Gentamicin, tobramycin, amikacin, ceftriaxone	As for *Enterobacter* and *E. coli*
Proteus mirabilis	Ampicillin	As for *Enterobacter* and *E. coli*
Proteus, indole-positive (*Providencia, Morganella*, and *P. vulgaris*)	Gentamicin, tobramycin, amikacin, ceftriaxone	As for *Enterobacter* and *E. coli*
Serratia	Gentamicin, tobramycin, amikacin, ceftriaxone	As for *Enterobacter* and *E. coli*
Other gram-negative bacilli		
Acinetobacter (Mima, Herellea)	Imipenem	Tobramycin,[c] gentamicin,[c] or amikacin, carbenicillin,[c] ticarcillin,[c] mezlocillin,[c] piperacillin,[c] minocycline, doxycycline
Brucella (brucellosis)	A tetracycline with streptomycin	Chloramphenicol with or without streptomycin, trimethoprim-sulfamethoxazole[c]
Francisella tularensis (tularemia)	Streptomycin or gentamicin[c]	Erythromycin,[c] tetracycline,[c] amoxicillin-clavulanic acid,[c] a tetracycline, chloramphenicol
Hemophilus ducreyi	Sulfonamide, chloramphenicol	Tetracycline, ampicillin, trimethoprim-sulfamethoxazole[c]

Infecting Organism	Drug of First Choice	Alternative Drugs
Hemophilus influenzae	Ampicillin, chloramphenicol, cefamandole	Trimethoprim-sulfamethoxazole, cefuroxime, a sulfonamide with or without erythromycin, amoxicillin-clavulanic acid, cefuroxime, cefaclor, cefotaxime, ceftizoxime, ceftriaxone, a tetracycline
Legionella pneumophila	An erythromycin	Trimethoprim-sulfamethoxazole
Pseudomonas aeruginosa	Carbenicillin, ticarcillin, mezlocillin, piperacillin, or azlocillin plus tobramycin, gentamicin, or amikacin	Tobramycin, gentamicin or amikacin with ceftazidime, imipenem, or aztreonam, ciprofloxacin
Actinomycetes		
Actinomyces israelii (actinomycosis)	Penicillin G	A tetracycline
Nocardia	Penicillin G or sulfonamides	Trimethoprim-sulfamethoxazole,[c] amikacin,[c] minocycline,[c] ampicillin,[c] erythromycin,[c] tetracycline
Chlamydiae		
Chlamydia trachomatis (trachoma)	A tetracycline (oral plus topical)	A sulfonamide (oral plus topical)
Chlamydia trachomatis (inclusion conjunctivitis, pneumonia)	Doxycycline, tetracycline, an erythromycin (oral or IV)	A sulfonamide
Chlamydia trachomatis (urethritis or pelvic inflammatory disease)	A tetracycline or an erythromycin	Sulfisoxazole
Rickettsia		
Rocky Mountain spotted fever, tick bite fever, typhus	A tetracycline	Chloramphenicol

Table 3-1. (continued)

Microorganism	First-choice drugs	Effective alternative drugs
Spirochetes		
Borrelia burgdorferi (Lyme disease)	A tetracycline[c]	Penicillin G[c] or V[c], ceftriaxone,[c] erythromycin[c]
Treponema pallidum (syphilis)	Penicillin G	A tetracycline, an erythromycin
Mycobacteria		
Mycobacterium tuberculosis	Rifampin[c]	Steptomycin
Mycobacterium fortuitum	Amikacin	Kanamycin, amikacin, rifampin

[a] Some drugs are available or may be made up for topical and systemic use; others are available for topical or systemic use only as indicated in other tables or text. All use should be confirmed as appropriate by sensitivity testing of clinical isolates.
[b] Coagulase + and − staphylococci resistant to penicillinase-resistant drugs are resistant to cephalosporins and imipenem as well.
[c] Not FDA approved for this indication.

Table 3-2. Dosage of systemic antimicrobial drugs used in ocular infections*

Drug	Adults		Children				Newborn (parenteral)	
	Oral daily dosage	Parenteral daily dosage	Oral daily dosage	Parenteral daily dosage	Usual divided dose interval	Usual maximum dose/day	Up to 1 week	1–4 weeks
Amikacin	—	15 mg/kg IM, IV	—	15 mg/kg IM, IV	q8–12h	1.5 g	15 mg/kg/d, q12h	15–22.5 mg/kg/d, q8–12h
Amoxicillin	0.75–1.5 g		20–40 mg/kg	—	q8h	3 g	Not recommended	Not recommended
Amoxicillin/clavulanic acid	0.75–1.5 g²		20–40 mg/kg	—	q8h	1.5 g	Not recommended	Not recommended
Ampicillin	2–4 g	2–12 g IM, IV	50–100 mg/kg	100–200 mg/kg IM, IV	q6–8h	12 g	50–100 mg/kg/d, q12h	100–200 mg/kg/d, q6–8h
Ampicillin/sulbactam		6–12 g IM, IV			q6h	12 g	—	—
Aztreonam^d		1–8 g IM, IV			q6–12h	8 g	—	—
Carbenicillin^b	4–8 tablets (382 mg/tab)	30–40 g IM, IV	50–65 mg/kg	100–600 mg/kg IM, IV	q4–6h	40 g	200–300 mg/kg/d, q8h	400 mg/kg/d, q6h
Cefaclor (1)^b,c	0.75–1.5 g		20–40 mg/kg		q8h	4 g	—	—
Cefadroxil (1)^b,c	1–2 g		30 mg/kg		q12–24h	2 g	—	—
Cefamandole (2)^b,c		1.5–12 g IM, IV		50–150 mg/kg IM, IV	q4–8h	12 g		50–150 mg/kg/d, q4–8h
Cefazolin (1)^b,c		1–6 g IM, IV		25–100 mg/kg IM, IV	q6–8h	6g	30 mg/kg/d, q12h	30–60 mg/kg/d, q8–12h
Cefotaxime (3)^b,c		2–12 g IM, IV		100–200 mg/kg IM, IV	q4–8h	12 g	100 mg/kg/d, q12h	150 mg/kg/d, q8h

Table 3-2. (continued)

Drug	Adults Oral daily dosage	Adults Parenteral daily dosage	Children Oral daily dosage	Children Parenteral daily dosage	Usual divided dose interval	Usual maximum dose/day	Newborn (parenteral) Up to 1 week	Newborn (parenteral) 1–4 weeks
Cefoxitin (2)[b,c]	—	3–12 g IM, IV	—	80–160 mg/kg IM, IV	q4–8h	12 g	—	—
Ceftazidime (3)[b,c]	—	0.5–6 g IM, IV	—	90–150 mg/kg	q8–12h	6 g	30 mg/kg/d, q12h	30 mg/kg/d, q12h
Ceftizoxime (3)[b,c]	—	2–12 g IM, IV	—	150–200 mg/kg	q6–12h	12 g	—	—
Ceftriaxone (3)[b,c]	—	1–4 g IM, IV	—	50–100 mg/kg	q12–24h	4 g	125 mg IM once (Neisseria)	125 mg IM once (Neisseria)
Cefuroxime (2)[b,c]	0.25–1 g	2.25–9 g IM, IV	250–500 mg	50–100 mg/kg	q8h	9 g	Not recommended	Not recommended
Cephalexin (1)[b,c]	1–4 g	—	25–50 mg/kg	—	q6h	4 g	Not recommended	Not recommended
Cephalothin (1)[b,c]	1–4 g	2–12 g IM, IV	—	80–160 mg/kg	q4–6h	12 g	40 mg/kg/d, q12h	60 mg/kg/d, q8h
Cephradine (1)[b,c]	1–4 g	2–8 g IM, IV	25–50 mg/kg	50–100 mg/kg	q6h	8 g	Not recommended	Not recommended
Chloramphenicol	50–100 mg/kg	50–100 mg/kg, IV	50–100 mg/kg	50–100 mg/kg, IV	q6h	4 g	25 mg/kg, q24h, IV	25–50 mg/kg, q12–24h, IV
Ciprofloxacin	0.5–1.5 g	—	—	—	q12h	2 g	—	—
Clindamycin	0.6–1.8 g	0.6–3.6 g IM, IV	10–25 mg–kg	10–40 mg/kg IM, IV	q6–8h	4–8 g	Unknown	Unknown
Cloxacillin	2–4 g	—	50–100 mg/kg	—	q6h	4 g	Not recommended	Not recommended
Dicloxacillin	1–2 g	—	12.5–25 mg/kg	—	q6h	4 g	Not recommended	Not recommended

Doxycycline	100–200 mg	100–200 mg, IV	1–2 mg/kg	1–2 mg/kg, IV	q12–24h	200 mg	Not recommended	Not recommended
Erythromycin	1–2 g	1–4 g, IV	30–50 mg/kg	15–50 mg/kg, IV	q6h	4 g	Not recommended	Not recommended
Gentamicin	Not recommended	3–5 mg/kg	Not recommended	3–7.5 mg/kg	q8h	5 mg/kg	5 mg/kg/d, q12h	7.5 mg/kg/d, q8h
Imipenem[d]	—	1–4 g IV	—	—	q6–8h	4 g	—	—
Kanamycin	—	15 mg/kg IM, IV	—	15–20 mg/kg	q8–12h	1.5 g	15–20 mg/kg/d, q12h	15–20 mg/kg/d, q8–12h
Methicillin	—	4–12 g IM, IV	—	100–200 g	q4–6h	12 g	50–75 mg/kg/d, q8–12h	100–150 mg/kg/d, q6–8h
Metronidazole	30 mg/kg	30 mg/kg IV	30 mg/kg	30 mg/kg IV	q6h	4 g	15 mg/kg once, then 7.5 mg/kg, q12h	15 mg/kg once, then 7.5 mg/kg, q12h
Mezlocillin	—	6–18 g IM, IV		300 mg/kg	q4–6h	24 g	150–225 mg/kg/d, q8–12h	225–300 mg/kg/d, q6–8h
Minocycline	100 mg	—	2 mg/kg	—	q12h	200 mg	Not recommended	Not recommended
Moxalactam	—	2–12 g IM, IV		150–200 mg/kg	q8h	12 g	100 mg/kg/d, q12h	150 mg/kg/d, q8h
Nafcillin	2–4 g	2–9 g IM, IV	50–100 mg/kg	100–200 mg/kg	q6h	12 g	40 mg/kg/d, q12h	60–80 mg/kg/d, q6–8h
Norfloxacin	800 mg	—	—	—	q12h	1200 mg	—	—
Oxacillin	2–4 g	2–12 g IM, IV	50–100 mg/kg	100–200 mg/kg	q6h	12 g	50–75 mg/kg/d, q8–12h	100–150 mg/kg/d, q6–8h
Oxytetracycline	1–2 g	0.75–1 g IM	20–50 mg/kg	10–20 mg/kg	q12h	2 g	10 mg/kg, q12h IV	10–20 mg/kg, q12h IV

Table 3-2. (continued)

Drug	Adults		Children				Newborn (parenteral)	
	Oral daily dosage	Parenteral daily dosage	Oral daily dosage	Parenteral daily dosage	Usual divided dose interval	Usual maximum dose/day	Up to 1 week	1–4 weeks
Penicillin G potassium	1–2 g	1.2–24 million U IM/IV: Potassium penicillin IV/subconj/intraoc: Sodium penicillin IM: procaine or benzathine penicillin	25–50 mg/kg	100,000–250,000 U/kg	q6h	24 million U	50,000–150,000 U/kg/d, q8–12h	75,000–250,000 U/kg/d, q6–8h
Penicillin V	1–2 g	—	25–50 mg/kg	—	q6h	4 g	Not recommended	Not recommended
Piperacillin	—	12–24 g IM, IV	—	200–300 mg/kg IM, IV	q4–6h	24 g	—	—
Rifampin[e]	0.6 g	—	10–20 mg/kg	—	q12–24h	0.6 g	—	—
Spectinomycin	—	2 g IM	—	40 mg/kg IM	—	4 g	Not recommended	Not recommended
Streptomycin	—	1–2 g IM	—	20–30 mg/kg IM	q12h	2 g	Not recommended	Not recommended
Sulfisoxazole	1–2 g	—	100 mg/kg	—	q6h	4 g	100 mg/kg	100 mg/kg
Tetracycline HCl	1–2 g	0.75–1 g IM, IV	25–50 mg/kg	10–20 mg/kg IM, IV	q6h	2 g	Not recommended	Not recommended

Ticarcillin	—	200–300 mg/kg IM, IV	—	200–300 mg/kg IM, IV	q4–6h	24–30 g	150–225 mg/kg/d, q8–12h	225–300 mg/kg/d, q8h
Ticarcillin/clavulanic acid	—	9–18 g IM, IV	—	200–300 mg/kg IM, IV	q4–6h	18 g	Not recommended	Not recommended
Tobramycin	—	3–5 mg/kg IM, IV	—	6–7.5 mg/kg IM, IV	q8h	5 mg/kg	4 mg/kg/d, q12h	6–7.5 mg/kg/d, q6–8h
Trimethoprim-sulfamethoxazole (TMP-SMX)	4 tablets (80 TMP + 400 SMX/ tab)	8–20 mg/kg (TMP) IV	8–20 mg (TMP + SMX)	8–20 mg/kg (TMP)	q6–12h	1200 mg TMP with 600 mg SMX, IV	Not recommended	Not recommended
Vancomycin	0.5–2 g	2 g IV	50 mg/kg	40 mg/kg IV	q6–12h	2 g	20 mg/kg/d, q12h	30 mg/kg/d, q8h

a Dosage should be adjusted down in patients with renal failure in consultation with an internist or infectious disease consultant. Parenteral routes are IM or IV unless only one route is stated.

b Number in parentheses indicates cephalosporin generation.

c Second- and third-generation cephalosporins are less active than first-generation against staphylococci and streptococci, but more active against gram-negative bacilli and anaerobes.

d A beta lactam. Imipenem is the most active drug against all pathogenic bacteria; aztreonam is very active against gram-negative aerobic bacilli only.

e Not FDA approved.

* Adapted from Handbook of Antimicrobial Therapy, New Rochelle, NY: The Medical Letter, 1989.

Because of the need for less frequent systemic dosage, the cephalosporin is less expensive and less inconvenient to the patient, thus encouraging better compliance. Another factor favoring the use of penicillins and cephalosporins where systemic therapy is required is the favorable therapeutic index, ie, a wide margin between therapeutic and toxic blood levels. Conversely, drugs such as the aminoglycoside family have a very narrow therapeutic index, which requires much closer patient monitoring. As a rule, agents with wide therapeutic indices may be given systemically in a standard dose such as cefazolin 3–4 times daily. Drugs with narrow therapeutic indices, eg, gentamicin, are given in doses calculated on the basis of patient body weight, thus minimizing risk of toxic overdosing. Therapy of specific microbial disease is discussed further under "Management of Clinical Ocular Infections" (Sec. **VI**).

3. **Prophylaxis.** Prophylactic antibiotics may be used preoperatively, intraoperatively, and after penetrating injury or perforation.

   a. **Preoperative topical antibiotics** appear to be effective in reducing but not totally preventing the incidence of postoperative endophthalmitis. Although the available data come from studies that may be criticized for lack of control groups, variation in surgical technique and surgical environment, retrospective nature, and inconsistency in the antibiotics used, the results indicate an incidence of endophthalmitis of 0.71–3.05% if antibiotic prophylaxis is not used and only 0.05–0.11% if it is. Although no reasonably practical regimen will completely sterilize the lids and conjunctiva, 48–72 hours of topical broad-spectrum antibiotic such as gentamicin drops or polymyxin-bacitracin ointment 4 times daily will greatly reduce the bacterial count without significant risk of toxicity or emergence of resistant strains. Most ocular surgeons now use preoperative prophylactic antibiotics before intraocular (cataract, glaucoma), retinal detachment, and even strabismus surgery to reduce the risk of infection. If there appears to be preoperative evidence of active infection, such as blepharitis, conjunctivitis, or dacryocystitis, elective surgery should probably be postponed until longer, more specific therapy can be given.

   b. **Intraoperative subconjunctival antibiotics.** As an adjunct to preoperative topical prophylaxis, a single subconjunctival-subtenon antibiotic injection given at the end of the procedure is also commonly used after intraocular procedures. If such an injection is used after a glaucoma filtering procedure, the drug should be placed as far away from the filtering site as possible to prevent toxic intraocular levels entering through the opening into the anterior chamber. For routine postoperative injection, a cephalosporin or aminoglycoside is often used. For a penetrating injury or perforation, combination cephalosporin-aminoglycoside for broadest coverage possible is advisable, as the potential offending agent usually is not known. Although there is no definitive study showing that postoperative subconjunctival antibiotics actually reduce the incidence of endophthalmitis, the mode of access of organisms to the eye is usually via the anterior chamber. Subconjunctival subtenon drug delivery achieves very high aqueous therapeutic levels very quickly. This has at least the potential of obviating a potential source of infection, thus making such prophylaxis a popular, probably effective, albeit not entirely proven therapeutic modality.

   c. **Prophylactic systemic antibiotic therapy** is reserved largely for penetrating injury or ocular perforation as in a melting corneal ulcer (chemical burn, herpes). On occasion, however, systemic therapy may be indicated to prevent endophthalmitis from the spread of a deeply invading bacterial keratitis, particularly in an aphakic eye without an intact posterior capsule. In any event, the drugs should not be given until appropriate smears and cultures have been taken from the site of injury or perforation.

B. **Routes of administration.** In the face of an ocular infectious process, the physician must make two key decisions concerning therapy: the antibiotics to be used, and the routes of administration. The four primary means of administering drugs are **topical** drops and ointments, **subconjunctival** injection of systemic drug preparations, **intravitreous** injection of systemic antibiotic preparations, and **intramuscular (IM) or intravenous IV** drug administration. The use of one or several of these routes depends on the diagnosis and on the virulence of the organism and the disease process. Recommended routes of administration will be discussed in further detail under specific clinical diagnoses. As a rule, however, topical treatment is used for infections of the lids, conjunctiva, and cornea, with the exception of certain organisms such as the *Neisseria* and chlamydial (TRIC) agents or extension of an infection beyond the cornea, which require additional systemic therapy. Intraocular infections usually require both intravitreal and systemic therapy, with topical drugs added if the infection was acquired through anterior segment trauma or a spreading corneal infection. Orbital and periorbital infections require systemic therapy. Subconjunctival injection may be used as an adjunct to any of the other three routes of antibiotic administration and often depends largely on disease severity and patient compliance.

   1. **Topical antibiotics.** Drugs delivered via topical drops and ointments enter the eye primarily through the cornea. Drug penetration depends on the chemical properties of the drug (qualities of biphasic solubility), integrity of the corneal epithelium, presence or ab-

Table 3-3. Commercial single-agent ophthalmic antibiotic preparations

Drug	Solution	Ointment	Commercial name
Bacitracin	−	+	Bacitracin (Lilly, Pharmafair, Pharmaderm)
Chloramphenicol	+	−	AK-Chlor (Akorn)
	+	+	Chlorofair (Pharmafair)
	+	+	Chloromycetin (Parke-Davis)
	+	+	Chloroptic (Allergan)
	+	+	Ocu-chlor (Ocumed)
	+	−	Ophthochlor (Parke-Davis)*
Chlortetracycline	−	+	Aureomycin (Lederle)
Erythromycin	−	+	AK-Mycin (Akorn)
	−	+	Erythromycin (Pharmafair, Pharmaderm)
Gentamicin	+	+	Garamycin (Schering)
	+	+	Genoptic (Allergan)
	+	+	Gentacidin (IOLAB)
	+	+	Gentafair (Pharmafair)
	+	+	Gentak (Akorn)
	+	−	I-Gent (Americal)
	+	+	Ocu-mycin (Ocumed)
Sulfacetamide (10,15,30%)	+	+	Many
Sulfisoxazole	+	−	Gantrisin (Roche)
Tetracycline	+	+	Achromycin (Lederle)
Tobramycin	+	−	Tobrex (Alcon)

*Preservative-free. Reconstituted by pharmacist.

sence of ocular inflammation, drug concentration, and frequency of administration. Tables 3-3 through 3-5 list the commercially available single and combination antibiotics and antibiotic-steroid combinations for topical use.

a. **Chemical properties** that influence drug penetration and concentration in the cornea and anterior chamber are related to the lipophilicity, hydrophilicity, and molecular weight of the compound. The epithelium and endothelium are lipid-rich layers that allow the passage of lipophilic drugs. The stroma, on the other hand, is primarily a water-based structure that favors the passage of hydrophilic agents. Passage of any antibiotic across the cornea requires biphasic solubility, with nonpolar regions enhancing lipid solubility and polar groups enhancing water solubility. The pH and buffering system of the drug formulation may have a notable effect on these factors and, therefore, on drug penetration. Antibiotics of small molecular weight pass

Table 3-4. Commercial combination ophthalmic antibiotic preparations

Drug	Solution	Ointment	Commercial name
Neomycin-polymyxin B-bacitracin	−	+	AK-Spore (Akorn)
	−	+	Bacitracin-Neomycin-Polymyxin (Pharmaderm)
	−	+	Neosporin (Burroughs Wellcome)
	−	+	Ocuspor B (Ocumed)
	−	+	Ocutricin (Pharmafair)
Neomycin-polymyxin B-gramicidin	+	−	AK-Spore (Akorn)
	+	−	Neosporin (Burroughs Wellcome)
	+	−	Ocuspor G (Ocumed)
	+	−	Ocutricin (Pharmafair)
Polymyxin B-bacitracin	−	+	AK-Poly-Bac (Akorn)
	−	+	Ocumycin (Pharmafair)
	−	+	Polysporin (Burroughs Wellcome)
Trimethoprim-polymyxin B	+	−	Polytrim (Allergan)

more easily across the corneal barriers. Larger drugs such as bacitracin and polymyxin penetrate the anterior segment structures poorly, resulting in low corneal and aqueous drug concentrations.

b. **Drug concentration and vehicle.** Tactics used to enhance corneal and aqueous concentrations of drugs that would otherwise have poor ocular penetration include (1) the use of fortified or high-concentration solutions made up from systemic antibiotic drug preparations, (2) use of antibiotic ointments or viscous agents to increase contact time and decrease rapidity of drainage through the nasolacrimal system, and (3) increasing the frequency of drug administration.

(1) A significant **increase in the concentration** of an antibiotic solution will greatly enhance the diffusion gradient across the corneal tissues and thus increase intraocular and intracorneal levels. Although the concentrations are limited by solubility and toxicity of any given antibiotic, these fortified solutions are more effective in eliminating infectious organisms than are commercially available antibiotic solutions. Their use should, however, be confined to more serious anterior segment infections. They are not commercially available and must be made

Table 3-5. Commercial combination ophthalmic antibiotic-steroid preparations

Drugs	Solution	Ointment	Commercial name
Chloramphenicol-hydrocortisone	+*	−	Chloromycetin-hydrocortisone (Parke-Davis)
Chloramphenicol-polymyxin B-hydrocortisone	−	+	Ophthocort (Parke-Davis)
Fluoromethalone 0.1% = sulfacetamide 10%			FML-S (Allergan)
Gentamicin-prednisolone 1%	+	−	Pred G (Allergan)
Neomycin-polymyxin B-hydrocortisone	+	−	AK-Spore, HC (Akorn)
	+	−	Cortisporin (Burroughs Wellcome)
	+	−	Ocutricin HC (Pharmafair)
Neomycin-polymyxin B-bacitracin-hydrocortisone	−	+	AK-Spore, HC (Akorn)
	−	+	Cortisporin (Burroughs Wellcome)
	−	+	Ocutricin HC (Pharmafair)
Neomycin-polymyxin B-prednisolone 0.5%	+	−	Poly-Pred (Allergan)
Neomycin-dexamethasone 0.1%	+	+	NeoDecadron (Merck Sharp & Dohme)
	+	−	Ne Dexair (Pharmafair)
	+	+	AK-Trol (Akorn)
Neomycin-polymyxin B-dexamethasone 0.1%	+	+	Dexacidin (IOLAB Pharmaceuticals)
	+	+	Maxitrol (Alcon)
	+	+	Ocutrol (Ocumed)
Sulfacetamide 10%-prednisolone 0.5–0.25%	+	+	Many
Tobramycin-dexamethasone 0.1%	+	−	Tobradex (Alcon)

* No preservative.

up in hospital pharmacies. Methods of preparation and dosages are listed in Table 3-6.

(2) **Ointments and viscous vehicles** increase drug contact time and, therefore, offer superior bioavailability compared with commercially available solutions. However, hydrophilic drugs may crystallize within the carrying base, resulting in decreased bioavailability. Because ointments may interfere with absorption of eye drops, they should be given after any concomitantly administered solutions. Fortified ointments are not available commercially and are not usually made in hospital pharmacies, as there is no apparent advantage over fortified solutions. Viscous vehicles are less effective than ointments in increasing tissue contact time and penetration and appear to work primarily by reducing rate of lacrimal drainage.

(3) **Aqueous suspensions,** as opposed to true solutions, require that the patient shake the bottle vigorously before use to assure delivery of the suspended drug particles to the eye. Even with shaking, however, bioavailability and tissue penetration of suspensions are variable and are dependent on dissolution of drug in the tear film. The ultimate therapeutic efficacy is dependent on both competent delivery to the eye and the state of the host tear film, ie, an inflamed, tearing eye will wash drug out much more quickly than a normal eye.

(4) An increase in the **frequency of drop delivery** greatly elevates drug concentration in the cornea and aqueous humor. Although drops given more closely than every 4–5 minutes wash the preceding drug out, a rapid loading dose of 1 drop every minute for 5 minutes repeated in an hour will produce extremely high therapeutic drug concentrations within the cornea. Therapy may then be reduced to 1 drop every 30 minutes to 1 hour around the clock initially for severe anterior segment infections, eg, bacterial keratitis. When more than one drug is being used, 4–5 minutes must be allowed to elapse between delivery of the two drugs at any given time. There appears to be little advantage of continuous topical lavage with dilute antibiotic solution through an irrigating contact lens. The recent advent, however, of spontaneously dissolving **collagen contact lenses** may offer an alternative means of delivery of high doses of antibiotic to the cornea. Soaking these contact lenses in antibiotic before placement on the eye results in continuous passage of drug across the cornea for several hours. Antibiotic dosage using these lenses

Table 3-6. Preparation of antibiotics for fortified topical and subconjunctival use

Antibiotic (IM or IV formulation)	Commercial solution	Fortified topical drops			Subconjunctival		
		Diluent[a] (ml) added to 1.0 ml commercial solution	Final concentration	Shelf life 4°C[b]	Diluent[a] (ml) added to 1.0 ml commercial solution	Final concentration	Final dose
Amikacin	1.0 g/10 ml	9.0	10 mg/ml	30 ds	3.0	50 mg/ml	25–50 mg
Ampicillin	250 mg/ml	4.0	50 mg/ml	4 hrs	—	250 mg/ml	125 mg
Bacitracin	50,000 U/5 ml	—	10,000 U/ml	7 ds	—	10,000 U/ml	5,000 U
Carbenicillin	1.0 g/10 ml	24.0	4 mg/ml	3 ds	—	100 mg/ml	100 mg
Cefamandole	1.0 g/5 ml	3.0	50 mg/ml	4 ds	1.0	100 mg/ml	100 mg
Cefazolin	1.0 g/10 ml	2.0	33 mg/ml	10 ds	—	—	—
Cefazolin	1.0 g/10 ml	1.0	50 mg/ml	10 ds	4.0	100 mg/ml	100 mg
Cefazolin	1.0 g/2 ml	2.75	133 mg/ml	10 ds	—	—	—

Ceftriaxone	1.0 g/10 ml	1.0	50 mg/ml	10 ds	—	100 mg/ml	100 mg
Chloramphenicol	1.0 g/10 ml	19.0	5 mg/ml	7 ds	—	100 mg/ml	100 mg
Gentamicin	80 mg/2 ml	1.8	14 mg/ml	30 ds	—	—	—
Gentamicin	80 mg/2 ml	1.0	20 mg/ml	30 ds	—	40 mg/ml	20 mg
Methicillin	1.0 g/10 ml	1.0	50 mg/ml	4 ds	—	100 mg/ml	100 mg
Moxalactam	1.0 g/10 ml	1.0	50 mg/ml	4 ds	—	100 mg/ml	100 mg
Penicillin G	5 million U/5 ml	—	—	—	—	1 million U/ml	1 million U
Penicillin G	1 million U/10 ml	—	100,000 U/ml	7 ds	—	—	—
Polymyxin B	5000,000 U/ml	9.0	50,000 U/ml	3 ds	—	—	—
Ticarcillin	1.0 g/10 ml	16.0	6 mg/ml	14 days	—	—	—
Tobramycin	80 mg/2 ml	1.8	14 mg/ml	30 ds	—	40 mg/ml	20–40 mg
Vancomycin	500 mg/ml	9.0	50 mg/ml	14 ds	9.0	50 mg/ml	25 mg
Vancomycin	500 mg/ml	19.0	25 mg/ml	14 ds	—	—	—

[a] With the exception of carbenicillin and vancomycin (sterile water for injection only) and bacitracin (normal saline for injection only), diluent may be sterile water or saline for injection (USP), or sterile artificial tears, using the original tears bottle to administer the reconstituted topical drug solution.

[b] Freezing (−20°C) extends expiration time to 12 weeks for aminoglycosides, cephalosporins, and vancomycin; 4 weeks for ticarcillin.

new and drug-soaked daily will, with drops, be very high.

2. **Subconjunctival (anterior subtenon) injection** (see Table 3-6). Antibiotics administered by injection in the subconjunctival and anterior subtenon space enter the eye through leakage into the precorneal tear film and then across the cornea, and by direct penetration through the cornea and sclera. The latter route is probably of greater importance, as drug concentrations are highest in the injection region. Extremely high corneal drug concentrations are achieved through subconjunctival injection, but these decline rapidly over 3–6 hours, necessitating repetition every 12–24 hours to maintain high therapeutic doses.

The use of subconjunctival injection is currently the subject of some controversy for several reasons: the injections may be painful, even when given with concomitant Xylocaine and after pre-anesthetizing the tissues with cocaine-soaked pledgets (recommended if the injection is to be given); they may induce subconjunctival and subtenon scarring and focal necrosis; and they are no more effective therapeutically than frequent fortified antibiotic drops. This route is less used now than previously and is generally reserved for cases in which extremely high local tissue levels of drug are required immediately, for infants in whom drug administration may be difficult, and for unreliable or uncooperative patients. Subconjunctival injections are generally not used alone as therapy but in combination with fortified topical antibiotic drops with or without concomitant systemic antibiotics. Despite the high corneal tissue drug levels, aqueous levels achieved with subconjunctival injection are significantly lower, although they are in the therapeutic range for most antibiotics. Subconjunctival injection is also being replaced by intravitreal injection as part of the therapeutic approach to bacterial endophthalmitis.

3. **Intravitreal antibiotic injection.** In the management of endophthalmitis, the use of combined topical subconjunctival and intravenous antibiotics has failed in most cases to produce sustained therapeutic levels of intravitreal drug. As a result, direct injection of diluted antibiotics into the vitreous has become a more favored therapeutic approach.

Appropriate and safe concentrations of intravitreal antibiotics have now been worked out and are listed in Table 3-7. Water-soluble drugs diffuse freely within the aqueous and pass out of the eye via the trabecular meshwork or by passive and active transport across the retina. The aminoglycosides, which are cleared primarily through the trabecular meshwork, have a half-life of approximately 30 hours, although intraocular inflammation and aphakia will shorten this half-life. Concomitant use of probenecid prolongs the half-life of carbenicillin from 10 to 20 hours and that of cefazolin from 7 to 30 hours in the vitreous. The third-genera-

Table 3-7. Intravitreous antibiotic preparations

	Initial Solution Mix		Final Solution Mix			
Drug	Commercial preparation (IV)	First diluent[a] added to 1.0 ml commercial preparation	Initial solution (ml)	Plus second diluent[a] (ml)	Final drug concentration	Injected dose (0.1 ml)
Amikacin	1.0 g/10 ml	—	0.4	9.6	4.0 mg/ml	0.4 mg
Amikacin	1 g/10 ml	—	0.2	18.8	1.0 mg/ml	0.1 mg
Ampicillin	1.0 g/5 ml	1.0	1.0	1.0	50 mg/ml	5.0 mg
Carbenicillin	5 g/10 ml	1.0	1.0	9.0	25 mg/ml	2.5 mg
Cefamandole	1.0 g/5 ml	1.0	1.0	4.0	20 mg/ml	2.0 mg
Cefazolin	500 mg/ml	1.0	1.0	9.0	25 mg/ml	2.5 mg
Ceftriaxone	1.0 g/5 ml	1.0	1.0	4.0	20 mg/ml	2.0 mg
Chloramphenicol	1.0 g/5 ml	1.0	1.0	4.0	20 mg/ml	2.0 mg
Clindamycin	150 mg/ml	2.0	1.0	4.0	10 mg/ml	1.0 mg
Clindamycin	150 mg/ml	2.0	1.0	9.0	5 mg/ml	0.5 mg
Gentamicin	80 mg/2 ml	6.0	1.0	9.0	1.0 mg/ml	0.1 mg
Gentamicin	80 mg/2 ml	6.0	2.0	8.0	2.0 mg/ml	0.2 mg
Methicillin	1.0 g/5 ml	—	1.0	9.0	20 mg/ml	2.0 mg
Tobramycin	80 mg/2 ml	3.0	1.0	9.0	1.0 mg/ml	0.1 mg
Vancomycin	500 mg/ml	9.0	1.0	4.0	10 mg/ml	1.0 mg
Vancomycin	500 mg/ml	9.0	0.4	0.6	20 mg/ml	2.0 mg

[a] With the exception of carbenicillin and vancomycin (sterile water for injection only), diluent may be sterile water or saline for injection (USP).

tion cephalosporin, ceftriaxone, remains in the vitreous and aqueous for up to 2 days after intravitreal injection. Human studies have shown aminoglycoside (gentamicin) levels as long as 24–48 hours after intravitreal administration.

Intravitreal preparations must be made accurately, as retinal toxicity from antibiotics is the chief limiting factor in their use and the main source of potential adverse effects. Drug dilution should be made in large solutions to minimize dilution errors, and injections made gently into the anterior midvitreous area to avoid high concentrations near the retina.

4. **Systemic administration.** Systemic antibiotics are used in infections of the external eye caused by certain organisms such as *Neisseria, Hemophilus,* and *Chlamydia,* in the treatment pf preseptal and orbital cellulitis, dacryocystitis, and endophthalmitis. Intravenous injection is superior to intramuscular or oral administration in achieving therapeutic tissue levels. Systemic drugs are usually not indicated in therapy of corneal infections, as tissue levels achieved by this route are insignificant. They are indicated only in the face of impending or actual perforation, extension of the infectious process beyond the limits of the corneal limbus, or in aphakia where there is a deep corneal infection and no intact posterior capsule. Aqueous concentrations in therapeutic levels are achieved after systemic administration and parallel the concentration in cerebrospinal fluid for most drugs, thus reflecting the similarity between the blood–brain barrier in the CNS and in the eye. Significant vitreous levels are not well achieved even by intravenous therapy, however, although ocular inflammation, either anterior or posterior, enhances penetration of drug administered by any systemic route. Lipophilic antibiotics such as chloramphenicol and the tetracyclines have a greater ocular penetration than do systemically administered nonlipophilic drugs.

As reviewed later under "Specific Antibiotics," systemic administration of these drugs should take into consideration a patient's hepatic and renal function, as their metabolism and excretion are a function of one or both of these organ systems. **Assessment of renal and liver function before and during the course of systemic drug therapy is paramount,** and drug dosages and frequency of administration should be adjusted accordingly. Many of these drugs have significant neural, hepatic, and renal toxicity if systemic levels are allowed to rise too high.

C. **Allergic reactions to antibiotics**
   1. **History.** The validity of a patient's report of drug allergy should be investigated by more extensive history and, if warranted and possible, communication with the patient's physician at the time. Many patients are not, in fact, truly allergic to many drugs to which they may have had an unpleasant reaction. The exact drug,

route of administration, and type of reaction should be ascertained and judgment made as to whether the event was an allergic one. Frequently, patients may have taken the same drug at a later date and had no problem, thus implying the former reaction was not allergic.

2. **Severe allergic reactions** to antibiotics are more commonly seen after parenteral administration. The penicillins may cause delayed reactions such as skin rash, serum sickness, and drug fever, with ampicillin and amoxicillin causing maculopapular rashes more frequently than other members of this drug group. Oral medication resulting in a rash is likely to produce the same type of reaction again if given by the same route. Anaphylaxis with oral penicillin is rare, particularly in children. Injected drug resulting in swelling of the tongue or shortness of breath, however, is a serious warning of a potentially serious, even anaphylactic, reaction if the drug is given again. Allergy to one penicillin presumes allergy to all. Although cephalosporins are occasionally used as alternative therapy in penicillin-allergic patients, it should be remembered that there may be cross-allergenicity (5%–10%) between these two drug groups because of molecular similarity of the beta lactam rings.

3. Allergic reactions to **other antibiotic drugs** are not as commonly encountered as with penicillins but may occur with the sulfonamides, trimethoprim-sulfamethoxazole, nitrofurantoin, demeclocycline, flucytosine, nalidixic acid, and novobiocin.

4. **Skin testing.** If doubt persists about allergy and the drug in question is critical to best patient care, skin testing is of some use. Unfortunately, patients may react to the skin test itself, and a few who tested negatively to the skin test may still have a severe reaction when therapeutic drug doses are given. If true allergy is suspected, every effort should be made to substitute a non–cross-reacting drug.

IV. **Specific Antibiotics.** The methods of use and the dosages of the following antimicrobial agents are indicated in Tables 3-1, 3-2, 3-6, and 3-7.

A. **Aminoglycosides.** The aminoglycoside antibiotics of importance in ophthalmology are **gentamicin, tobramycin, amikacin, neomycin,** and occasionally **streptomycin.** These bactericidal polycationic drugs are amino sugars bound by glycosidic linkage. Their polarity results in poor absorption after oral administration, low cerebrospinal and, therefore, potentially low intraocular concentrations after systemic administration, and rapid renal clearance. Much of the gentamicin that does enter the eye after systemic, topical, or subconjunctival administration is bound in the iris and choroidal pigment epithelium, thus reducing bioavailability.

1. **Spectrum of activity.** With the exception of neomycin, all aminoglycosides may be given systemically as well as topically. These drugs are used primarily in

treating external, periocular, and intraocular infections with aerobic gram-negative bacilli, alone or in combination with a cephalosporin or a penicillin. Aminoglycosides should **not** be mixed directly with a penicillin, as the former drug may be inactivated. Susceptible organisms include *Pseudomonas aeruginosa, Escherichia coli, Herellea (Mima), Enterobacter, Proteus, Klebsiella,* and *Serratia marcescens.* Tobramycin is somewhat more active than gentamicin against *P. aeruginosa.* Unlike gentamicin and amikacin, tobramycin has poor activity against *Enterococcus* and *Mycobacterium.* Amikacin is a drug of choice for the atypical mycobacterium, *M. fortuitum.* Tobramycin and neomycin are also active in vitro against 95% of strains of *S. aureus* and *S. epidermidis,* but neither should be used alone as the primary drug against serious ocular infections with these aerobic gram-positive cocci. *Streptococcus pneumonia (Pneumococcus)* and *Streptococcus pyogenes* are highly resistant to all aminoglycosides. However, gentamicin, and to a lesser extent tobramycin and amikacin, are synergistic with penicillin G, a cephalosporin, or with vancomycin in treatment of *Streptococcus faecalis* and *Streptococcus viridans.*

2. **Mechanism of action and resistance.** The aminoglycosides interfere with bacterial protein synthesis through ribosomal inhibition. Resistance against these drugs may emerge rapidly, either through mutations affecting proteins in the bacterial ribosomes or through plasmid transfer of genetic information conferring ability to produce drug-metabolizing enzymes. Bacteria resistant to one aminoglycoside may be resistant to others. Fortunately, most gentamicin- and tobramycin-resistant microorganisms are susceptible to amikacin because of its unique resistance to drug-inactivating enzymes.

3. **Adverse side effects**
   a. **Topical use** of the aminoglycosides may produce transient irritation, burning, or stinging with either drug or ointment. A reversible toxic superficial punctate keratitis and conjunctivitis may develop within 2 weeks or longer of topical treatment. Hypersensitivity reactions, usually skin rashes, are seen much more commonly with neomycin than with other aminoglycosides; this adverse effect develops in 6–8% of patients after topical use. Pseudomembranous conjunctivitis has been reported with topical administration of gentamicin.
   b. **Systemic drug** reactions include reversible and irreversible renal and vestibular/cochlear ototoxicity. Prolonged or successive courses of therapy enhance the chances of significant irreversible auditory/vestibular dysfunction. Renal function impairment is almost always reversible, however, because of the regenerative capacity of the proximal

renal tubules. The incidence of ototoxicity is approximately 25% and renal impairment 8–26% when aminoglycosides are given for more than several days. Patients should be monitored for these effects with audiometry at baseline and every 2–3 weeks thereafter until levels are stable after the drug has been stopped; serum creatinine levels taken within 24 hours of starting therapy and monitored 2–3 times weekly. Serum drug levels are taken at 72 hours (optimal peak, 4–10 mcg/ml; trough, <2 mcg/ml). Pre-existing renal insufficiency will enhance toxicity through elevated serum levels, and appropriate dosage adjustments should be made. The concomitant use of cephalosporin will also enhance both ototoxicity and renal toxicity, as these drugs themselves are damaging to these organ systems.

   c. **Rare systemic side effects** include hypersensitivity reactions such as rash, fever, and eosinophilia. A neuromuscular blockade is rare, but can produce muscle weakness or respiratory failure. Other toxic side effects include hemolytic anemia, agranulocytosis, depression of clotting factor 5 levels, and myocarditis.

B. Bacitracin and gramicidin

  1. Spectrum of activity and mechanism of action. These bactericidal polypeptide antibiotics are comparably effective against a variety of gram-positive cocci and bacilli. Gramicidin alters cell wall permeability; bacitracin, a neutrophil chemotactic agent and a chelating agent, alters cell wall peptidosynthesis. Susceptible organisms include *S. aureus, S. epidermidis, Neisseria, Haemophilus influenzae,* and *Treponema pallidum,* all of which are sensitive to 0.1 U or less of bacitracin/ml. *Actinomyces* and *Fusobacterium* are inhibited by concentrations of 0.5–5.0 U/ml.

  2. Routes of administration. The use of commercial topical preparations of either drug or of subconjunctival bacitracin will produce excellent therapeutic external ocular drug levels. Therapeutic aqueous levels are achieved only in the presence of an epithelial defect or inflammation. As a fortified solution, bacitracin may be used in therapy of keratitis due to susceptible organisms. Gramicidin is used only as a topical preparation in combination with neomycin and polymyxin B, a preparation most commonly used for blepharoconjunctivitis or marginal keratitis.

  3. Adverse side effects. Because bacitracin is highly nephrotoxic and gramicidin is a potent hemolytic agent, these drugs can not be used systemically. Hypersensitivity reactions are very rarely seen with topical bacitracin, thereby giving it an advantage over other antibiotics of similar therapeutic spectrum. Both fortified drops and subconjunctival injection of bacitracin are, however, locally toxic and irritating, but are indicated in certain more severe ocular infections such as methicillin-resistant staphylococcal keratitis. The drugs are not indicated for therapy of endophthalmitis, as vitreous levels are poor regardless of the route of administration.

C. **Cephalosporins.** The cephalosporins, like the structurally related penicillins, are all classified as beta lactams owing to the common presence of a lactam ring in all drugs of these groups. This rapidly expanding drug family is now categorized into first-, second-, and third-generation agents (see Table 3-2). These drugs are widely used, often empirically, because of their broad spectrum, good bactericidal activity, and low toxicity.

1. **Spectrum of activity.** The cephalosporins have therapeutic activity against many gram-positive, gram-negative, and anaerobic organisms. As a rule the first-generation drugs such as cefazolin are most effective against the gram-positive staphylococci and streptococci (except *Strep. faecalis*), whereas second- and third-generation drugs such as cefoxitin, cefamandole, and cefotaxime are most effective against the gram-negative bacilli, *P. aeruginosa* and Enterobacteriaceae (*E. coli, Klebsiella, Proteus mirabilis, Serratia*).

   a. **Gram-positive organisms.** For staphylococci sensitive to cephalosporins, first-generation drugs are preferred, with cefazolin being the drug of choice. It has the advantage over semisynthetic penicillins in reduced frequency of dosage, thus making it more convenient and cost effective. With the exception of ceftizoxime and cefotaxime, the third-generation cephalosporins have limited activity against staphylococci. No available cephalosporins are therapeutically effective against methicillin-resistant *S. aureus,* penicillin-resistant *Strep. pneumoniae* or *Listeria monocytogenes.* If **methicillin-resistant staphylococcus** is isolated, vancomycin and bacitracin are the drugs of choice. With the exception of enterococci (*Strep, faecalis*), streptococci as a group are sensitive to most cephalosporins. Cefazolin has the highest activity against streptococci, and, of third-generation agents, ceftizoxime is the most effective. Cefazidime, moxalactam, cefsulodin, and aztreonam have little or no activity against these microorganisms.

   b. **Gram-negative organisms.** *H. influenza* (bacillus) and *Neisseria gonorrhoeae* (coccus) are generally susceptible to most second-generation drugs with the exception of cefoxitin. Third-generation cephalosporins show good activity against these organisms.

      The gram-negative bacillus family, or Enterobacteriaceae, may be classified into two drug-senstivity groups. *E. coli, P. mirabilis,* and *Klebsiella* are generally sensitive to all cephalosporin drugs with the exception of cefsulodin. The *Enterobacter* species,

Serratia and some other Enterobacteriaceae, are more resistant to first- and second-generation cephalosporins. Third-generation cephalosporins, imipenem, and aztreonam, however, are highly active against *Enterobacter, Serratia,* and gram-negative bacilli resistant to multiple other antibiotics.

P. aeruginosa is resistant to first-, second-, and some third-generation cephalosporins. There is, however, considerable therapeutic activity against this organism by the third-generation agents ceftazidime (most active), cefsulodin, and cefoperazone. Imipenem has high activity comparable to that of ceftazidime, and the monobactam aztreonam is comparable to the other third-generation cephalosporins with activity against this organism. Of all the cephalosporins, cefsulodin is unique in that it shows considerable activity against only *Staphylococcus* and *P. aeruginosa.* **Imipenem is the most active broad-spectrum antibiotic currently available.**

2. **Mechanism of action.** Cephalosporins inhibit bacterial cell wall synthesis in a manner similar to that of penicillin. The beta-lactam antibiotics cross the bacterial cell wall, resist degradation by beta-lactamases, and then bind to penicillin-binding proteins. This process interferes with cell wall construction, resulting in death of the organism.

3. **Microbial resistance** to these drugs is almost invariably due to hydrolytic degradation of the antibiotics by bacterial beta-lactamase enzymes. Enzymatic disruption of the beta-lactam ring inactivates the antibiotic. Newer cephalosporins have been synthesized with alterations directed toward stabilizing the beta-lactam ring or with side chain substitutions that preserve antimicrobial activity by protecting the drug from enzymatic inactivation by bacterial enzymes. Such drugs include cefotaxime, ceftizoxime, and ceftriaxone. More radical changes of the drug nuclear structure have resulted in beta-lactamase–resistant carbapinem (imipenem) and the monobactam, aztreonam. Some cephalosporins, such as cefoxitin, may induce beta-lactamase production and cause broad microbial resistance to other antimicrobials. Other agents, such as aztreonam and imipenem, do not induce beta-lactamase activity and are poor substrates for drug-destructive enzymes.

4. **Adverse side effects.** Compared with other antimicrobial agents, the cephalosporins are relatively nontoxic.

   a. **Topical** administration of fortified cephalosporin eye drops may produce transient stinging or burning, but significant drug toxic reactions to topical agents have not been a major problem with this drug family.

   b. **Systemic drugs** may produce hypersensitivity or

allergic reactions in the form of maculopapular rash, urticaria, drug fever, or eosinophilia in 1–5% of patients. Severe reactions such as anaphylaxis and angioedema are extremely rare. Although hypersensitivity cross-reactions may occur between penicillins and cephalosporins, the latter may usually be safely given to patients with a history of only a penicillin-induced skin rash. They should not be used in patients with a history of anaphylaxis or other severe penicillin reactions. Immunologic studies have demonstrated cross-reactivity in up to 20% of patients who are allergic to penicillin, but most reports indicate a frequency in the range of 5–10%.

  c. **Other adverse side effects of systemic drugs** include hemorrhagic complications due to platelet dysfunction or prothrombin deficiency, particularly with third-generation cephalosporins and moxalactam. Disulfiram-like reaction after alcohol ingestion, diarrhea, superinfection with *Pseudomonas, Candida,* and enterococci, seizures (imipenem) and nausea, hypotension, dizziness, and sweating have all been reported after systemic administration.

  Cephalosporins are potentially nephrotoxic agents, and their concomitant administration with aminoglycosides such as gentamicin or tobramycin appears to cause nephrotoxicity synergistically. Patients on these drug combinations should be carefully monitored for renal dysfunction.

D. **Chloramphenicol** is a broad-spectrum bacteriostatic antibiotic active against many gram-positive, gram-negative, and anaerobic organisms. The drug is absorbed well orally and intravenously and is metabolized by the liver before renal excretion. Systemic administration results in a 60% protein binding in the serum, and because of its high lipid solubility compared with other antibiotics, systemic administration results in excellent aqueous humor penetration. Good therapeutic aqueous levels are also achieved after topical administration of commercially available chloramphenicol solution or ointment. No route of administration results in therapeutically adequate vitreous levels.

  1. **Spectrum of activity.** Susceptible organisms include *S. aureus,* streptococci including *Strep. pneumoniae,* the gram-negative bacilli *E. coli, H. influenza, Klebsiella,* Enterobacteriaceae spp., *Moraxella lacunata,* and *Neisseria* spp. The drug is **not** adequately effective against *P. aeruginosa* or *S. marcescens.*

  2. **Mechanism of action.** Chloramphenicol acts by inhibiting bacterial protein synthesis through interference with transfer of amino acids from soluble RNA to ribosomes. This is achieved primarily by reversible drug binding to the 50S ribosomal subunit. Chloramphenicol also may inhibit mitochondrial protein synthesis in mammalian cells, perhaps because of

similarities between bacterial and mammalian mito-
chondria. Red blood cells appear to be particularly sensitive to this drug.

3. **Resistance** to chloramphenicol by both gram-positive
and gram-negative microorganisms is a problem of increasing importance clinically. The resistance of gram-
negative organisms is usually through plasmid transfer of genetic information that codes for resistance not
only to chloramphenicol but also to tetracycline and to
a beta-lactamase, resulting in penicillin resistance. Up
to 50% of hospital-strain staphylococci are also resistant to chloramphenicol as a result of microbial enzymatic degradation of the drug, decreased permeability
of the microorganism to drug entry, and insensitivity
to chloramphenicol through ribosomal mutation.

4. **Adverse side effects. Because of potential life-
threatening toxicity, therapy with chloramphenicol must be limited to those infections in which
the benefits of the drug outweigh the toxic risk. If
other antimicrobial drugs of equal efficacy and
less potential toxicity are available, they should
be used in place of chloramphenicol.**

   a. **Topical.** Ophthalmic use of chloramphenicol is reserved almost entirely to topical administration.
   Local drug toxicity is negligible and true allergic
   reactions are extremely rare. Bone marrow hypo-
   plasia, including aplastic anemia and death, have
   been reported after topical application of chloramphenicol. The drug's ability to produce a fatal aplastic anemia is extremely rare, in the range of
   1:50,000, and is considered idiosyncratic. Bone marrow suppression with pancytopenia appears to be
   dose related, with leukopenia being an early indication. Monitoring the blood count is essential during full therapy longer than 1 month; full bone
   marrow recovery is common within 3 weeks of discontinuing the drug if leukopenia is noted. Four
   instances of agranulocytosis, two fatal, were reported after prolonged topical use (40–690 days). It
   should be noted that these patients had been taking
   other concomitant systemic medication.

   b. **Systemic** long-term chloramphenicol therapy has
   caused acute bilateral optic neuritis in certain patients with cystic fibrosis. Some patients recover
   hearing after discontinuation of the medication.
   High doses or overdose of chloramphenicol may result in acute circulatory collapse in any age group.
   Oral administration may also result in gastrointestinal symptoms, including cramping and diarrhea,
   and superinfection with resistant bacteria or fungi.

   c. **Concomitant administration** of chloramphenicol
   with other drugs, including the sulfonylureas, coumarin, and diphenylhydantoin, may potentiate
   their effects.

E. **Clindamycin** is a bacteriostatic congener of lincomycin.

It is active against a wide variety of gram-positive and gram-negative organisms including anaerobes. The drug may be administered orally, IM, or IV, and although aqueous levels are negligible after systemic administration, clindamycin is actively concentrated in the retina and choroid. The drug is 25% protein bound in the serum and is metabolized in the liver before renal and gastrointestinal clearance. Topical clindamycin penetrates the cornea to reach the aqueous in therapeutic levels; the hydrochloride form produces aqueous levels twice those of the phosphate.

1. **Spectrum of activity.** Clindamycin is active against *Strep. pneumoniae, Strep. pyogenes,* and *Strep. viridans.* It is also active against many strains of *S. aureus,* with the exception of methicillin-resistant organisms. Strains resistant to clindamycin are often resistant to erythromycin and chloramphenicol, as all three drugs have a similar mechanism of action despite the fact that they are not structurally related. Clindamycin is superior to erythromycin in therapy of anaerobic bacteria, especially *Bacteroides fragilis* and *Actinoymces*; it is also effective against *Toxoplasma gondii* (see Chap. 6, Antiparasitic Drugs). Essentially all aerobic gram-negative bacilli are resistant, as are Enterococci (*Strep. faecalis*) and *N. meningitidis,* to drug concentrations that can be achieved clinically.

2. **Mechanism of action and resistance.** Like erythromycin and chloramphenicol, clindamycin binds exclusively to the 50S subunit of bacterial ribosomes. Because these three drugs all work by similar mechanisms, combination therapy with two or more may result in **inhibition of the therapeutic efficacy** of one or both agents. Resistance to clindamycin via plasmid-mediated methylation of bacterial ribosomal RNA has been reported in *B. fragilis.*

3. **Adverse side effects.** Diarrhea, possibly due to alteration of intestinal flora, is the most common side effect of clindamycin therapy. Other gastrointestinal side effects include abdominal pain, esophagitis, nausea and vomiting, and, rarely, pseudomembranous colitis, which is potentially fatal. Abnormal liver function tests, jaundice, transient neutropenia, and eosinophilia have all been reported during clindamycin treatment. Hypersensitivity reactions as manifested by maculopapular skin rashes and urticaria may occur, and, very rarely, erythema multiforme and anaphylaxis.

F. **Erythromycin** is a macrolide antibiotic that may be either bacteriostatic or bactericidal, depending on the organism and drug concentration. The drug may be given as a topical ointment or oral systemic preparation. Despite the excellent systemic absorption of oral erythromycin ethylsuccinate or stearate and the high systemic levels achieved by erythromycin lactobionate and gluceptate, the drug does not penetrate ocular tissues well. It is rapidly metabolized by the liver and excreted in the bile.

Systemic preparations, therefore, have little or no place in the treatment of serious corneal or intraocular infections.

1. **Spectrum of activity.** Erythromycin is most effective against gram-positive cocci such as *Strep. pyogenes* and *Strep. pneumoniae*. Although some staphylococci are sensitive to erythromycin, drug-resistant strains of *S. aureus* are frequently encountered in hospitals. Many gram-positive bacilli are sensitive to erythromycin, including *Clostridium perfringens, Corynebacterium diphtheriae,* and *Listeria monocytogenes.* The drug is not active against aerobic gram-negative bacilli and has only moderate activity against *H. influenza* and *Neisseria meningitidis* although it has excellent activity against most strains of *N. gonorrhoeae. Chlamydia trachomatis* is also susceptible to easily achieved therapeutic levels of erythromycin.

2. **Mechanism of action.** Erythromycin inhibits bacterial protein synthesis by reversible competitive binding to the 50S ribosomal subunits of sensitive organisms. The drug may interfere with the binding of chloramphenicol or clindamycin, both of which also act at the 50S site. Mutational changes in the ribosomal subunit result in failure of drug binding and thus confer drug resistance on the microorganism.

3. **Adverse reactions. Topical** erythromycin ointment is the least toxic antibiotic preparation commerically available. Toxic or allergic reactions to this drug are extremely rare. **Systemic** erythromycin may on occasion induce abdominal cramping, nausea, vomiting, or diarrhea, but this is uncommon with the usual oral dose. True allergic reactions are uncommon; they range from mild maculopapular skin rash to anaphylactic shock.

G. **Penicillins.** The penicillins, like the cephalosporins, are a constantly expanding antibiotic family with at least 21 different natural and semisynthetic drugs currently available. The original penicillin drugs are as useful today against many bacteria as they were when initially introduced 40 years ago. Semisynthetic penicillins, with changes in the acyl side chain on the drug nucleus, have conferred penicillinase resistance and extended the antimicrobial spectrum of this drug family to include not only the original gram-positive organisms but aerobic gram-negative bacilli such as *P. aeruginosa.* The penicillins, like their close relatives the cephalosporins, all possess a beta-lactam ring. In ocular infections the drugs may be given effectively as topical fortified solutions by subconjunctival or intravitreal injection, and systemically with excellent bactericidal activity and low toxicity. Although most penicillins are cleared from the body via the renal system in active form, the new ureidopenicillins are cleared through both the biliary system and urinary tract.

1. **Spectrum of activity.** Penicillin G is the drug of choice for almost all *Streptococcus* infections of the eye,

including *Strep. pneumoniae,* group A, B, C, G, *Strep. viridans, Strep. faecalis,* and *Peptostreptococcus* (anaerobic), as well as non–penicillinase-producing, coagulase-negative *S. aureus* and *N. meningitidis.* Numerous other organisms of little importance in ophthalmology are also susceptible to penicillin G. The emergence of **penicillinase-producing staphylococci** resulted in the development of penicillinase-resistant drugs in which the acyl side chain prevented disruption of the beta-lactam ring. These drugs include methicillin, oxacillin, nafcillin, cloxacillin, and dicloxacillin. Unfortunately, **methicillin-resistant staphylococci** have now become a major clinical problem, and methicillin-resistant strains of this organism should be treated with vancomycin.

The amino penicillins, ampicillin and amoxicillin, were developed to achieve **gram-negative** antimicrobial activity with a therapeutic spectrum that included *E. coli, P. mirabilis, Hemophilus, Listeria,* and other gram-negative bacilli. The carboxy penicillins, carbenicillin and ticarcillin, and the ureido- and piperazine penicillins, mezlocillin and piperacillin and others, were developed to extend even greater antimicrobial efficacy against the Enterobacteriaceae and *P. aeruginosa.* The most recent development in the penicillins is the combination of amoxicillin and ticarcillin with clavulanate, and ampicillin with sulbactam, both additives being beta-lactamase inhibitors, thus further extending the antimicrobial spectrum with microbial resistance-protected agents. The addition of clavulanate or sulbactam confers penicillinase resistance against beta-lactamase–producing strains of *S. aureus* and *S. epidermidis, H. influenza, E. coli, Proteus,* and *Klebsiella.*

2. **Mechanism of action and resistance.** The antimicrobial efficacy of the penicillins is dependent on the presence of a bacterial cell wall that contains peptidoglycans accessible to the drug. Penicillins are most active, therefore, against actively growing organisms, and interfere with the biosynthesis of the peptidoglycan structure, preventing development of the normal structural support of the cell wall, leading to lysis. These drugs may also activate bacterial autolysis, thus disrupting the structural integrity of the cell wall.

Development of microbial resistance to the penicillins is similar to that described above under cephalosporins. The target site in the drug is the beta-lactam ring, which may be susceptible to bacterial beta-lactamases unless protected by semisynthetic alterations in the acyl side chain.

3. **Adverse drug reactions**
   a. **Hypersensitivity.** A hypersensitivity reaction develops in 3–10% of patients treated with a penicillin, and the reaction extends to all penicillins. The most common allergic reactions are maculopapular

skin rash, fever, serum sickness, and nephropathy, with anaphylaxis being rare but more common than with other antimicrobial families. Atopic patients have a higher incidence of penicillin hypersensitivity. In contrast to drops or to topical application followed by IM injection, topical application of penicillin G ointment to the eye is particularly prone to producing a hypersensitivity reaction. Skin testing will identify many, but not all, penicillin-allergic patients. From 5–20% of penicillin-allergic patients also display a cross-allergenicity with the cephalosporins. This drug family should, therefore, be used with caution as an alternative to penicillin. **Alternative drugs** for the penicillins and cephalosporins include erythromycin, vancomycin, and clindamycin in the treatment of gram-positive infections. The aminoglycosides are alternatives for gram-negative disease.

   b. Toxic reaction to penicillins include diarrhea, neutropenia, anemia, drug fever, and pseudomembranous colitis. High doses may produce a nephropathy, neuromuscular irritability with or without seizures, and potassium or sodium overload. Hematologic disorders have been reported with carbenicillin and methicillin and include platelet dysfunction, thrombocytopenia, and hemorrhagic cystitis. Oxacillin and ticarcillin have occasionally produced neurologic reactions with aberrant psychological behavior.

H. Polymyxins. The polymyxins B and E (colistin) are bactericidal, peptide cationic detergents that are highly effective against certain gram-negative organisms. Neither drug is absorbed orally or through mucous membranes. Polymyxin B sulfate is commercially available for ophthalmic topical use in ointment form combined with bacitracin or bacitracin and neomycin. Parenteral use is not advised, although subconjunctival injection of polymyxin B may be useful adjunctive therapy in certain gram-negative bacterial corneal ulcers.

   1. Spectrum of activity. The antimicrobial activity of the polymyxins is confined to gram-negative bacteria, including *Enterobacter, E. coli, Klebsiella,* and other Enterobacteriaceae, as well as most strains of *P. aeruginosa.*

   2. Mechanism of action. Sensitivity to the polymyxins is related to the phospholipid content of the cell wall–membrane complex. The detergent action of the drugs interacts with the cell wall phospholipids, with subsequent drug penetration into and disruption of the structure of cell membranes. Resistance to polymyxins is rare, but when seen is the result of bacterial cell wall resistance to drug penetration to the level of the cell membrane.

   3. Adverse side effects
   a. Topical polymyxin B produces virtually no sys-

temic reactions because of almost complete lack of absorption of the drug. Hypersensitivity is, therefore, extremely uncommon or perhaps nonexistent. Rarely, topical use in the eye may result in a reversible superficial punctate keratitis. Subconjunctival injection of polymyxin B may result in severe conjunctival chemosis, so its use by this route should be done with caution and only with informed patient consent.

    b. **Systemically** administered drug may produce severe neural and renal toxicity and results in no significant penetration into the aqueous humor. Topical and subconjunctival administration results in corneal and aqueous therapeutic levels only in the presence of ocular inflammation or an epithelial defect. Therapeutic vitreous levels are not achieved by any route of administration. The drug is too toxic for intravitreal injection.

I. 4-Quinolones. In recent years a number of antimicrobial compounds structurally related to nalidixic acid have been synthesized. These 4-quinolones are broad-spectrum bactericidal agents and include **ciprofloxacin, norfloxacin, ofloxacin, temofloxacin, perfloxacin,** and **enoxacin.** Ciprofloxacin is a very active 4-quinolone with the broadest spectrum against many common ocular pathogens. After oral administration this drug achieves aqueous humor levels therapeutically effective against *S. aureus* and *P. aeruginosa.* Both norfloxacin and ciprofloxacin are FDA approved for systemic use, and ofloxacin is approved in certain foreign countries. Several pharmaceutical firms are currently studying the topical use of 4-quinolones in external ocular infections.

    1. Spectrum of activity. The 4-quinolones demonstrate good to excellent therapeutic activity against a large number of gram-negative and gram-positive microorganisms. Susceptible bacteria include the gram-positive coccus *S. aureus,* and the gram-negative bacilli *H. influenza, P. aeruginosa, E. coli, Klebsiella,* and other Enterobacteriaceae, anaerobes, and *Legionella.* The drugs also have excellent activity against *N. gonorrhoeae* and *Chlamydia trachomatis.*

    2. Mechanism of action. The 4-quinolones are believed to act on bacteria through inhibition of DNA gyrase, an enzyme involved in chromosomal supercoiling, a function vital to the replication of bacterial DNA. Human DNA gyrase is not susceptible to inhibition by these drugs. At present, little data is available on resistance to this drug group.

    3. Adverse side effects. Side effects of topical application of 4-quinolones include occasional transient burning or stinging.

J. Rifampin is a bactericidal macrocyclic antibiotic with activity against most gram-positive and many gram-negative microorganisms. Its primary use, however, is as a systemic drug against *Mycobacterium.* Although topical application of 1% rifampin every 15 minutes produces therapeutic concentrations in rabbit corneas, the drug is currently not in use as a topical ophthalmic preparation.

1. **Spectrum of activity.** Rifampin inhibits the growth of *M. tuberculosis* and other mycobacterial species. It also increases the in vitro activity of streptomycin and isoniazid but not of ethambutol against *M. tuberculosis*. This antibiotic very effectively inhibits the gram-negative organisms *E. coli, Pseudomonas, Proteus, Klebsiella, H. influenza,* and *N. meningitidis* as well as *S. aureus, Chlamydia,* and *Candida.*

2. **Mechanism of action.** Rifampin inhibits DNA-dependent RNA polymerase in mycobacteria and other organisms with the resulting suppression of RNA synthesis. The drug is bactericidal for both intracellular and extracellular microorganisms. Because resistance to rifampin may develop during therapy, this drug is often used in combination with a second antibiotic.

3. **Adverse side effects.** The drug is metabolized in the liver and excreted via the biliary and renal systems, and therefore is potentially toxic. It decreases the anticoagulant effects of coumarin and decreases the half-life of many drugs, including prednisone, digitoxin, quinidine, and ketoconazole. Rifampin colors the tears, saliva, urine, and sweat orange, and patients may experience gastrointestinal and neurologic symptoms. Hypersensitivity is more common with high-dose therapy, and rashes, drug fever, and hematologic, renal, hepatic, and joint dysfunction may occur. Pulmonary anaphylaxis is extremely rare.

K. **Sulfonamides.** The sulfonamides are all derivates of para-aminobenzenesulfonamide (PABA). They have a wide range of antimicrobial activity against gram-positive and -negative microorganisms as bacteriostatic agents. The drugs are well absorbed orally, metabolized in the liver, and excreted intact through the kidney. Their use in the eye, however, is confined to topical application.

1. **Spectrum of activity.** The organisms generally susceptible to sulfonamides include *Strep. pyogenes, Strep. pneumoniae, H. influenza,* some strains of *Bacillus anthrax, Corynebacterium, Nocardia, Actinomyces,* and *Chlamydia trachomatis.* Most strains of *Staphylococci* and *Neisseria* are now resistant to these drugs. Pyrimethamine and sulfonamides are given systemically as combined therapy for **toxoplasmosis** (see Antiparasitic Agents).

2. **Mechanism of action.** Sulfonamides are structural analogs and, therefore, competitive antagonists of PABA. Their activity interferes with normal bacterial utilization of PABA in the synthesis of folic acid. Resistant organisms can synthesize their own folic acid precursor and are not dependent on PABA. Exogenous administration of PABA will counteract the bacteriostatic effect of concomitant sulfonamide administration. Other modes of resistance are through alteration

in the enzyme that uses PABA, increased inactivation of the drug, or development of alternative bacterial metabolic pathways that bypass the PABA mechanism.

3. **Adverse side effects.** Topical use of sulfonamides may induce hypersensitivity reaction in approximately 5% of patients. This is manifested by itching, hyperemia, and lid edema and is reversible with discontinuation of the drug. Systemic administration may result in crystalluria, hematuria, and anuria. The risk of these side effects is reduced by increased fluid intake and ingestion of sodium bicarbonate. Rarely, erythema multiforme and folate deficiency anemia may occur after these oral preparations. Other side effects include agranulocytosis, hemolytic anemia, drug fever, photosensitization, peripheral neuropathy, hepatotoxicity, myopia, transient toxic amblyopia, and acute psychosis. Sulfonamides also increase the prothrombin time in patients on coumarin and the hypoglycemic properties of sulfonylureas.

L. **Tetracyclines.** The tetracyclines are bacteriostatic antibiotics with a broad spectrum of antimicrobial activity against gram-positive and -negative bacteria overlapping that of many other antimicrobials. Although the agents are given orally, they vary in their gastrointestinal absorption. **Tetracycline** and **oxytetracycline** are incompletely absorbed, whereas **doxycycline** and **minocycline** are almost completely absorbed through the gut. Inhibition of oral absorption occurs after ingestion of dairy products, iron pills, cimetidine (Tagamet), antacids, and calcium- or magnesium-containing compounds. These antibiotics are metabolized in the liver and concentrated in the gall bladder before excretion via the kidneys and GI tract. Because of their minimal accumulation in the serum, doxycycline and minocycline are preferable to tetracycline in patients with renal insufficiency. As tetracyclines are highly lipid soluble, they penetrate ocular tissues better than do many antimicrobials. Doxycycline and minocycline are bound less to plasma proteins than is tetracycline, and aqueous levels of minocycline are approximately 50% of those achieved in the serum after oral administration.

1. **Spectrum of activity.** In general, gram-positive microorganisms are more susceptible to the tetracyclines than are gram-negative species. These agents are, however, less useful for the gram-positive organisms because of the high number of resistant bacteria. In order of diminishing activity, the drugs are minocycline, doxycycline, tetracycline, and oxytetracycline. The tetracyclines are of extremely limited use in treating gram-positive cocci, but are therapeutically effective against many strains of *N. gonorrhoeae* and *N. meningitidis* as well as highly effective against *H. influenza*, *Actinomyces*, many **gram-negative bacilli** with the notable **exception** of *P. aeruginosa* and En-

terobacteriaceae, which are all resistant. These drugs, like chloramphenicol, are all highly effective against **rickettsiae** and the spirochete *Borrelia burgdorferi,* agent of **Lyme disease.** The tetracyclines (tetracycline 250 mg po qid or doxycycline 100 mg po bid for 10–21d) are the primary drugs of choice for this latter infection, however. Penicillin V, amoxicillin, or erythromycin are used in children under 8 years of age.

2. **Mechanism of action and resistance.** Being lipophilic, the tetracyclines pass easily through the lipid bilayer of susceptible microorganisms and reach the inner cytoplasmic membrane. Once inside the cell, they inhibit protein synthesis through a specific binding to the 30S ribosomes. Resistance to the tetracyclines usually is mediated by a plasmid carrying genetic information that confers resistance to drug transport.

3. **Adverse side effects.** Toxic reactions with **topical** tetracyclines are extremely rare and may be manifested by mild conjunctival hyperemia or punctate keratitis. **Systemic** tetracyclines may induce gastrointestinal irritation, pseudomembranous colitis, or diarrhea. Phototoxicity and hepatic and renal toxicity have all been reported with systemic administration of the tetracyclines. Doxycycline is a particular offender in phototoxicity. Oxytetracycline and tetracycline are less hepatotoxic than other drugs of this group, and doxycycline is the least nephrotoxic.

M. **Trimethoprim** is a broad-spectrum antibiotic now available in combination with polymyxin B as a topical ophthalmic solution. It is also available as a systemic preparation (Tables 3-1 and 3-2).

1. **Spectrum of activity.** Trimethoprim is active against a variety of gram-positive and gram-negative bacteria. The gram-positive organisms include *S. aureus, S. epidermidis, H. influenzae, Strep. pneumoniae* and *Strep. viridans.* Sensitive gram-negative bacteria include *E. coli, Klebsiella pneumoniae, Proteus mirabilis,* and other enterobacters; *Pseudomonas aeruginosa* is usually *resistant,* as are anerobes and *Neisseria* species. Because trimethoprim is chemically related to pyrimethamine, it also possesses antimalarial activity. The combination of trimethoprim with polymyxin B as an ophthalmic drop expands and enhances the gram-negative coverage to include the enterobacter, *E. coli, Klebsiella, H. influenzae, Salmonella, Pasteurella, Bordetella, Shigella* and, in particular, *Pseudomonas aeruginosa. Proteus* species and *Serratia marcescens* are less suceptible. The drug has been recommended in the pediatric literature as effective in the frequent occurrence of *Haemophilus influenzae* conjunctivitis. Available data suggest this combination drop is most useful in treating blepharoconjunctivitis or conjunctivitis due to the more common causative organisms as noted under specific ocular infections.

2. **Mechanism of action.** Trimethoprim blocks conversion of dihydrofolic acid to tetrahydrofolic acid, which is essential to bacterial purine and DNA synthesis. This interference with dihydrofolate reductase is far more selective in bacterial than mammalian cells. Because sulfonamides inhibit the subsequent conversion of para-aminobenzoic acid to dihydrofolic acid, antibacterial synergy appears to occur when these drugs are used in combination.

3. **Adverse side effects.** No significant ocular side effects have been reported in clinical studies other than a low incidence of local irritation and stinging. Systemic absorption of the ocular drop is extremely low.

N. **Vancomycin.** Vancomycin is a bactericidal glycopeptide with primary activity against gram-positive bacteria. Because of its toxicity, vancomycin's primary uses in ophthalmic infectious disease are in topical and subconjunctival administration for serious corneal bacterial infections and intravitreal injection in endophthalmitis. Therapeutic aqueous levels are achieved after both topical and conjunctival injection, but vitreous levels are achieved only by direct injection into the posterior segment of the eye. Because subconjunctival vancomycin may induce tissue necrosis and sloughing, patients should be informed of this potential side effect before the procedure is done. The drug is excreted unchanged.

1. **Spectrum of activity.** Vancomycin should be used primarily in treating serious infections due to **methicillin-resistant staphylococci** or for treatment of *Strep. viridans* infections in patients allergic to penicillin.

2. **Mechanism of action.** Vancomycin inhibits bacterial cell wall synthesis by binding with protein precursors of this structure. It is, therefore, rapidly bactericidal for actively dividing organisms. Antimicrobial resistance to vancomycin has not been encountered in ophthalmic infections.

3. **Adverse side effects.** Hypersensitivity reactions to topical vancomycin are rare, but the fortified drops may induce a diffuse punctate keratitis and leathery dermatitis in atopic patients. Systemic reactions include macular skin rashes and anaphylaxis, along with ototoxicity and nephrotoxicity. Other hypersensitivity reactions include drug fever, eosinophilia, and urticaria after systemic administration.

V. **Topical Anesthetics: Effect on Bacterial Cultures.** All topical anesthetics contain preservatives with antibacterial and antifungal properties. The anesthetic benoxinate (Fluress) itself has considerable bactericidal efficacy, particularly against *Pseudomonas,* hence its combination with fluorescein. Proparacaine 0.5% and tetracaine 0.5% with preservative have greater antimicrobial activity than benoxinate 0.4% and cocaine 5%, especially against *S. aureus, P. aeruginosa,* and *Candida.* Because of the potential interference with accurate cultures, all lid and conjunctival swabs should be taken before instillation of anesthetics. Unless a cornea is naturally anesthetic, eg, superinfected herpes, topical anesthetic must be used, but it is probably prudent to wait 5–10 minutes for drug washout before taking the culture.

VI. **Management of Clinical Ocular Infections.** The external ocular infections treated with **topical** antimicrobial therapy include **blepharitis, conjunctivitis,** and **corneal marginal ulcers. Ophthalmia neonatorum, dacrycystitis,** and adult **trachoma-inclusion conjunctivitis** are treated by **topical and systemic** antibiotic therapy, usually with single drug forms. **Central corneal ulcers, endophthalmitis, preseptal cellulitis,** and **orbital cellulitis** also are treated with various combined antibiotic preparations, topical, intravitreal, and systemic, as these are potentially vision- and even life-threatening conditions. A brief clinical description and the general therapeutic guidelines for each of these conditions will be given, as well as more details about specific therapeutic agents.

A. **Blepharitis**

1. **Clinical disease and causative agents.** Bacterial blepharitis is an infecion of the lids with or without underlying seborrheic dermatitis. *Staphylococcus aureus* is the prime cause of acute blepharitis, but *S. aureus, S. epidermidis, Propionibacterium acnes, Corynebacterium* spp., or the yeast *Pityrosporum* are commonly associated with chronic blepharitis; the staphylococci predominate. In acute blepharitis, patients complain of ocular discomfort with mucopurulent discharge and sticking of the lids, particularly in the morning on arising. Examination reveals lid swelling and erythema with papillary conjunctivitis, often hard brittle scales on the lid margins, particularly around the canthi, and mucopurulent exudate. Chronic blepharitis is commonly associated with seborrhea and is characterized by lid thickening, madarosis (loss of lashes), poliosis (lash whitening), crusted collarettes at the base of lashes, trichiasis (misdirected lash growth), chalazia (styes), and hordeola (acute meibomian gland infections). Systemic manifestations of seborrhea include dandruff of the scalp, eyebrows, lashes, nasolabial folds, and external ears, as well as acne rosacea. Either acute or chronic blepharitis may be associated with conjunctivitis, phlyctenule growth on the cornea, superficial punctate keratitis, marginal or central corneal bacterial infection, and corneal neovascularization.

2. **Therapy.** Treatment of blepharitis is directed at both the infection and any underlying seborrheic dermatitis, using antibiotic drugs coupled with a good lid hygiene regimen.

   a. **Antimicrobials in acute blepharitis,** or acute blepharitis superimposed on the chronic form, may be treated with single-drug ointments or drops such as erythromycin, bacitracin, or drug combinations containing   neomycin-polymyxin-bacitracin   ointment (or gramicidin in drop form), trimethoprim-polymyxin B drops, or polymyxin-bacitracin ointment 3–4 times daily for 7–10 days (see Tables 3-3 and 3-4). Most staphylococci are resistant to sulfonamides.

In particularly **severe acute staphylococcal blepharitis,** systemic therapy with the semisynthetic penicillinase-resistant penicillins, oral cloxacillin, or dicloxacillin may be useful. Oxacillin and nafcillin are also effective, but provide lower blood levels. A cephalosporin, erythromycin, or clindamycin may be used to control the acute infectious process, if penicillin cannot be used. See Table 3-2 for doses. For chronic smoldering blepharitis, systemic tetracycline or erythromycin, 250 mg po every day for several months or clindamycin 75 or 150 mg po every day is most useful in controlling the chronic disease state and in preventing recurrence of hordeola or styes.

b. **Lid and skin hygiene.** Warm wet compresses and lid scrubs with baby shampoo or commercial lid scrub preparations (OcuScrub, I-Scrub) to remove scales and mattering should precede instillation of the antibiotics. A cotton-tip applicator or lathered fingertips may be used to apply shampoo and remove the oil and scales. Warm soaks using a facecloth soaked in tap water or saline (1 tablespoon table salt/quart of tap water) for 10 minutes before lid scrubs are also therapeutically useful for both cleaning the lids and allowing meibomian gland secretions to drain. If the meibomian gland secretions are excessive, the lids may be expressed by the physician using cotton-tip applicators placed on either side of the lid margin and gently compressed. An additive to lid hygiene is daily hand- and face-washing with pHisoHex soap to lower the germ count on the skin. Once or twice weekly shampooing of the hair with pHisoHex is also useful, in addition to the use of a dandruff shampoo such as selenium sulfide to the scalp once weekly in patients with seborrhea.

c. **Chronic blepharitis.** In cases of chronic inflammatory blepharitis, topical ophthalmic steroid ointment or drops once or twice daily for 1–2 weeks will decrease the inflammatory reaction. Tetracycline or erythromycin 250 mg po every day for 3 months or longer as needed controls fatty acid secretion. Phlyctenulosis and marginal keratitis will also respond to topical steroids, but all such agents should be used in combination with antibiotics and antimicrobials and under the obervation of a physician familiar with the use of steroids in the eye (see Table 3-5). Daily lid and skin hygiene are instituted and continued for seveal months or as long as needed.

3. **Surgical intervention.** Hordeola or chalazia may be present with either acute or chronic blepharitis and frequently require surgical incision and curettage or injection of 0.1 ml aqueous dexamethasone 24 mg/ml if persistent after 2–3 weeks of topical antibiotic therapy.

B. **Conjunctivitis**

1. **Clinical disease and causative agents.** Bacterial conjunctivitis is the most frequent infectious ocular disease in adults. Like blepharitis, it may be acute or chronic and may resolve spontaneously, only to recur later despite adequate therapy.

   a. **Acute** bacterial conjunctivitis develops fairly rapidly over a day or two. Patients complain of external ocular discomfort, mucopurulent discharge with sticking of the lids, and a red eye. Causative agents include *S. aureus, Strep. pneumoniae, Haemophilus influenzae,* and *Moraxella* spp.

   b. **Hyperacute** bacterial conjunctivitis has a more threatening clinical presentation, with marked ocular pain, massive lid edema, lid and conjunctival hypermia, and copious and purulent discharge. This less common form of conjunctivitis is caused by vision-threatening organisms that include *N. gonorrhoeae, N. meningitidis,* and *C. diphtheriae.* Treatment of acute conjunctivitis is topical and administered on an outpatient basis, whereas treatment of hyperacute conjunctivitis is an emergency and requires systemic and secondarily, topical antibiotic, which may be administered on an inpatient basis depending on the severity of the presenting disease.

   c. **Chronic** bacterial conjunctivitis is characterized by mild to moderate ocular irritation, redness, mucopurulent mattering with micropapillary hyperplasia, and conjunctival thickening. This form of conjunctivitis may be caused by a variety of gram-positive and gram-negative organisms, the most common being staphylococci and the coliforms.

2. **Diagnostic tests.** Bacterial cultures and sensitivities are usually not taken in routine acute or chronic conjunctivitis patients but reserved for hyperacute cases or for refractive cases that have not responded to simple broad-spectrum antibiotic topical therapy. If cultures are to be taken, the procedures for lid and conjunctival cultures as described under Central bacterial ulcerative keratitis (see Sec. **VI. D.**) and Ophthalmia neonatorum (see Sec. **VI. E.**) should be followed. The diagnosis of neisserial conjunctivitis should be suspected in all cases of hyperacute purulent external ocular infection. Gram-staining will reveal typical gram-negative intracellular and extracellular diplococci, and culture of the copious exudate on Thayer-Martin selective medium will grow the typical oxidase-positive, gram-negative diplococci. Sugar fermentation

reactions may then be used to differentiate *N. gonorrhoeae* from *N. meningitidis.*

3. **Therapy.** Commonly used topical anti-infectious agents for **acute or chronic** bacterial conjunctivitis are the single drug agents erythromycin, or bacitracin, as well as neomycin combinations and polymyxin-B combinations. Gentamicin, tobramycin, and particularly chloramphenicol should be reserved for those cases where culture reports indicate that this is the drug of choice for a given infectious state. The therapeutic agent selected is commonly given 4 times daily for 7–10 days along with once or twice daily warm compresses as described under blepharitis (see Tables 3-3 and 3-4).

   a. **Topical.** Patients with **hyperacute conjunctivitis** due to *N. gonorrhoeae, N. meningitidis,* or *Streptococcus* spp. should be treated with penicillin G 100,000 U/ml eye drops, or, for penicillin-resistant *Neisseria,* erythromycin, bacitracin, or gentamycin ointment q3–6h as adjunct to systemic therapy. Those with *Hemophilus* or *Moraxella* infections are treated with topical 0.5% chloramphenicol or polymyxin B-trimethoprim drops. Gram-negative bacillus infections are amenable to 0.3% gentamicin or tobramycin drops unless culture and sensitivity tests indicate use of another agent. Topical drops for conjunctivitis should be administered every 2 hours for 2–3 days until the process is under control and then 4 times daily for another 7–10 days. Frequent irrigation of the eyes with sterile saline is a therapeutic adjunct highly useful in washing away infected mucopurulent discharge.

   b. **Systemic therapy** for infectious conjunctivitis is indicated for *N. gonorrhoeae,* and *N. meningitidis* and in children with *H. influenzae.* Adult uncomplicated (no corneal involvement) neisserial infections due to non-penicillinase producers should be treated for 5 days with 10 million U/d of aqueous penicillin G IV plus 1 g probenecid po daily. Alternative highly effective alternative therapy for uncomplicated adult neisserial conjunctivitis due to penicillinase producers or nonproducers, however, is ceftriaxone 1 g or 50 mg/kg IV once on an outpatient basis. More severe cases are admitted and treated with bid ceftriaxone 1.0 g for 3–5 d. Newborn dosage is 125 mg IM once. Rifampin 600 mg po q12h × 4 is effective for *N. meningitidis* prophylaxis in contacts. **Penicillin-allergic** patients may be treated with spectinomycin 2.0 g IM once, or, for more severe cases, 2.0 g IM bid for 3–5 d. Norfloxacin 1200 mg po once is also a good alternative in uncomplicated cases in penicillin-allergic or -nonallergic patients and against penicillinase-producing organisms. The isolation of *H. influenzae* type B in children warrants treatment with systemic ampicillin unless the strain proves drug resistant, in which case systemic cefamandole, trimethoprim or, as last choice, chloramphenicol may be substituted with appropriate hematologic monitoring (see Tables 3-1 and 3-2).

4. **Failure to respond to treatment.** If a patient with hyperacute or acute purulent conjunctivitis fails to respond to what is deemed appropriate therapy, an alternative process should be suspected. The infection may be viral, due to a **chlamydial** agent, or noninfectious, such as in erythema multiforme or Reiter's syndrome. Persistent unilateral purulent discharge warrants a search for a foreign body lodged in an upper or lower conjunctival cul-de-sac. Poor patient compliance with the therapeutic regimen must also always be considered in the face of therapeutic failure.

C. **Corneal marginal ulcers**
   1. **Clinical disease and causative agents.** As noted under blepharitis, corneal limbal white infiltrates are commonly associated with acute and chronic staphylococcal infections. *Moraxella* may also induce these lesions, especially inferiorly. The infiltrates are sterile inflammatory hypersensitivity reactions to the staphylococcal or *Moraxella* toxins. They may be single, multiple, or confluent almost to forming a 360° ring just inside the limbus, and may or may not have overlying ulcers with positive fluorescein or rose bengal staining. The conjunctiva and lids are moderately to markedly inflamed with sticky discharge.
   2. **Diagnosis.** Classification of corneal ulcers has traditionally been on an anatomic basis, central versus marginal, because of the predisposition of organisms such as *Staphylococcus* and *Moraxella* for producing toxic marginal reaction, but many infectious ulcer-inducing organisms can produce either type of ulceration. Diagnosis should not, therefore, be based solely on anatomic location but on the basis of clinical cultures and scrapings.
   3. **Therapy.** Because of this mixed infectious-immune origin, the illness may be treated either with antibiotic agents alone as described under blepharitis and conjunctivitis, or with combination steroid-antibiotic drugs, in which case the infiltrates will clear more rapidly but physician surveillance must be more stringent (see Tables 3-3–3-5). **Steroids should not be used in patients with acne rosacea** except by a physician specializing in ophthalmic care. Adjunctive therapy for marginal keratitis includes lid hygiene and warm wet compresses, as well as the antibiotic drops or ointment 4–6 times daily for 1–2 weeks as indicated under blepharitis.

D. **Central bacterial ulcerative keratitis.** Bacterial infections are second only to herpes simplex as the cause of central corneal ulcers. Unlike herpetic infections, these represent true emergencies, as the bacterial process may progress rapidly, over a matter of hours, with significant tissue destruction and visual loss.

1. **Etiologic agents.** Bacterial keratitis is almost invariably an opportunistic infection, as the vast majority of organisms are unable to penetrate an intact healthy epithelium. The exceptions to this rule are *N. gonorrhoeae, Corynebacterium diphtheriae, Hemophilus* spp. and *Listeria* spp., all of which can invade normal corneal epithelium. Once the infectious process is underway, corneal tissue is destroyed through a combination of released microbial exotoxins (living organisms) and endotoxins (released on microbial death) as well as the host response to this insult. Host polymorphonuclear leukocyte (PMN) and macrophage toxins include collagenase, elastase, proteoglycanase, myeloperoxidase, and several cathepsins. Enzymes from both invading microorganisms and the host white cell response can rapidly degrade corneal collagen and proteoglycans, leading to loss of tissue substance, scarring, and potential perforation in the absence of adequate therapy. Geographic location and patient population influence the potential causative agent, with *Staphylococcus* more common in the northern United States and other temperate climates and *Pseudomonas* more common in the southern United States. It has recently become apparent that a corneal ulcer associated with **contact lens wear** must also be considered secondary to *P. aeruginosa* until proved otherwise, and managed accordingly. *Moraxella* infections are encountered more frequently in alcoholics and debilitated patients. Other common causative agents of central bacterial keratitis include *Streptococcus,* the Enterobacteriaceae (*Klebsiella, Proteus, Enterobacter, Serratia, Citrobacter, Providencia*), and *N. gonorrhoeae* or *meningitidis.*

2. **Clinical disease.** Most patients present with ocular pain, photophobia, decreased visual acuity, redness, lid swelling, and mucopurulent or copious watery discharge. The severity and course of the corneal infection depend largely on the virulence of the microorganism. Relatively speaking, infections with *Staphylcoccus, Moraxella, Klebsiella, Nocardia,* and *Mycobacterium fortuitum* proceed more slowly over a 3- to several-day period, respectively, whereas *Pseudomonas,* β-hemolytic *Streptococcus, Pneumococcus,* and *Neisseria* progress extremely rapidly with extensive damage within a matter of several hours. Additionally, a severe chemotic conjunctivitis is often associated with gonococcal, pneumococcal, and *Hemophilus* infections. Pseudomembranes may be present. The tear film frequently is filled with cells and tissue debris, and the corneal epithelium is ulcerated over areas of active infection. The underlying white corneal infiltrate may be localized to the area of epithelial absence or extend beyond it. Anterior chamber inflammatory reaction may be minimal with the slower organisms, or intense with

Table 3-8. Initial treatment of bacterial keratitis or endophthalmitis[a] of unknown origin or based on gram's stain of smear

Smear results	Drugs of choice (topical, subconjunctival,[b] IV)	Alternative drugs[c]
1. No organism identified	Cefazolin plus tobramycin	Gentamicin or amikacin, cefamandole, moxalactam, vancomycin, or bacitracin
2. Gram-positive cocci	Cefazolin	Vancomycin, cefamandole, bacitracin
3. Gram-positive bacilli	Penicillin G	Erythromycin, chloramphenicol
4. Gram-positive rods	Gentamicin	Tobramycin, amikacin
5. Gram-negative cocci	Ceftriaxone	Penicillin G, norfloxacin
6. Gram-negative rods	Tobramycin	Gentamicin, amikacin
7. Acid-fast bacilli	Amikacin	Rifampin, streptomycin

[a] See Table 3-7 for intravitreal drugs and dosages.
[b] For endophthalmitis, deep keratitis with threatened or actual perforation or scleral extension of infection.
[c] See text and Table 3-1 for use of other antibiotics.

hypopyon formation in the more rapidly progressive microorganisms.

3. **Diagnosis.** Despite certain characteristic appearances of bacterial ulcers, the definitive diagnosis as to the causative agent can be arrived at only by an adequate microbiologic evaluation, which includes scrapings and cultures before any therapy is started. Although scapings taken for gram-staining of smears identify the causative agent reliably only 70% of the time, a positive smear may influence the initial therapeutic approach more specifically than the usual broad-spectrum cephalosporin-aminoglycoside shotgun therapy (Tables 3-8 and 3-9). Nonetheless, cultures are significantly more sensitive than smears, and, if positive, should be relied on more heavily in determining any alteration in the initial treatment.

4. **Antibiotic therapy**
   a. **Outpatient.** Most patients with central bacterial keratitis are admitted to the hospital. Patients with mild ulcers, defined as less than 2 mm in diameter with less than ⅕th corneal thickness loss and confinement of the infiltrate to the anterior stroma may be treated on an outpatient basis. They must be seen daily or every other day and treated with fortified topical antibiotic instilled every ½–1 hour while awake and every 1–2 hours during sleep,

waiting 5 minutes between drop instillations. Tapering usually begins in 2–3 days when the patient has stabilized or improved.

b. **Inpatient.** The initial management of moderate to severe bacterial keratitis includes hospital admission and the institution of fortified antibiotics every ½–1 hour around the clock until the patient is stabilized, at which time tapering may begin. The usual course of treatment at a 1–2-hour frequency commonly lasts for 5–10 days, depending on the clinical presentation and organism isolated.

c. **Fortified drugs.** Fortified antibiotic solutions themselves are not commercially available and must be made up in the hospital pharmacy (see Table 3-6). Antibiotic ointments are often not used initially, as they cannot achieve the therapeutic levels associated with fortified ophthalmic drops.

d. **Subconjunctival antibiotics** are generally reserved for severe infiltrative ulcers, corneal abscess, associated endophthalmitis, scleral extension of the infection, presence of infected descemetocele or perforation, and in poorly cooperative patients. Additionally, involvement of the sclera or corneal perforation requires parenteral antibiotic (see Table 3-2) as indicated under therapy of endophthalmitis. Adequate analgesics should be given both before and after such injections (see Table 3-6).

e. **Systemic therapy,** like subconjunctival injection, is indicated in infected endophthalmitis and pending or actual perforation, or scleral extension of the infection. The *maximum recommended daily dose* is usually used in these situations unless renal function is impaired.

(1) **Initial treatment.** Antibiotics are usually given intravenously initially, using the broad-spectrum cephalosporin-aminoglycoside approach (see Tables 3-1 and 3-8). Exceptions are the *Neisseria* and *Hemophilus* spp., which must not only be treated with systemic as well as topical antibiotic, but also with penicillin or a third-generation cephalosporin, eg, cephtriaxone, or with chloramphenicol, respectively, until cultures indicate a causative agent other than that suspected by smear. See Hyperacute conjunctivitis.

The cephalosporins provide coverage of gram-positive cocci and some gram-negative rods. The addition of an aminoglycoside provides additional therapy of gram-positive organisms and most important gram-negative rods, including many *Pseudomonas* spp. Because *Neisseria* is not covered by this regimen, the finding of gram-negative diplococci on the gram-stained smear should redirect even the initial therapy toward the use of topical fortified penicillin or bacitracin drops along with subconjunctival and intravenous penicillin G or as indicated (see Tables 3-1, 3-2, and 3-6).

(2) **Therapeutic modification to higher specificity.** When the results of cultures and sensitivities are available, the initial broad-spectrum therapy may be continued unchanged or altered as indicated. If gram-negative organisms such as *Pseudomonas* are recovered, treatment is usually modified to include topical and subconjunctival aminoglycosides plus ticarcillin or carbenicillin, and probenecid, a synergistic combination for gram-negative infections. Similarly, the recovery of a **methicillin-resistant** *Staphylococcus* would indicate a switch to treatment with vancomycin and bacitracin, usually the only drugs to which this mutant organism is sensitive.

Antibiotic therapy is continued every $1/2$–1 hour until the patient has stabilized, usually over several days, and then gentle tapering is begun over 7–14 days. Certain organisms, such as *Pseudomonas,* may require therapy for as long as 3–4 weeks, as premature discontinuation of treatment may result in rebound growth of this organism.

5. **Nonantibiotic concomitant therapy.** Additional therapy variously employed in bacterial keratitis includes cycloplegics, corticosteroids, therapeutic soft contact lenses, tissue adhesive and patch graft or penetrating keratoplasty, collagenase inhibitors, and cryosurgery.

E. **Ophthalmia neonatorum.** Ophthalmia neonatorum may be defined as any conjunctivitis occurring during the first month of life; it may be caused by any of a variety of agents.

1. **Causative agents.** The noninfectious cause of conjunctivitis of the newborn is Crede's prophylaxis with 1% silver nitrate; the most common infectious cause in the United States is *Chlamydia trachomatis* (**TRIC,** inclusion conjunctivitis, or inclusion blennorrhea). The TRIC agent, an obligate intracellular parasite, is derived from but is not a true bacterial agent. The bacterial organisms most commonly causing ophthalmia neonatorum include *S. aureus, Pneumococcus, Streptococcus* spp., *Neisseria gonorrhoeae,* and *Hemophilus* spp.

2. **Clinical manifestations.** Purulent exudate out of proportion to erythema and edema is characteristic of this illness. The ocular findings may vary in severity from mild conjunctivitis secondary to silver nitrate to the fulminating, chemotic, purulent conjunctivitis with secondary corneal invasion, perforation, and panophthalmitis of *Neisseria* or *Pseudomonas.* With inclusion conjunctivitis, the lids are red and inflamed, with hy-

peremia, conjunctival chemosis, and exudative discharge. Untreated TRIC infection in infants may resolve within 5–9 months or persist for years, resulting in chronic follicular conjunctivitis, vascular pannus overgrowth of the cornea, and conjunctival scarring. Unfortunately, even mild or moderate ocular infection in the newborn may be associated with significant systemic findings not immediately apparent unless actively investigated by the attending physician. Newborns may fail to raise a febrile response to sepsis and have an immature defense system against microbial invasion.

3. **Diagnosis.** Both eyes should be cultured with calcium alginate swabs and smears taken by conjunctival scraping to identify the offending organism and sensitivity testing. Where indicated, nasopharyngeal cultures may be taken as well.

4. **Therapy.** Treatment is begun based on the suspected causative agent (see Tables 3-1–3-4).

   a. **Chemical conjunctivitis** secondary to silver nitrate will begin to clear spontaneously within 24 hours. The eyes may be gently irrigated and accumulated exudate removed from the fornices by gentle swabbing.

   b. **Inclusion conjunctivitis (TRIC)**

   (1) **Systemic** therapy is the prime mode of management for inclusion conjunctivitis, with topical agents used only if patients can not tolerate full systemic therapeutic doses. This regimen is not only for effective therapy of the eyes, but because 10–20% of exposed infants have concomitant chlamydial pneumonia as late as 6 months after birth and may have gastrointestinal involvement as well. Both the parents (presumptive carriers of the **TRIC** agent) and the infant must receive full therapy. Infants are treated effectively with erythromycin 40 mg/kg po daily in four divided doses for 3 weeks. Adult therapy is discussed below in more detail but, in brief, is doxycycline, tetracycline, or erythromycin 500 mg po for 3 weeks. **Children under 8 years of age should not receive systemic tetracycline unless there is no alternative.** Alternative drug for newborns, children, or adults is sulfisoxazole (see Table 3-2).

   (2) **Topical** antimicrobial therapy with tetracycline or erythromycin ointment is useful but not absolutely necessary for patients receiving full systemic therapy. Topical treatment alone is slow and only partially effective in treatment of either adult or newborn conjunctivitis, with relapses being a frequent consequence.

   (3) **Corticosteroids** are contraindicated in all but adult patients who develop anterior iritis and who are on full systemic antimicrobial therapy.

(4) **Rifampin** topical ointment has been reported as successful in ocular TRIC infections, but is available only as an investigational drug in the United States.

(5) **Silver nitrate prophylaxis** does **not** prevent inclusion conjunctivitis infection in the newborn.

c. **Bacterial conjunctivitis in the newborn**

(1) **Infection due to gram-positive cocci and diplococci** may be treated with 0.5% erythromycin ointment q2h for the first day and qid for 1 week. Acute purulent conjunctivitis caused by gram-negative organisms is treated with fortified tobramycin (14–20 mg/ml) or gentamicin (14–20 mg/ml) hourly for the first 24 hours and then every 4 hours for the next 10–14 days. The initiation of this treatment is particularly crucial in the face of a *Pseudomonas* infection. Mucopurulent materials should be irrigated from the eyes before instillation of antimicrobials.

(2) *Hemophilus* spp. should be treated both systemically and topically. Topical therapy is either sulfacetamide, trimethoprin, chloramphenicol, ampicillin, or other drugs (see Tables 3-1–3-3). Drops are given hourly until improvement is noted and then tapered to every 4 hours for 5–7 additional days. This is coupled with systemic ampicillin in doses indicated in Table 3-2. If the *Hemophilus* strain is **ampicillin-resistant,** the physician may use systemic trimethoprin, cefamandole or, last, turn to systemic chloramphenicol. In particularly severe infections the physician may use chloramphenicol both topically and systemically. The usual initial adult ampicillin dose is 400 mg/kg IV or 3 gm po q6h daily for 10–14 days. Trimethoprim (TMP)-sulfamethoxozole is given as 4 tablets po q6h or TMP 10–20 mg/kg IV q6h for 10 days. Chloramphenicol dosage is 100 mg/kg IV or po, also for 10–14 days (see Table 3-2); use of this drug requires constant hematologic monitoring.

(3) **Gonococcal ophthalmia neonatorum** is, like inclusion conjunctivitis, indicative of probable venereal infection in the parents, thus indicating therapy for both adults and infant. In the infant this acute purulent conjunctivitis is treated under isolation with aqueous crystalline penicillin G, 50,000 U/kg in two divided doses IV daily for 7 days for nonpenicillinase-producing organisms. Neonates should not receive probenecid. Alternative therapy for penicillinase- and nonpenicillinase-producing organisms is ceftriaxone 125 mg IM once or gentamicin IV in doses listed in Table 3-2. Topical antibiotics are not indicated in the absence

of corneal infection, but the eyes should be irrigated immediately and hourly as long as necessary to wash out contaminated discharge. If there is ciliary spasm or secondary iritis, 1% atropine drops 2 times daily is advisable.

(4) **Adult neisserial infections** are discussed under hyperacute conjunctivitis, but, in brief, therapy is aqueous penicillin G, 10 million units IV daily for 3–5 days with 1.0 g probenecid po 1 hour before the initial dose of penicillin and daily thereafter (see Table 3-2). A single dose of ceftriaxone 1 g or 50 mg/kg IM once, spectinomycin 2 g IM once, ciprofloxacin 1 gm po bid for 1 day, or norfloxacin 1 g po once have also been reported as highly effective in therapy of uncomplicated clinical disease. Any one of the three drugs are indicated in penicillinase- or β-lactamase–producing organisms and the latter two in penicillin-allergic patients. Alternative drugs with secondary effective alternative antigonococcal drugs include chloramphenicol, ampicillin, cephaloridine, cephalexin, oleandomycin, and kanamycin. Topical gentamicin, erythromycin, or bacitracin q3–6h may be used in addition to systemic agents. See Hyperacute conjunctivitis.

F. **Adult chlamydial infections (trachoma-inclusion conjunctivitis, TRIC)**

1. **Causative agents.** The chlamydial agents, obligate intracellular organisms of bacterial descent, are divided into two groups, *Chlamydia trachomatis* and *C. psittaci*. Only *C. trachomatis* is a human pathogen and is the causative agent of both trachoma and inclusion conjunctivitis (IC) in adults and newborns.

2. **Inclusion conjunctivitis**

   a. **Clinical disease.** Adult IC infection is manifested as a chronic follicular conjunctivitis and keratitis that may present acutely with muco-watery discharge, sticking of the lids, foreign body sensation, conjunctival hyperemia, and lid swelling. There may be preauricular adenopathy and, invariably, follicular conjunctivitis and papillitis. A superficial keratitis may be present, including fine and larger macropunctate epithelial erosions, subepithelial infiltrates similar to adenoviral infections, and limbal infiltration with superficial pannus, particularly inferiorly.

   b. **Diagnosis.** In the adult the diagnosis is best made by scrapings taken from the conjunctiva and planted in cell culture for isolation of the organism or fluorescent antibody testing.

   c. **Therapy.** Adult inclusion conjunctivitis is treated **systemically** with doxycycline 100 mg po bid or tetracycline 500 mg po qid for 3 weeks. Alternative effective therapy is erythromycin 500 mg po qid daily in four divided doses for 3 weeks. Erythromycin is less well tolerated than the tetracyclines and carries a risk of toxic hepatitis. A very effective third-choice drug for therapy of adult IC is sulfisoxazole 100 mg po bid daily for 3 weeks (see Tables 3-1 and 3-2).

Topical ocular antimicrobial therapy with tetracycline or erythromycin ointment is optional if the patient can tolerate the full therapeutic dose systemically. Although corticosteroids are contraindicated in neonatal IC infections, they may be used in adults who develop acute iritis of IC, but only in those able to tolerate, and under therapy with, full systemic antimicrobial treatment. Topical corticosteroids are contraindicated in patients not on systemic antimicrobial therapy or on topical therapy alone.

3. **Trachoma.** Clinical features are a chronic keratoconjunctivitis manifested by papillae, follicles, scarring of the palpebral conjunctiva, superior corneal neovascular pannus, and corneal opacities with secondary severe scarring from superinfecting microorganisms. Trachoma may be associated with systemic manifestations, including rhinitis, otitis media, upper respiratory infections, and preauricular lymphadenopathy.

   a. **Diagnosis.** The diagnosis of trachoma is based on scrapings and with Giemsa stain, looking for intracytoplasmic inclusions, and, when available, fluorescent antibody testing or culture of scrapings on irradiated fibroblast tissue culture.

   b. **Therapy.** The therapy of trachoma is combined topical and systemic. Topical agents include the highly effective tetracyclines (chlortetracycline, oxytetracycline, or tetracycline, all on empty stomachs), erythromycin ointment, or 10% sulfacetamide tid for 6 (ointment) or 8 weeks (solution). Systemic agents coupled with topical therapy include either a tetracycline or erythromycin 15 mg/kg po daily in four divided doses for 3 weeks, or 1.5 mg/kg doxycycline or 30 mg/kg sulfamethoxazole for 3 weeks (see Tables 3-2 and 3-3).

G. **Dacryocystitis**
   1. **Etiologic factors.** Dacryocystitis is an inflammation of the lacrimal sac secondary to impaired drainage of the nasolacrimal system from the level of the sac and below. Contributing factors include systemic diseases such as diabetes, neighboring infections in the nose and paranasal sinuses, malignant lymphoma, sarcoidosis, facial fractures, and, in infants, congenital occlusion of the nasolacrimal duct. Acute dacryocystitis is associated with *Staphylococcus* and *Streptococcus,* whereas chronic adult disease may be associated with the hyphate fungus, *Streptothrix* (dacryoliths).
   2. **Clinical disease.** Acute suppurative dacryocystitis may develop with or without a preceding chronic con-

dition. It presents as swelling and hyperemia of the tissue overlying the lacrimal sac associated with intense pain and tenderness. Pressure over the sac may produce regurgitation of mucopurulent material through the canaliculi in the lid or spontaneous drainage into the nose, into the ethmoid sinuses, or through a pointing abscess in the overlying skin. Chronic dacryocystitis may be manifested by tearing and mild swelling and tenderness over the lacrimal sac region with regurgitation of mucopurulent material on pressure in this area. The chronic state is often associated with mycotic dacryoliths or stones in the canaliculus or sac. These mycotic infections appear as doughy or granular masses made up of degenerated cells, fungi, and other debris. They are noncalcific and, therefore, do not show up on X ray.

3. **Diagnosis** is based on clinical findings, culture, and, in chronic cases, dacryocystography.

4. **Therapy**

   a. **Infants** with nasolacrimal obstruction should be treated conservatively, as mature canalization of the lacrimal drainage system is usually incomplete until 6 months of age. The mother should be instructed in massaging of the tear sac from the canthal region down across the sac several times daily in an effort to push through the accumulated material within the nasolacrimal system and break open the membrane at the level of the inferior meatus. Antibiotic drops such as neomycin-polymyxin, trimethoprim-polymyin, or an aminoglycoside should be given 3–4 times daily for 2–3 weeks. The nasolacrimal system should be probed at 3–6 months of age if there is no evidence of improvement with massage. The probing should not be delayed for more than 1 year after birth, as this significantly reduces the chances of successfully opening the system.

   b. **Adults** with mild acute dacryocystitis may respond simply to irrigation of the sac with antibiotic or antibiotic-steroid combination solutions, as this may open up a partial obstruction of the duct. Systemic therapy is added in management of more severe acute infections because of the intense presentation and pain and risk of periorbital spread. Therapy includes a semisynthetic penicillin such as cloxacillin 1 g po qid, a cephalosporin such as cephalexin 1 g po qid for 7–10 days, or other drugs (see Tables 3-1–3-5).

   c. **Dacryoliths.** Patients suspected of having mycotic dacryoliths as manifested by chronic dacryocystitis, dilation of the lacrimal sac with pouting of the canaliculus, and mild deep tenderness should have systemic treatment with 1.2 million U penicillin G IM initially, followed by 250–500 mg penicillin V q6h po for 7–10 days. Systemic antifungal agents are ineffective in this condition. In instances where **Candida** or **other yeasts** are isolated, nystatin 20,000 U/ml topically, 1 drop tid for 2–3 weeks with irrigation of the affected canaliculus every other day for 1 week or until improvement is noted, is effective therapy. Alternative treatment is natamycin 5% drops q1–2h daily for 2–3 weeks. Any dacryoliths or concretions should be removed surgically, or all systemic treatment will be of only transient value.

H. Preseptal and orbital cellulitis and abscess. Preseptal cellulitis is an inflammation of the tissues anterior to the orbital septum separating them from the contents of the orbit and deeper structures. It is, therefore, less serious than a true orbital cellulitis, which by definition is located posterior to the orbital septal membrane and, therefore, in direct contact with the globe and potentially with the retro-orbital structures.

1. Preseptal cellulitis

    a. Clinical disease and causative agents. Preseptal cellulitis is usually manifested by a patient who is not particularly ill systemically but who has mild to moderate swelling of the periocular tissues and upper lid with erythema and mild tenderness. There is mild discharge and no ocular or periocular involvement. Microorganisms most frequently associated with this condition are *S. aureus* and occasionally *Pneumococcus*.

    b. Therapy. Patients with mild disease as described above may be treated on an outpatient basis with systemic erythromycin 500 mg po q6h or a broad-spectrum semisynthetic penicillin such as ampicillin at doses indicated in Table 3-2. Improvement should be noted within 1–2 days and followed up within that time by the physician to ascertain that the process has not spread to deeper structures and subsequently become a true orbital cellulitis. Any patient with preseptal cellulitis of moderate or greater degree and systemic signs and symptoms or fever higher than 100°F should be hospitalized and treated as noted under orbital cellulitis below.

2. Orbital cellulitis

    a. Clinical disease and causative agents. Orbital cellulitis is a vision- and potentially life-threatening process, which mandates admission to the hospital. The clinical findings include an acutely ill patient with fever, proptosis, external ophthalmoplegia, diminished vision, swelling and erythema of the lids, and an elevated white count. Progression of the illness is rapid in the absence of appropriate therapy, although chronic orbital infections may on occasion be seen and are due to nonpurulent bacterial, fungal, or parasitic infection. The causative agents of acute orbital cellulitis in children include most commonly *H. influenzae* and to a lesser extent *Staphylococcus*; in adults they include *Streptococcus,* anaerobes *(Peptostreptococcus, Clostridium, Bacterioides),* and *Staphylococcus.*

b. **Diagnosis** is based on the classical clinical presentation and sinus and orbit X rays, which often reveal an associated acute or chronic sinusitis or orbital foreign body, and culture of any ocular or orbital drainage.

c. **Therapy** (see Tables 3-1 and 3-2)

(1) **Children.** Therapy of orbital cellulitis caused by *H. influenzae* in children under 4 years of age is 100 mg/kg chloramphenicol IV daily with concomitant ampicillin 200 mg/kg IV daily for 1 week, followed by oral ampicillin 100 mg/kg for *Hemophilus* known not to be resistant to ampicillin or oral cefaclor 40 mg/kg in three divided doses for 7 days. If the organism is ampicillin sensitive on culture and sensitivity testing, the chloramphenicol may be discontinued and the child treated with ampicillin alone.

Children suspected of having staphylococcal infection, but in whom *H. influenzae* has not yet been ruled out, are treated with combined chloramphenicol IV 100 mg/kg in four divided doses q6h as above and oxacillin 100 mg/kg IV q4h. If *Staphylococcus* is isolated on culture, the chloramphenicol may be discontinued and the child treated with oxacillin alone.

For children older than 4 years of age, the incidence of *Hemophilus* infection is much lower, thus obviating the need for chloramphenicol as an initial mode of therapy. These children may be treated with combined oxacillin and ampicillin in doses indicated in Table 3-2, unless a culture and sensitivity testing of the isolated organism indicate that chloramphenicol should be used.

(2) **Adult** orbital infections are commonly treated with penicillinase-resistant drugs such as oxacillin or nafcillin in combination with penicillin G. Oxacillin is active against anaerobes and *Streptococcus,* but less so than penicillin. Penicillin G dosage is 2–4 million U IV q4h with oxacillin or nafcillin 1.5 g IV q4h for 7 days. Penicillin-allergic adults not prone to anaphylactic-type penicillin allergy may be treated with a cephalosporin such as cefazolin 1 g IV q8h. Although there may be cross-allergy between these two beta-lactam drugs, serious cross-reactions are rare. Patients with anaphylactic-type penicillin allergy may be treated alternatively with clindamycin, vancomycin, or chloramphenicol (see Table 3-2) IV or IM for 5–10 days.

If an orbital abscess is apparent clinically or

on radiologic study, prompt surgical drainage with exploration of the orbit is indicated. Concomitant drainage of infected sinuses should also be carried out at this time, and any orbital foreign body noted on X ray or at exploration should be removed. Orbital drains should be left in place for several days after surgery.

I. Bacterial endophthalmitis

1. **Clinical disease.** Bacterial endophthalmitis is an inflammatory response of the intraocular tissues secondary to microbial invasion. This highly urgent ocular entity is most commonly seen postoperatively (cataract and glaucoma surgery), but also after penetrating ocular trauma or as the result of endogenous spread via blood-borne organisms from a peripheral site of infection. Bacterial endophthalmitis should be suspected in any situation where the intraocular inflammation or discomfort is out of proportion to that anticipated in the particular postsurgical or post-traumatic situation. The infectious process usually presents clinically 1–4 days after surgery or trauma and commonly but not invariably presents with severe pain and the findings of lid and conjunctival edema, hyperemia, exudate, corneal haze, and anterior chamber inflammation with or without hypopyon and inflammatory response in the vitreous. The differential diagnosis of bacterial endophthalmitis includes postoperative retention of lens material, wound incarceration of iris or vitreous, reaction to intraocular lens-induced or other foreign body-induced inflammation, and an idiopathic postoperative iridocyclitis.

2. **Causative agents.** Microorganisms of acute bacterial endophthalmitis include *Staphylococcus aureus, Proteus,* and *Pseudomonas.* However, a low-grade endophthalmitis lasting weeks may be produced by less virulent bacteria such as strains of *S. epidermidis* and *Propionibacterium acnes.* **Fungal endophthalmitis** is also often indolent and is discussed under Antifungal Drugs. Post-traumatic endophthalmitis is commonly associated with *S. epidermidis* or the acute inflammatory response to *Bacillus subtilis, B. cereus,* or *Streptococcus. Streptococcus* is often associated with endophthalmitis seen in glaucoma patients who have undergone filtration surgery. The most common gram-negative organism isolated in this same group of patients is *H. influenzae.*

3. **Diagnosis** is based on clinical findings and on the results of culture and sensitivity tests taken on specimens removed by diagnostic vitrectomy (see Therapy).

4. **Therapy.** Management of patients with suspected bacterial endophthalmitis is initially broad spectrum with antibiotics delivered intravitreally at the time of vitrectomy and, if indicated, 1 and 2 days later combined with subconjunctival and systemic antibiotics for postoperative or endogenous endophthalmitis. Topical for-

tified antibiotics are added to this regimen if the endophthalmitis is secondary to a penetrating injury. See Tables 3-7 and 3-8.

a. **A diagnostic and therapeutic vitrectomy** is performed as an emergency procedure under local or general anesthesia. In aphakia, a keratotomy site is used for midvitreous aspiration and drug injection. In phakic patients, a sclerotomy is opened 4 mm posterior to the limbus. The vitreous aspirate is immediately inoculated onto appropriate culture media, and 0.1 ml drug is injected via the same site.

In general, it is suggested that until the specific causative agent(s) is known, **postoperative** endophthalmitis be treated with intravitreal vancomg. **Post-traumatic** endophthalmitis is best treated initially with intravitreal vancomycin 1.0 mg or clindamycin 0.5 mg (clindamycin if *Bacillus* is suspected—gram-positive rods) and tobramycin 0.2 mg or amikacin 0.1 mg. **Post-glaucoma filtration** endophthalmitis is treated with vancomycin 1.0 mg and a second- (cefamandole 2.0 mg) or third- (ceftriaxone 2.0 mg) generation cephalosporin, or tobramycin 0.2 mg intravitreally. Table 3-7 indicates alternative drugs and dosages that may be deemed appropriate for the suspected organism.

b. **Concomitant antibiotic therapy.** Immediately after vitreous cultures are obtained, broad-spectrum antibiotic therapy should be begun IV, subconjunctivally, and, if indicated, topically in the postoperative period (see Tables 3-1, 3-2, and 3-6). Subconjunctival injections of tobramycin 40 mg and cefazolin 125 mg, or other drugs as in Table 3-7, may be begun in the operating room and repeated daily for several days as indicated. Initial systemic treatment often includes amikacin 15 mg/kg IV or IM q8h coupled with cefazolin 1 g IV q6h for 10–14 days each. In the presence of a penetrating injury or if the route of entry of the organism is suspected to be from the external eye, topical fortified aminoglycoside (eg, tobramycin, gentamicin) and cefazolin drops are begun every hour postoperatively. Topical cycloplegics should be used to minimize ciliary spasm and synechia formation. Antimicrobial therapy may be readjusted according to microorganism sensitivities based on clinical isolates removed surgically (see Table 3-7). If the microorganism is particularly virulent, intravitreal injections may be repeated 24–48 hours after the initial dosing.

c. **Corticosteroids.** Twenty-four hours after an identified organism has been under therapy with appropriate antibiotics, systemic corticosteroids may be begun topically (for iritis), subconjunctivally, and systemically. **Intravitreous steroid** may be given at the time of a repeat intravitreal antibiotic injection. Dosage is 400 μg in 0.1 ml midvitreous. It is prepared by mixing 1 ml sterile aqueous dexamethasone for injection (24 mg/ml) with 5 ml sterile water for injection (USP) to give a concentration of 4 mg/ml. Additional steroid regimens are: topical, prednisolone 1% q4h; subconjunctival injection, 50 mg methylprednisolone; systemic, prednisone 40–80 mg po daily with meals for 7–14 days. If fungal endophthalmitis is at all suspected or the organism is not identified, corticosteroid therapy should **not** be initiated.

Information Sources and Suggested Reading (*Antibiotics*)

1. Antimicrobial susceptibilities at Massachusetts Eye and Ear Infirmary, Winter 1987. In *Massachusetts Eye and Ear Infirmary Infection Control Letter* 1(10), 1988.
2. Barr C., Recognizing and treating infectious endophthalmitis. National Eye Center Symposium, Focus on Cornea and Anterior Segment. 1:3&7, Slack Inc., Thorofare, N.J., 1989.
3. Baum, J., Preparation of antibiotics for topical, subconjunctival or subtenon use. In Lamberts, D.W., and Potter, D.E. (Eds.), *Clinical Ophthalmic Pharmacology.* Boston: Little, Brown, 1987, pp. 519–524.
4. Choice of antimicrobial drugs, in *The Medical Letter,* New Rochelle, NY, 30 (No. 762): 33–40, 1988.
5. Davis, J.L., Koidou-Tsiligianni, A., Pflugfelder, S.C., et al., Coagulase-negative staphylococcal endophthalmitis: increase in antimicrobial resistance. *Ophthalmology* 95:1404–1410, 1988.
6. Donowitz, G., and Mandell, G., Beta-lactam antibiotics. *N. Engl. J. Med.* 318:490–500, 1988.
7. Ellis, P., *Ocular Therapeutics and Pharmacology,* 7th ed. St. Louis: C.V. Mosby, 1985, pp. 42–59, 105–157, 187–198, 283–286 (principles of antibiotic therapy, therapy of infections of the lids, conjunctiva, lacrimal apparatus, cornea, intraocular infections).
8. Fraunfelder, F., and Roy, F.H. (Eds.), *Current Ocular Therapy 3,* 3rd ed. Philadelphia: W.B. Saunders, 1990, multiple contributing authors, pp. 3–49 (bacterial infections), pp. 53–67 (mycotic infections), pp. 50–52 (Chlamydia), pp. 402–403 (bacterial conjunctivitis), pp. 21, 32, 50, 416–418 (ophthalmia neonatorum), pp. 439, 445–448 (corneal ulcers), pp. 184, 422–423, 510, 522–524 (blepharitis), pp. 379, 533–537 (bacterial and fungal endophthalmitis), pp. 605–608 (dacryocystitis), pp. 641–643 (orbital cellulitis), pp. 68–71 (rickettsia).
9. Gentamicin, tobramicin and amikacin in the treatment of microbial keratitis. In *Ocular Therapy Report,* American Health Consultants, Atlanta, 1(2):5–8, 1988.
10. Glasser, D., and Hyndiuk, R., Antibiotics. In Lamberts, D.W., and Potter, D.E. (Eds.), *Clinical Ophthalmic Pharmacology.* Boston: Little, Brown, 1987, pp. 53–96.

11. Glasser, D., and Hyndiuk, R., Ocular penetration of antibiotics. In Lamberts, D.W., and Potter, D.E. (Eds.), *Clinical Ophthalmic Pharmacology*. Boston: Little, Brown, 1987, pp. 525–566.
12. Gleckman, R., and Czachor, J., Antibiotic concerns in the elderly. Geriatric Med. Today 7(1):45–60, 1988.
13. Haimovici, R., and Roussel, T., Treatment of gonococcal conjunctivitis with single-dose intramuscular ceftriaxone. Am. J. Ophthalmol. 107:511–514, 1989.
14. *Handbook of Antimicrobial Therapy*. New Rochelle, NY: The Medical Letter, 1989, pp. 5–92 (antibacterials).
15. Havener, W.H., Antibiotics, *Ocular Pharmacology*, 5th ed. St. Louis: C.V. Mosby, 1983, pp. 120–210.
16. Intravitreal antibiotics: vancomycin with aminoglycosides. Ocular Therapy Report, American Health Consultants, Atlanta, 2(9):33–36, 1989.
17. Kestelyn, P., Bogaerts, J., Stevens, A., Piot, P., and Meheus, A., Norfloxacin for adult gonococcal keratoconjunctivitis. Am. J. Ophthalmol., 108:516–523, 1989.
18. Laga, M., Plummer, F., Piot, P., et al., Prophylaxis of gonococcal and chlamydial ophthalmia neonatorum. N. Engl. J. Med. 318:653–657, 1988.
19. Leopold, I.H., Anti-infective agents. In Sears, M.L. (Ed.), *Pharmacology of the Eye*. Handbook of Experimental Pharmacology, Vol. 69. New York: Springer-Verlag, 1984, pp. 385–441 (antibacterials).
20. Liesegang, T., Bacterial and fungal keratitis. In Kaufman, H.E., McDonald, M., Barron, B., and Waltman, S. (Eds.), *The Cornea*. New York: Churchill Livingstone, 1988, pp. 217–270.
21. Mannis, M., (1) Bacterial conjunctivitis. (2) Chlamydial disease. In Kaufman, H.E., McDonald, M., Barron, B., and Waltman, S. (Eds.), *The Cornea*. New York: Churchill Livingstone, 1988, pp. (1) 189–200, (2) 201–216.
22. Meisler, D., and Mandelbaum, S., Propionibacterium-associated endophthalmitis after extracapsular cataract extraction. Ophthalmology 96:54–61, 1989.
23. Nussenblatt, R.B., and Palestine, A.G., *Uveitis: Fundamentals in Clinical Practice*. Chicago: Yearbook Medical Publ., 1989, pp. 388–406 (bacterial and fungal uveitis).
24. O'Brien, T., Sawusch, M., Dick, J., and Gottsch, J., Topical ciprofloxacin treatment of *Pseudomonas* keratitis in rabbits. Arch. Ophthalmol. 106:1444–1446, 1988.
25. Pavan-Langston, D., and Foulks, G., Cornea and external disease. In Pavan-Langston, D. (Ed.), *Manual of Ocular Diagnosis and Therapeutics*, 3rd ed. Boston: Little, Brown, 1990, pp. 65–116.
26. Reed, A., and Pachman, L., Lyme disease in children and adolescents. Compr. Ther. 15(1):31–36, 1989.
27. Sande, M., and Mandell, G., In Gilman, A.G., Goodman, L.S., Rall, T., and Murad, F. (Eds.). *The Pharmacological Basis of Therapeutics*, 7th ed. New York: Macmillan, 1985, pp. 1066–1094 (general considerations), pp. 1095–1218 (sulfonamides, penicillins, cephalosporins, aminoglycosides, tetracyclines, chloramphenicol, erythromycin, and miscellaneous antibacterial agents).

28. Smolin, G., and Thoft, R.A. (Eds.), *The Cornea*, 2nd ed. Boston: Little, Brown, 1987, pp. 141–153 (bacterial microbiology, Okumoto, M.), pp. 179–192 (antibiotic mechanisms, Baum, J.), pp. 193–224 (keratitis, Hyndiuk, R., Snyder, R.), pp. 154–155 (chlamydial microbiology, Okumoto, M.), pp. 285–295 (chlamydial disease, Whitcher, J.)

29. Tabbara, K.F., and Hyndiuk, R.A., (Eds.), *Infections of the Eye*. Boston: Little, Brown, 1986, pp. 107–114 (chlamydia diagnosis, Malaty, R.), pp. 421–436 (chlamydial conjunctivitis, Tabbara, K.F.), pp. 115–150 (diagnostic bacteriology, Brinser, J.), pp. 211–238 (antibacterial agents, Glasser, D., Hyndiuk, R.), pp. 293–302 (corticosteroids in ocular infections, Kleinert, R.), pp. 303–330 (bacterial keratitis, Hyndiuk, R.A., Skorich, D., Burd, E.), pp. 413–420 (bacterial conjunctivitis, Antonios, S., Tabbara, K.F.), pp. 461–468 (ophthalmia neonatorum, Flach, A.), pp. 499–510 (endogenous bacterial chorioretinitis, Weinberg, R.), pp. 517–562 (orbit, Gonnering, R., Harris, G.), pp. 543–550 (lacrimal apparatus, Tabbara, K.F.), pp. 551–562 (eyelids, Alvarez, H., Tabbara, K.F.), pp. 563–586 (endophthalmitis, Parke, D. II, Brinton, G.), pp. 601–612 (interstitial keratitis, Yee, R., Hyndiuk, R.A.).

30. Treatment of bacterial endophthalmitis: Part 1, Gram-positive micro-organisms: cefazolin, vancomycin. In Ocular Therapy Report, American Health Consultants, Atlanta 2(1):1–4, 1989.

31. Treatment of bacterial endophthalmitis: Part II, The aminoglycosides and gram-negative micro-organisms. In Ocular Therapy Report, American Health Consultants, Atlanta 2(2):5–8, 1989.

32. Wylkowske, C., and Hermans, P., Symposium on antimicrobial agents—Part 1: General principles of antimicrobial therapy. Mayo Clin. Proc. 62:789–798, 1987.

4

Antifungal Drugs

Mycotic infections constitute a small fraction of ocular or orbital disease, but are among the most difficult clinical entities both in terms of diagnosis and management. Antifungal therapy is limited to a few variably effective, toxic drugs and is often hampered by delayed diagnosis, insufficient clinical data on efficacy of drug regimens, and a multiplicity of adverse host factors. In vitro fungal drug sensitivities do not always correlate well with in vivo efficacy. The narrow therapeutic index is in large part because fungi, unlike bacteria but like human cells, are eukaryocytic, ie, have a true nucleus. Therefore, drug toxicity aimed at fungal cells is often toxic to the host.

I. Antifungal agents

The three primary **drug groups** used in antifungal therapy are the polyenes, imidazoles, and the antimetabolite, flucytosine. These will be reviewed along with the less often used hydroxystilbamidine, griseofulvin, and potassium iodide.

A. Polyenes are fungicidal drugs and include **amphotericin B, natamycin,** and **nystatin.** The last is no longer used with any frequency in ophthalmic disease.

1. **Amphotericin B** (Fungizone) is a broad-spectrum heptene that is poorly water soluble and of large molecular weight, both characteristics limiting tissue penetration.

   a. **Spectrum of activity.** Sensitive fungi include *Histoplasma capsulatum, Cryptococcus neoformans, Coccidioides immitis, Candida* spp., *Blastomyces dermatitidis, Aspergillus* spp., *Sporothrix schenckii,* and *Paracoccidioides brasiliensis.*

   b. **Drug synergy and antagonism.** Certain antimicrobials can increase the in vitro activity of amphotericin B. Rifampin, an agent without antifungal activity on its own, decreases the concentration of amphotericin required in vitro to inhibit growth of *Candida, Aspergillus,* and *Histoplasma.* Similarly minocycline, a semisynthetic tetracycline, increases amphotericin B activity in vitro against *Candida* and *Cryptococcus.* Although there is as yet no clinical data on the efficacy of the above combinations, it has been demonstrated both in vitro and clinically that the concurrent use of flucytosine with amphotericin B reduces the concentration of the latter required to inhibit growth of *Candida* and *Cryptococcus,* thus reducing the incidence and severity of toxic side effects. This **synergy** may result from increased flucytosine penetration into fungal walls damaged by amphotericin. Conversely, the combined use with ketoconazole, an antifungal imidazole, results in **antagonism** of amphotericin B efficacy.

   c. **Mechanism of action.** The primary effect of the polyenes is exerted through the binding of the agent preferentially to ergosterol, a steroid moiety found in the wall of fungal but not mammalian cells. This results in increased permeability of the fungal cell membrane, allowing leakage of intracellular contents and death by electrolyte imbalance.

d. Routes of administration and dosage (Table 4-1). Amphotericin B is supplied in vials containing 50 mg of the antifungal and 41 mg of sodium deoxycholate to effect colloidal dispersion in the 10 ml diluent of sterile water.

(1) **Drops** for therapy of keratomycosis are prepared from the above suspension in sterile water to final concentrations up to 0.3% for therapy of fungal keratitis. Topical administration of drops in concentrations greater than 0.3% is very poorly tolerated. Current clinical data indicate that concentrations of 0.075–0.15% are better tolerated and have comparable antifungal efficacy. **Initial therapy** is 1 drop q30–60min, 24 hours a day, with gradual tapering (q1–2h to q3–4h, etc.) after stabilization and initial improvement are noted. Topical therapy is usually continued 3–4 times daily for several weeks, even after apparent resolution of active infection. Preclinical studies on drug-soaked (0.5%) **collagen shields** show corneal levels higher than or equal to q1h 0.15% drops (after q 1 min × 5 doses) for 3 hours and high levels at 6 hours.

(2) **Subconjunctival injection** of more than 300 mg of amphotericin B is painful, poorly tolerated, discolors the conjunctiva yellow, and may cause tissue necrosis or module formation. Little is known about ocular penetration via this route.

(3) **Systemic administration** of amphotericin B is reserved for fungal infections of the choroid, retina, and orbit. Because of significant toxic side effects, an internist or infectious disease specialist should be involved in patient care. The drug is best given by the intravenous (IV) route, as this drug is poorly absorbed from the gastrointestinal tract. About 95% of drug is bound by plasma lipoproteins with aqueous humor levels being two-thirds that of plasma concentrations. Little drug penetrates the cerebrospinal fluid (CSF) or vitreous cavity. Once prepared, drug concentration is stable only for 48 hours at room temperature and 1 week in the refrigerator. The mixed solution for IV administration must be used immediately because of rapid deterioration after dilution.

Initial therapy should be a small test dose of 1 mg in 500 ml of 5% dextrose solution (D5W) IV over 2–4 hours. Vital signs should be recorded every half hour for 4 hours and adverse reactions noted. These include fever (see Adverse side effects below, Sec. **I.A.1.e.**), chills,

Table 4-1. Antifungal therapeutic regimen

Drug (Commercial)	Topical	Intravitreal	Subconjunctival	Systemic[a]	Efficacious against
1. Amphotericin B[b] (Fungizone)	0.075–0.3% drop, q1h; taper over several weeks. Collagen shield delivery.	5–10 µg	100–300 mg	1 mg in 500 ml D5W IV over 2–4 h test dose. Work up by 5–10 mg total dose/day to maintenance of 0.3–0.5 mg/kg (4–6 h infusion). Synergistic with Flucytosine po	Candida, Aspergillus, Cryptococcus, Coccidioides, Sporothrix, Blastomyces, Histoplasma, Paracoccidioides, Mucor
2. Clotrimazole[b] (Lotrimin, Mycelex)	1% cream or ointment for skin. 1% eye drop or ointment prepared by pharmacy[b]	—	—	—	See Miconazole. Dermal mycoses
3. Fluconazole (Diflucan)	—	—	—	200–400 mg po initial dose, 100–200 mg/d po × 3w (Candida) and × 10–12 w (Cryptococcus)	Candida, Cryptococcus
4. Flucytosine[b] (5FC, Ancobon)	—	—	—	150–200 mg/day po in 4 divided doses, q6h	Candida, Aspergillus, Cryptococcus, Cladosporium
5. Griseofulvin[b] (Grifulvin)	—	—	—	500 mg–1.0 g/day po in 4 divided doses,	Microsporum, Epidermophyton, Tricho-

				q6h		*phyton* (Tinea) *Blastomyces*
6. Hydroxystilbamidine isethionate[b]	—	—	—	25–50 mg/500 ml D5W test dose, then 225 mg in 200 ml IV D5W/day over 2–4h, q24h		*Blastomyces*
7. Ketoconazole (Nizoral)[b]	—	—	—	200–400 mg/day po in single dose		See Miconazole. Dermal mycoses
8. Miconazole[b] (Monistat)	10 mg/ml drop, q1h	40 µg	10 mg, q48h	0.2–0.6 g IV, q8h (4–6 h infusion)		*Candida, Fusarium, Penicillium, Aspergillus, Alternaria, Rhodotorula, Histoplasma, Cladosporium, Coccidioides, Mucor, Paracoccidioides, Phialophora, Actinomycetes*
9. Natamycin (Pimaricin)	5% drop, q1h; 1% ointment[c]	—	—	—		*Candida, Fusarium, Cephalosporium, Aspergillus*
10. Potassium iodide[b] (saturated solution)	—	—	—	10 drops po tid working up to daily total of 120 drops in 3 divided doses		*Sporotrichosis*

[a] Gradual taper with clinical improvement.
[b] Not FDA approved for ocular disease.
[c] On comparssionate plea from Shearing Corp., Kenilworth, NJ, after obtaining emergency FDA–IND number; (301) 443-4310.

dyspnea, and hypotension. If the patient has only a mild reaction and cardiopulmonary function is good, 12 hours later a second dose of 5 mg amphotericin B in 500 ml of D5W IV over 4–6 hours may be given. In the absence of a significant adverse reaction, in 24 hours dosage may be moved to 10 mg and then 15 mg in each 24-hour period as the physician moves to establish maintenance daily dose of 0.4–0.5 mg/kg of amphotericin B IV in 500 ml of D5W over 4–6 hours. If the initial test dose reaction is severe, a smaller dose such as 0.5 mg total over 6 hours or 1.0 mg over 12 hours may be given. Dosage is increased daily by 2–5 mg total dose with slower infusion to a final daily dose of 0.3–0.5 mg/kg as tolerated. Once maximum daily dose is reached, the patient may be given a double dose every other day (not to exceed 70 mg/day in **alternate-day regimen** even if daily dose was greater than 35 mg/day) without loss of therapeutic efficacy.

Maintenance doses in excess of 1 mg/kg/day may cause renal toxicity without added therapeutic benefit. The customary total IV dose for intraocular *Candida* is 2–3 g, although the absolute dose requirement is not established. The drug is eliminated via the biliary tract and very slowly via the urine for up to 8 weeks after treatment is stopped.

(4) **Intravitreal** amphotericin B is given for progression of disease into the vitreous cavity, whether postsurgical, post-traumatic, or breakthrough of a chorioretinitis. Doses of 5–10 µg have apparent beneficial effect, especially when coupled with vitrectomy. Retinal toxicity may occur even on recommended doses, however, thus necessitating accurate documentation of disease. Table 4-2 gives the method of preparation of the intravitreal drug.

e. **Adverse side effects** are the result of the combined toxicity of amphotericin B and Na^+ deoxycholate. Table 4-3 lists suggested management to minimize these complications.

(1) **Topical amphotericin B drops** can be very irritating and tissue toxic especially at concentrations higher than 0.3%. This may result in conjunctival hyperemia, delayed corneal epithelial wound healing (which may enhance drug penetration and be of benefit during the first 7–10 days), and iridocyclitis. **Collagen shield** delivery may minimize toxicity.

(2) **Subconjunctival toxicity** is discussed under Routes of administration (Sec. **I.A.1.d.**) above.

(3) **Systemic drug** may, in addition to the fever, cause chills, hypotension, and dyspnea already mentioned, produce flushing, headache, anorexia, generalized pain, anaphylaxis, convul-

Table 4-2. Preparation of topical and intravitreal amphotericin B[a]

Route	Vial size	Amount of initial diluent	Initial concentration	Aliquot	Water added	Final concentration	Dose given
Intravitreal	50 mg	10 ml	5 mg/ml	0.1 ml	9.9 ml	50 µg/ml	5 µg/0.1 ml
				0.2 ml	9.8 ml	100 µg/ml	5 µg/0.1 ml
Topical[b]	50 mg	50 ml	1 mg/ml	0.3 ml	99.7 ml	0.3%	0.3%/gtt
				0.75 ml	199.25 ml	0.075%	0.075%/gtt

[a] Use lyophilized drug powder for parenteral use.
[b] Stable for 7 days at 4°C and 48 h at room temperature.

Table 4-3. Management of adverse reactions to systemic amphotericin B*

Reaction	Management
Fever and chills, myalgia, headache	Aspirin 300–600 mg or aceta-minophen (Tylenol) 375 mg–1.0 g po plus chlorpheniramine 4 mg po q6–8h prn
Nausea and vomiting, anorexia	Chlorpromazine (Compazine) 10–25 mg po, pr, or IM (painful) and hydroxyzine pamoate (Vistaril) 25–50 mg po (pill or oral suspension) or IM for associated anxiety q8–12h.
If above symptoms persist:	Add 5–20 mg/day hydrocortisone sodium succinate (Solu-Cortef) to IV fluid
Thrombophlebitis	Add 5 mg heparin to each IV bottle; use pediatric scalp vein needles alternating veins daily or an indwelling catheter with keep-open D5W drip in as distal veins as possible.
Hypokalemia (may cause paralysis or cardiac arrhythmias)	BIW to TIW K^+ levels. If low, give 20–60 mEq po qd prn
Azotemia	BIW to TIW BUN. Withhold drug if BUN rises to >50. IV mannitol may decrease renal toxicity
Anemia	Transfuse packed cells

* Vary dose and/or rate of administration if any of these reactions are moderate to severe or not controlled by above suggestions.

sions, thrombocytopenia, phlebitis, anemia, and decreased renal function. Fever and chills usually decrease with sequential injections and are often prevented by the concurrent addition of 5–10 mg of hydrocortisone to the IV solution. Adequate hydration is essential to minimizing renal toxicity.

2. **Natamycin (Pimaricin)** is a macrolide polyene that is currently the drug of choice for most cases of keratomycosis because it has less ocular toxicity than amphotericin B. **It is the only antifungal that is FDA approved for topical use in the eye.** However, recent clinical and experimental work indicate that amphotericin B concentrations of 0.15–0.75% may be more effective than natamycin in keratomycosis therapy without the toxic side effects seen at higher concentrations.

   a. **Spectrum of activity.** Sensitive fungi include *Candida* species, *Fusarium, Cephalosporium,* and *Aspergillus.*

   b. **Mechanism of action.** Like amphotericin B and nystatin, this drug works primarily by binding ergosterol in the fungal cell wall, thus altering cell membrane permeability and causing death by electrolyte imbalance.

c. **Routes of administration and dosage** (see Table 4-1). Natamycin is too toxic to be given systemically or subconjunctivally. Its use is confined to topical administration as a 5% drop or 1% ointment (ointment not available in the United States). The drug is poorly water soluble but does form a stable, bland microsuspension that is viscous, adhering to areas of epithelial defects and in the conjunctival fornix. Despite this prolonged contact time, drug penetration into the ocular tissues is poor, making it less effective in deeper keratomycoses. Initial treatment with the 5% natamycin suspension is hourly by day and every 2 hours during sleep, with gradual tapering over several weeks as stabilization and signs of improvement appear.

d. **Adverse side effects.** Topical suspension is bland and causes no conjunctival or corneal toxicity.

B. **Imidazoles** are synthetic, broad-spectrum, fungistatic drugs with good potency but less than amphotericin B. The compounds available in the United States include **miconazole,** which may be given parenterally, topically, and subconjunctivally, **ketoconazole** and **fluconazole,** which are given orally, and **clotrimazole,** which is available as a skin cream or powder. The **indications** for imidazole therapy are not well established in the absence of adequately controlled clinical trials. The polyenes remain the drugs of choice in many situations, but their established efficacy and toxicity must be weighed against the greater convenience and lower toxicity of the imidazoles.

1. **Spectrum of activity.** Sensitive fungi include *Candida* species (spp.), *Fusarium* spp., *Penicillium* spp., *Alternaria* spp., *Rhodotorula* spp., *Aspergillus* spp., *H. capsulatum, Cladioporum* spp., *C. immitis, Mucor* spp., *Paracoccidioides brasiliensis, Phialophora* spp., and *Actinomycetes* spp. Gram-positive bacteria and certain anaerobes such as *Bacteroides fragilis* are also susceptible. Very rarely, acquired resistance may be seen with *Candida albicans.*

2. **Mechanism of action.** Imidazoles inhibit ergosterol synthesis in the fungal cell membrane causing disorganization and thickening of the plasmalemma and interference with nutrient uptake.

3. **Routes of administration and dosage** (see Table 4-1).

a. **Miconazole (Monistat),** using the parenteral preparation as eye drops has been used successfully in keratomycosis.

(1) **Topical drops** (10 mg/ml) are given hourly around the clock coupled with **subconjunctival injections** (10 mg) every 48 hours. The injections are discontinued on clinical improvement and the drops gradually tapered over 6–12 weeks. As drug penetration is poor in the face of intact corneal epithelium, early healing

of the ocular surface may warrant repeated debridement to assure continued therapeutic levels in the deeper tissues.

(2) **Intravitreal injection** of 40 μg of miconazole for *Candida* endophthalmitis may be a reasonable therapeutic choice based on limited data, despite the marked potential for drug-induced retinal toxicity.

(3) **Intravenous therapy** with a regimen of 200–1200 mg q8h has met with only limited success and a number of failures in therapy of keratomycosis, but miconazole is considered a reasonably good therapeutic agent in certain fungal endophthalmitides. Drug is given IV q8h for total daily doses of 0.6–1.8 g over 4–12 weeks.

(4) **Adverse side effects** of IV miconazole include nausea, vomiting, anemia, phlebitis, thrombocytopenia, hyponatremia, sudden cardiac arrhythmia or arrest, blurred vision, seizures, arthralgias, and confusion. The drug appears to be benign topically and subconjunctivally.

b. **Ketoconazole (Nizoral)** is a water-soluble imidazole that achieves good corneal and aqueous drug levels following oral administration. Successful resolution of human keratomycosis using ketoconazole as adjunctive therapy has been reported with a single dose of 400 mg/day po over several weeks. Ketoconazole is used in the United States primarily in patients who have developed toxicity to amphotericin B or who must undertake chronic therapy for ocular fungal disease prone to recurrence.

(1) **Absorption and metabolism.** Drugs that reduce gastric acidity such as H_2 blockers and antacids interfere with the systemic absorption of the drug; the effects of taking the pills with meals are conflicting, but suggest that side effects may be reduced without reduction in drug levels. The drug is metabolized in the liver and has a half-life of 90 minutes after 200 mg and 4 hours after 800 mg. Dosage is usually 200–400 mg/day po for several weeks.

(2) **Adverse side effects** include nausea and vomiting (may be reduced by taking drug with meals), anorexia, headache, epigastric pain, photophobia, paresthesias, gingival bleeding, rash, thrombocytopenia, and, rarely, hepatotoxicity.

c. **Clotrimazole (Lotrimin, Mycelex)** may be used directly on the eye as a 1% ointment or suspension for *Candida* keratomycosis. Ocular drug should be prepared from pure clotrimazole powder. It is available on a compassionate plea basis from, Schering Corp., Kenilworth, N.J., after M.D. has obtained **emergency IND number** (Investigational New Drug) **from the FDA (tel. 301-443-4310).** The ointment or suspension is more commonly used for periocular dermatophytosis (*Tinea* spp.) and chronic cutaneous candidiasis. Efficacy for therapy of keratomycosis is not well established. Other agents should be used as first choice. Clotrimazole is applied to the eye 8–12 times daily or to the skin 4–6 times daily for 3–4 weeks. Adverse side effects by this route are negligible.

d. **Fluconazole** is FDA approved for therapy of Candidiasis and Cryptococcal meningitis. Initial studies suggest that it may be superior to Amphotericin B for *Candida* infections, including chorioretinitis (not FDA approved for ocular use). For *Candida,* initial dosage is 200–400 mg po, then 100–200 mg/d po for 3 weeks. For *Cryptococcus,* it is 400 mg po once, then 200 mg/d for 10–12 weeks.

C. **Flucytosine (5FC, Ancobon)** is a halogenated pyrimidine that achieves good aqueous levels after oral administration.

1. **Spectrum of activity.** 5FC inhibits *Candida* species, *Cryptococcus neoformans,* and some *Cladosporium* and *Aspergillus.* The resistance rate of *Candida* before treatment is about 50%, and more may become resistant during treatment.

2. **Mechanism of action.** The drug is enzymatically converted within susceptible fungi to 5-fluorodeoxyuridilic acid, an inhibitor of thymidylate synthetase, essential to DNA synthesis. Similar drug conversion by mammalian cells is minimal, thus limiting potential drug toxicity.

3. **Route of administration and dosage** (see Table 4-1). 5FC is rapidly and well absorbed after oral administration, minimally bound by plasma proteins, and excreted unchanged in the urine. Cerebrospinal fluid and aqueous levels are approximately 65–90% those of plasma levels. In ocular disease the drug is used concurrently with amphotericin B in treatment of retinal *Candida* or *Candida* endophthalmitis. Dosage is 150–200 mg/day po in four divided doses q6h with reduced dosage in renal insufficiency. Duration of treatment is usually several (4–8) weeks; emergence of resistant organisms may be avoided by concurrent use of another antifungal agent such as Amphotericin B.

4. **Adverse side effects** from this antimetabolite are bone marrow depression with anemia, leukopenia, and thrombocytopenia. Other side effects are nausea, vomiting, diarrhea, and enterocolitis. All these untoward effects are increased in azotemic patients, including those on amphotericin B and especially when drug levels exceed 100 µg/ml.

D. **Griseofulvin (Grifulvin)** is an antifungal used orally for treatment of periocular dermatophytes.

1. **Spectrum of action** is a fungistatic effect on *Microsporum, Epidermophyton,* and *Trichophyton* (ringworm). The agent is ineffective against yeast or other fungi.

2. **Mechanism of action** is through inhibition of fungal mitosis, resulting in multinucleate giant fungal cells

incapable of replication.
3. **Route of administration and dosage** (see Table 4-1). After oral administration, the drug is well absorbed, especially if given with a fatty meal, and subsequently selectively deposited in keratin precursor cells. It is tightly bound to keratin, making this substance resistant to fungal growth. As old hair and skin are shed, they are replaced by disease-free tissues. Very little drug is found in body fluids or tissues other than skin, and the drug is excreted in the urine. The drug is available as capsules (125–250 mg), tablets (250–500 mg), and oral suspension (125 mg/5 ml). The pediatric daily dose is 10 mg/kg and for adults 500 mg–1.0 g in four divided doses q6h for several weeks.
4. **Adverse side effects** include transient but sometimes severe headache, nervous system manifestations such as blurred vision and macular edema, lethargy, vertigo, and augmented alcohol effect. Other side effects are nausea, vomiting, dry mouth, heartburn, and angular stomatitis. Hepatotoxicity, hematologic effects such as leukopenia, neutropenia, and monocytosis, and renal toxicity may also occur, thus requiring that liver, blood, and kidney function be monitored weekly for at least the first month of treatment.
E. **Hydroxystilbamidine isothionate** is an aromatic diamidine given intravenously, primarily for cutanous **blastomycosis.** This dermal mycosis may be periocular. After a test dose of 25–50 mg IV, therapeutic dosage is 225 mg in 200 ml D5W infused over 2–4 hours every 24 hours for 1–2 weeks or as indicated by disease severity (see Table 4-1). Side effects include anorexia, malaise, nausea, rash, and hepatotoxicity.

II. **Diagnosis and Therapy of Ocular and Periocular Mycotic Infections**
A. **Keratomycosis** is an uncommon clinical entity in the United States. Even when suspected, it is difficult to diagnose and treat. Successful therapy is often the result of early diagnosis and appropriate medical and, if warranted, surgical management.
1. **Causative agents** reported in keratomycosis are listed in Table 4-1. Of the yeasts, *Candida albicans* is the most common, causing 5–7% of cases in the South and 32–43% of cases in the northern United States. *Fusarium,* the most common of the filamentous fungi, causes 45–61% of the cases of filamentous keratitis. Other important fungi causing this disease are *Aspergillus, Cephalosporium, Currilaria,* and *Alternaria.*
2. **The clinical features** of keratomycosis are only moderately pathognomonic. Similarity with other forms of microbial keratitis, especially stromal herpes interstitial keratitis and some less virulent bacterial infections, may delay diagnosis and make ultimate control of the disease far more difficult. Initial workup of any suspected microbial keratitis should include evaluation for fungus. Nontraumatic filamentous forms of disease may present as an ulcer anywhere on the cornea, whereas post-traumatic keratomycosis may ini-

tially appear as a discrete intrastromal infiltrate or plaque without an overlying epithelial defect. Characteristically the infiltrate is slowly progressive and grayish white with hyphate margins and adjacent but distinct smaller satellite lesions. If an ulcer is present, the margin is usually elevated with delicate linear infiltrates extending into stroma. Additional findings are endothelial plaques (inflammatory cells, stromal immune rings, and hypopyon), even with small ulcers.

3. **Laboratory diagnosis** is made by scraping for stained smears (gram, Giemsa, periodic acid-Schiff [PAS], Grocott-Gomori) and cultures on Sabouraud's or blood agar plates at room temperature.

4. **Therapy of keratomycosis** is as outlined under specific antifungal agents and in Table 4-1. **Steroids are contraindicated** in any known fungal infection until well after the disease process is controlled and resolving, and even then, with extreme caution if at all.

   a. **Filamentous organisms** are most often treated with topical natamycin or amphotericin B. Epithelium should be partially debrided during the first several days to enhance drug penetration. Cases refractory to one of the above polyenes may well respond to topical and subconjunctival miconazole. Ketoconazole is usually reserved for patients intolerant of amphotericin B or on long-term therapy of disease prone to recurrence.

   b. **Yeast: Candida infections** are usually responsive to topical and subconjunctival miconazole or the synergistic combination of oral flucytosine and topical amphotericin B with the epithelium kept partially debrided for the first several days to enhance drug penetration. Ketoconazole orally is an effective adjunctive anti-Candida drug, but is an antagonist of amphotericin B and therefore should not be used concurrently with it. Ketoconazole po may, however, be used adjunctively with miconazole drops and subconjunctival injection or with clotrimazole cream.

   c. **Surgical intervention** is a difficult decision to make. Therapeutic penetrating keratoplasty is often delayed for longer than is advisable and should be done if disease is progressive despite maximum tolerated therapy and before fungal elements penetrate the anterior chamber or extend to the corneal periphery.

B. **Fungal chorioretinitis** is discussed under Fungal endophthalmitis below. Systemic therapy with IV amphotericin B alone or in combination with oral flucytosine or IV miconazole are the antifungal agents of therapeutic efficacy in this disease. If there is no fungal breakthrough into the vitreous cavity, vitrectomy is not indicated.

C. **Fungal endophthalmitis** may result from breakthrough of an endogenous chorioretinitis (chronically ill or immunosupressed patients, patients on IV hyperalimentation, IV drug abusers), postoperatively, or after penetrating injury. The first entity is almost invariably due to

Candida, the postsurgical to either yeast or filamentous forms, and the post-traumatic usually to filamentous.

1. **Clinical characteristics** of fungal endophthalmitis are delayed onset (7–30 days), indolence, mild discomfort and hyperemia (excluding that due to trauma), occasional hypopyon, blurred and then slowly progressive loss of vision, localized but progressive vitreous gray-white patches, vitreal and anterior chamber satellite lesions, and focal, yellow-white, round, posterior pole retinal infiltrates with overlying vitritis.

2. **Diagnosis** is made by clinical history, knowledge of pre-existing fungal chorioretinitis, and, in many cases, diagnostic vitreous aspiration. (See Bacterial endophthalmitis and keratomycosis.)

3. **Therapy of fungal endophthalmitis.** None of the currently available antifungal agents penetrate the vitreous cavity, but once the diagnosis is confirmed by vitreous aspiration of the intravitreal extension of an endogenous chorioretinal fungal infection, the treatment should be as aggressive as is tolerable to the patient. Intravitreal administration of 5–50 μg of amphotericin B or 40 μg of miconazole has, by limited data, been therapeutically useful in yeast and filamentous infections. After the therapeutic/diagnostic core or subtotal vitrectomy is performed, care must be taken to place the needle for drug injection in the midvitreous cavity as far from the retina as possible because of the notable retinal toxicity of these agents. Intravitreal injection may be repeated in 24–48 hours, but in such eyes the prognosis is very poor based on disease alone. (See Treatment of bacterial endophthalmitis.) Adjunctive systemic therapy is often concurrent oral flucytosine and IV amphotericin B, or IV and subconjunctival miconazole and oral flucytosine in the doses and regimen described under specific antifungal agents.

D. **Other mycotic infections,** besides keratomycosis, fungal chorioretinitis, and fungal endophthalmitis, may involve almost any ocular, adnexal, or orbital structure. Although all are relatively rare, the more common diseases are summarized below in terms of clinical presentation and therapy. Where pertinent, **additional diagnostic tests** other than scraping and culturing accessible lesions will be mentioned under each specific fungal agent. **Drug doses** are as discussed under specific antifungal agents and in Table 4-1.

1. **Actinomycosis.** Although referred to as a mycotic infection, the causative anaerobic organism is not a true fungus. This is a disease seen in rural areas, primarily affecting cutaneous, cervicofacial, thoracic, and abdominal sites. It reaches the eye and orbit by spread from the mouth or nasal passages.

   a. **Ocular manifestations** include: lid abscesses, fibrosis, canaliculitis, dacryocystitis; angular, catarrhal, or pseudomembranous conjunctivitis with mucopurulent discharge, yellow nodules, keratomycosis, orbital abscess, infiltration, proptosis.

    b. Therapy of blepharitis, conjunctivitis, or keratitis is penicillin drops, 100,000 U/ml, as described under specific antifungal drugs. For corneal ulcers, adjunctive therapy is subconjunctival penicillin G 0.5–1.0 million U. Orbital or larger lid lesions are treated with surgical drainage or scraping and several weeks of IV penicillin therapy, 2–6 million U q4h.

2. **Aspergillosis** is a filamentous, saprophytic fungal disease seen most commonly in farming communities. Ocular and orbital diseases usually result from trauma, sinus disease, IV drug abuse, or immunosuppression. This fungus accounts for nearly 50% of all cases of keratomycosis.

    a. Ocular manifestations include keratitis, keratoconjunctivitis, endophthalmitis, proptosis, canaliculitis, dacryocystitis, and cranial nerve palsy.

    b. Therapy of keratitis includes topical natamycin, topical and subconjunctival miconazole, or amphotericin B, as described under specific antifungal agents. Drugs used in endophthalmitis are intravitreal and systemic miconazole or amphotericin B; those for orbital or other periocular infection are IV amphotericin B, miconazole, or ketoconazole.

3. **Blastomycosis** is a chronic filamentous fungal infection that produces granulomatous lesions anywhere on the body. Ocular disease is by direct spread of adjacent infection or by hematogenous spread from the lungs.

    a. Ocular manifestations include: lid granulomas, abscesses, entropion; keratomycosis, nodular anterior uveitis, focal choroiditis, orbital abscess, or cellulitis.

    b. Therapy is IV hydroxystilbamidine as the least toxic drug of choice, IV amphotericin B, or IV miconazole at the highest tolerated doses. Subconjunctival and intravitreal miconazole or topical forms of this drug or amphotericin B are used for keratomycosis or endophthalmitis as indicated. Surgical drainage or curettage of focal lesions should also be carried out.

4. **Candida** is discussed earlier under keratomycosis and endophthalmitis. Candida meibomitis (blepharitis) is treated with meibomian gland expression by compressing the lid between cotton-tip applicators, and Candida canaliculitis by curettage, both along with topical antifungal therapy.

5. **Coccidiomycosis,** a disease endemic to the semiarid regions of the United States, is caused by a dimorphic fungus capable of infecting any organ of the body, with most ocular lesions being choroidal.

    a. Ocular manifestations include: lid granulomas, erythema multiforme, conjunctival palpebral granulomas, ulcers, and phlyctenules, scleritis, episcleritis, keratomycosis as necrotic inflammatory foci, granulomatous iridocyclitis, hypopyon, retinal edema, exudates, hemorrhages, perivascular sheathing, choroidal scars, granulomas, choroiditis, vitritis, endophthalmitis; orbital granulomas, and sixth nerve palsy.

b. **Additional diagnostic tests** include coccidioidin skin testing, serologic studies, chest X rays, complete blood count, erythrocyte sedimentation rate, and knowledge of geographic exposure.

c. **Therapy** of ocular coccidiomycosis is even less effective than that of other ocular fungal disease. Amphotericin B IV is still the drug of choice and usually must be given over several months. Subconjunctival doses of 0.75–5.0 mg in 1.0-ml aqueous suspension have been used, but its efficacy in intraocular coccidiomycosis is unknown. Similarly, intravitreal injections at the time of diagnostic/therapeutic vitrectomy or for cases of severe anterior uveitis have been used with dubious benefit and notable toxicity.

Miconazole is approved for therapy of various forms of coccidiomycosis but is used IV and subconjunctivally for ocular disease only in patients who fail to respond to amphotericin B. Effects of intravitreal miconazole are unknown in this disease, but therapeutic response appears very limited regardless of route of administration.

Ketoconazole po is effective in pulmonary coccidiomycosis, but has not yet been used in therapy of ocular or periocular disease.

6. **Cryptococcus** is a yeast-like fungus found in soil; it is the most common cause of CNS mycosis. It usually occurs in chronically ill or immunosuppressed patients, but may cause disease in otherwise healthy people.

a. **Ocular manifestations** are associated with cryptococcal meningitis and include: blurred vision to visual loss, conjunctival hyperemia, photophobia, focal or multifocal chorioretinitis with progression to retinitis, vitritis, and anterior segment inflammation, papilledema or optic atrophy, and extraocular muscle palsy.

b. **Additional diagnostic tests.** Presumptive diagnosis of cryptococcosis may be made in the absence of direct demonstration of the organism in ocular fluid or tissue. Cerebrospinal fluid abnormalities are elevated protein, low glucose, and mononuclear pleocytosis. Cerebrospinal fluid or aqueous fluid cryptococcal antigen titer by latex fixation may be positive even when an India ink preparation is negative.

c. **Therapy** of choice is IV amphotericin B for up to 3 months. Intravitreal amphotericin B may be given where indicated for intraocular involvement.

7. **Dermatophytoses (tinea, epidermophytosis),** fungal infections of keratinized tissue only, cause ringworm and athlete's foot. Ocular or periocular involve-

ment is rare and results from spread of facial infection.

a. **Ocular findings** are red, circular, scaly patches on the lids with minimal inflammation, marginal blepharitis, lid ulcers, and lash loss. Rarely conjunctivitis, and very rarely, corneal ulcers may develop.

b. **Additional diagnostic tests.** Most dermatophytes fluoresce under ultraviolet light, thus indicating the diagnosis in situ.

c. **Therapy** is twice daily application of 1% clotrimazole, 2% miconazole, 1% tolnaftate, or 1% haloprogin cream, taking care to avoid direct contact with the eyes because of the irritating potential of these agents.

8. **Histoplasmosis (*Histoplasma capsulatum*),** a yeast-like organism, is considered the causative agent of presumed ocular histoplasmosis syndrome (POHS). "Presumed" refers to the fact that although the organism has been recovered from the eyes of patients with disseminated histoplasma with endophthalmitis, it has never been isolated from eyes with the actual syndrome.

a. **Ocular findings** of POHS are bilateral, disseminated, atrophic scars ("histo spots"), peripapillary scarring, serous and hemorrhagic maculopathy, and clear media. Optic disc edema is rare. Early symptoms are those of macular involvement, blurred vision, and metamorphopsia.

b. **Additional diagnostic tests.** Histoplasmin skin testing has minimal diagnostic value.

c. **Therapy.** Recurrent inflammation in the scars usually resolves spontaneously, although some physicians believe that 1–2 weeks of oral prednisone 40–60 mg/day may be indicated. Because of the tendency for development of subretinal neovascularization to within 200 μm of the foveal avascular zone after 10–20 years of disease, however, existing central vision may be lost if not monitored by fluorescein angiography and laser therapy for total destruction of the vascular net applied when indicated. Red krypton is somewhat better than blue-green photocoagulation and both better than the natural course of disease. Photocoagulation of histo spots is not indicated and may activate them. Systemic antifungals are without effect in POHS.

9. **Mucormycosis,** caused by a filamentous fungus, is an opportunistic, acute, often fatal disease of chronically debilitated patients such as the ketoacidotic diabetic, uremic, immunosuppressed, malnourished, or burn patient.

a. **Ocular findings** are the result of spread from adjacent upper respiratory structures. Classically a chronically ill patient, often with a history of unilateral nosebleed, presents with the orbital apex syndrome of proptosis, blurred or lost vision, corneal venous engorgement anesthesia, central retinal artery thrombosis, exudative retinitis, internal or external ophthalmoplegia, and ptosis. There also may be associated orbital cellulitis, anhidrosis, facial pain, or facial palsy.

b. Additional diagnostic tests. A black, necrotic patch on the nasal mucosa is pathognomonic, and smears and cultures of this area or other skin lesions often reveal the organism. Orbital and sinus tomograms and CT scans reveal total ocular/orbital involvement, and carotid arteriography, EEGs, and lumbar puncture assist in diagnosing and monitoring disease progress.

c. Therapy has three guiding principles: (1) correction, if possible, of predisposing factors such as acidosis; (2) surgical debridement of all necrotic or involved areas, including drainage and irrigation of sinuses with amphotericin B; and (3) antifungal therapy, with IV amphotericin B being the drug of choice. The antifungal regimen is as described under specific antibiotics, and the total dose over the course of treatment of most patients is 3.0 g, with a few going to 4.0 g but sustaining renal damage.

10. **Nocardiosis** is caused by a filamentous organism (*N. asteroides*). Predisposing factors include autoimmune, malignant, or immunosuppressive disease or therapy.

    a. Ocular infection may range from iridocyclitis to severe panophthalmitis. Findings may include a single, unilateral chorioretinal lesion with focal vitritis, multiple choroidal abscesses with retinal necrosis and detachment, and diffuse iridocyclitis with heavy keratic precipitates.

    b. Additional diagnostic tests include culture of the organism from sputum or tracheal aspirate.

    c. Therapy is both medical and surgical. Systemic sulfonamides are the treatment of choice: 6–10 g sulfadiazine or sulfisoxazole po for 6 weeks in immunocompetent patients and for up to 1 year in the immunosuppressed. Surgically, a diagnostic/therapeutic vitrectomy is recommended for vitritis and focal chorioretinitis. If, however, retinal necrosis is apparent and retinal detachment considered inoperable, enucleation is advisable. The prognosis for life may depend on this.

11. **Sporotrichosis (*S. schenckii*)** is a chronic fungal disease usually initiated by traumatic inoculation of spores into the skin or eye.

    a. Ocular findings include one or more lid nodules that progress to purulent, ulcerative blepharitis with secondary preauricular adenopathy, dacryocystitis, orbital abscess, keratitis, and scleritis. Intraocular disease is usually a granulomatous iris tumor and, very rarely, endophthalmitis.

    b. Additional diagnostic tests. Other than scrapings and culture of lesions, there are none.

    c. Therapy of ocular disease is 10 drops of a saturated solution of potassium iodide (KI) po tid progressively, increasing to a total dose of 120 drops po daily and continued for 1 month after lesions have cleared. Systemic treatment with KI is supplemented with topical natamycin or amphotericin B q1h initially for keratomycosis and then as described under specific antifungals and keratomycosis. For noncorneal external involvement, topical treatment may start at lower doses such as q2h, with curettage of lesions as indicated. If endophthalmitis is present, diagnostic/therapeutic vitrectomy should be done and 5–10 µg amphotericin B injected intravitreally. Systemic treatment with po KI and IV amphotericin B are maintained for several weeks to months, particularly if there is disseminated disease. (See specific antifungals, amphotericin B.) Flucytosine is ineffective against this organism, and ketoconazole has produced inconsistent results.

Information Sources and Suggested Reading (*Antifungals*)

1. Cobo, L.M., Antifungals. In Lamberts, D.W., and Potter, D.E. (Eds.), *Clinical Ophthalmic Pharmacology.* Boston: Little, Brown, 1987, pp. 97–107.
2. Fraunfelder, F., and Roy, F.H. (Eds.), *Current Ocular Therapy 3,* 3rd ed. Philadelphia: W.B. Saunders, 1990, multiple contributing authors, pp. 53–67, 445–447 (mycotic infections).
3. Liesegang, T., Bacterial and fungal keratitis. In Kaufman, H.E., Barron, B., McDonald, M., and Waltman, S. (Eds.), *The Cornea.* New York: Churchill Livingstone, 1988, pp. 217–270.
4. Nussenblatt, R.B., and Palestine, A.G., *Uveitis: Fundamentals in Clinical Practice.* Chicago: Yearbook Medical Publ., 1989, pp. 379–387 (histoplasmosis), pp. 399–407 (fungal).
5. Pavan-Langston, D., and Foulks, D., Cornea and external disease, in Pavan-Langston, D. (Ed.), *Manual of Ocular Diagnosis and Therapy,* 3rd ed. Boston: Little, Brown, 1990, pp. 65–116.
6. Sande, M., and Mandell, G., Antifungal and antiviral agents. In Gilman, A.G., Goodman, L.S., Rall, T., and Murad F. (Eds.), *The Pharmacological Basis of Therapeutics,* 7th ed. New York: Macmillan, 1985, pp. 1219–1239.
7. Schwartz, S., Harrison, S., Engstrom, R. J., et al., Collagen shield delivery of Amphotericin B, Am. J. Ophthalmol. 109:701–704, 1990.
8. Smolin, G., and Thoft, R.A. (Eds.), *The Cornea,* 2nd ed. Boston: Little, Brown, 1987, pp. 169–176 (fungal microbiology, Okumoto, M.), pp. 228–239 (fungal ocular disease, Forster, R.).
9. Tabbara, K.F., and Hyndiuk, R.A. (Eds.), *Infections of the Eye.* Boston: Little, Brown, 1986, multiple contributing authors, pp. 151–166 (diagnostic mycology, Halde, C.), pp. 239–256 (antifungal agents, Hyndiuk, R., Yee, R.), pp. 331–342 (fungal keratitis, Koenig, S.), pp. 511–516 (endogenous *Candida,* Tabbara, K.).

5

Antiglaucoma Drugs

I. **Glaucoma** is a condition in which the intraocular pressure is sufficiently high to cause optic nerve damage and potential visual field loss. The goal of therapy is to reduce the pressure such that nerve damage and field defects are prevented or arrested. Because of the chronicity of the disease and the wide variety of drugs available, the pressure reduction should be achieved using the least amount and fewest number of drugs that are efficacious, to minimize the risk of local and systemic adverse side effects.

A. **Before initiating therapy:** Because a diagnosis of glaucoma often means a lifelong commitment to multiple ocular medications, it is extremely important to instruct the patient well from the start to attain optimal clinical efficacy.

1. Ascertain any **history** of **drug allergy** or **cardiopulmonary** or **renal** disease, as certain antiglaucoma drugs will aggravate one or more of these.

2. **Instruct** the patient in finger **compression over the nasolacrimal** area after drop instillation to limit drainage and systemic absorption of drug through the nasolacrimal mucous membrane and the associated systemic side effects.

3. **Timing of multiple drops** should allow for 5 minutes between drugs to allow adequate ocular absorption, allow tearing to dissipate, and prevent washout of the first drug by the second.

4. **Compliance problems** should be anticipated and dealt with appropriately. Most such problems stem from the frequent need for long-term multiple drug therapy by patients with limited economic resources and the age-related problems of decreased vision, memory failure, arthritic hands, and tremors.

B. **In initiating treatment** it is best, in non-urgent situations, to:

1. **Start only one medication** at a time to ascertain its therapeutic effect.

2. On **addition of a second drug,** consider discontinuing the first to ascertain if both or only one is needed to achieve the same level of control.

3. **Minimize local and systemic side effects** by starting with the lowest drug concentrations deemed appropriate and working the patient up to higher doses as necessary. Adverse reactions are directly correlated with the amount of drug and metabolite present in the tissues.

C. **Parameters** followed in glaucoma patients include periodic tonometry, visual fields, and disc examination. Tonography, stereophotography of the discs, red-free photographs of the nerve fiber layer, and diurnal curves to determine time of peak pressure from 8:00 A.M. are useful if available.

D. **Susceptibility to progressive nerve damage** is increased in patients with high myopia, congenitally large disc cupping, asymmetry of cup/disc ratio greater than 0.2, family history of glaucoma (both primary open and angle-closure), vascular insufficiency, diabetes mellitus, and anemia.

E. **Aims of pressure control.** As a rule, IOP in the mid-teens (16–18 mm Hg) will be adequate control in patients with disc cupping of 0.8 or less and no or minimal field loss (enlarged blind spot, nasal steps, early Bjerrum's scotomas not threatening central vision). For more advanced disc cupping of 0.9 to near-total and field losses encroaching on the central 10–15 degrees or more, IOP should be in the low teens (11–13 mm Hg). Total cupping or field loss below 10 degrees is usually only stabilized with pressures less than 10, control usually achieved only with filtering surgery. The reader is referred to more comprehensive texts for more detailed information on diagnosis and criteria for determining the adequacy of a selected management course.

II. **Antiglaucoma drugs** may be classified into four categories: (1) the parasympathomimetic cholinergics and anticholinesterases (miotics); (2) alpha- and beta-adrenergic agents; (3) carbonic anhydrase inhibitors; and (4) hyperosmotic agents.

A. **The cholinergics, pilocarpine** and **carbachol,** are still among the most frequently used antiglaucoma medication, despite the advent of newer classes of drugs.

1. **Pilocarpine** is a natural alkaloid available as the nitrate or hydrochloride. There is no significant difference in their therapeutic effect (Table 5-1).

a. **The mechanism of action** is via increased outflow facility. Pilocarpine molecules adhere to the small muscle fibers of the ciliary body, stimulate the muscarinic receptors, cause contraction of the longitudinal muscle fibers inserting in the scleral spur, and thus widen the drains of the trabecular meshwork. There also may be a direct effect on the cholinergic receptors in the meshwork itself. The associated stimulation of pupillary sphincter receptors and consequent miosis is not associated with any lowering of IOP and may even be considered an adverse side effect of the drug (see Thymoxamine).

b. **Intraocular penetration** is excellent because of the biphasic solubility of the pilocarpine molecules. Nonionized drug is lipid-soluble and easily crosses epithelium. Ionized molecules are water-soluble, thus readily crossing the stromal barrier before reconverting to the nonionized form and crossing the endothelium. Although high levels of pilocarpine are detectable in the aqueous 5 minutes after topical instillation, the binding of drug by serum proteins and ocular melanin alters drug availability at receptor sites. A dark brown iris will bind more drug than a blue iris, resulting in less lowering of pressure, but longer duration of action in the darker eyes.

Table 5-1. Medications for glaucoma management: miotics

Drug commercial names	Mechanism of action	Common dosages	Major clinical indications	Adverse side effects
Miotics-cholinergics				
Pilocarpine: Adsorbocarpine, Akarpine, Almocarpine, Isopto Carpine, Pilocar, Pilocel, Pilomiotin, Piloptic, P.V. Carpine, Ocusert P20 or 40, Pilopine Gel	Increased outflow facility via ciliary muscle pull on trabecular meshwork (direct stimulation muscarinic neuroreceptors)	• 1, 2, 4% drops bid to qid (1–2% q15min acute angle closure) • Ocular inserts 20–40 μg, 1 insert q7d • 4% gel qHs	Primary open-angle glaucoma, acute and chronic angle closure glaucoma certain noninflammatory secondary glaucomas	*Ocular:* miosis, aching, and myopia (ciliary spasm), cataract, ? ocular pemphigoid *Systemic:* hiccoughs, tearing, nausea, vomiting, diarrhea, tenesmus, bronchospasm, pulmonary edema
Carbachol: Carbacel, Isopto Carbachol	Increased outflow facility via ciliary muscle pull on trabecular meshwork (direct stimulation muscarinic neuroreceptors and cholinesterase inhibition)	• 0.75, 1.5, 2.25, or 3.0% drops bid or qid • 0.01% intracameral solution	As per pilocarpine. Longer duration of action, less fluctuating miosis and myopia. Intraoperative miosis and postoperative IOP control	See pilocarpine
Miotics-anticholinesterases				
Echothiophate iodide (phospholine iodide):	Increased outflow facility via ciliary	0.03–0.25% drops qd–q12h	As per pilocarpine. Longer duration of	*Ocular:* allergic conjunctivitis, contact dermatitis, chronic

	Mechanism	Dosage	Indications	Side Effects
Echodide Phospholine Iodide	muscle pull on trabecular meshwork (cholinestrerase inhibitor)		action, less fluctuating miosis, and myopia. Accommodative esotropia.	conjunctival hyperemia, ocular pemphigoid, iritis, miosis, aching and myopia (ciliary spasm), pupillary cysts, anterior chamber shallowing, cataracts, ? retinal detachment, and vitreous hemorrhage *Systemic:* asthma, diarrhea, tenesmus, nausea, vomiting, systemic hypertension, bradycardia, sweating, salivation, tearing, muscle weakness, twitching, paralysis, prolonged respiratory depression after succinylcholine
Isoflurophate: Fluoropryl	As per echothiophate iodide	0.01–0.1% drops in anhydrous vegetable oil or ointment qd–q12h	As per echothiophate iodide except not used for accommodative esotropia	As per echothiophate iodide
Demecarium bromide: Humorsol	As per echothiophate iodide	0.125–0.25% drops qd or less. IOP decrease up to 4 days after 1 drop	As per echothiophate iodide except not used for accommodative esotropia	As per echothiophate iodide
Physostigmine: Eserine sulfate Isopto Eserine	As per echothiophate iodide	0.25–0.5% drops q6–12h or ointment qHs	As per echothiophate iodide except not used for accommodative esotropia	As per echothiophate iodide

   c. **Pilocarpine preparations** may lower pressure in both glaucomatous and normal eyes.

     (1) **Drops.** The drug is available in drop form under a variety of trade names and ranging in concentration from 0.25–10% (see Table 5-1). Intraocular pressure begins to fall within 40–60 minutes of drop instillation, reaching peak effect at about 75 minutes and dropping below therapeutic levels by 5–6 hours after application. There is a clear dose–response curve for drug concentrations up to 4%. Higher dosage does not result in further lowering of IOP, but will result in a prolonged hypotensive effect compared with the 4% concentration. The therapeutic efficacy also is influenced by drug vehicle, eg, dehydroxymethylcellulose base results in less IOP-lowering effect than the same drug concentration in the more viscous Adsorbobase. Although pilocarpine has a reduced pressure-lowering effect when combined with acetylcholinesterase inhibitors such as phospholine iodide because of reduced sensitivity of the aqueous outflow system, the **combination** of pilocarpine with nonparasympathomimetics is usually synergistic. Particularly effective are combined pilocarpine and sympathomimetics, β-blockers, or carbonic anhydrase inhibitors. Pilocarpine drops are commonly given bid to qid.

     (2) **Diffusion membranes (Ocusert).** The Ocusert unit is a thin, pliable oval (5.5 × 12.2 × 0.4 mm) membrane that is worn under the lower or upper lid for a week at a time. The core of the unit is a pilocarpine base that diffuses across the surrounding copolymeric membrane delivering a steady, low, but therapeutic level of drug to the eye. **Advantages** of the system are reduced fluctuating myopia and miosis with greater stability of vision, especially in younger patients with accommodative power, absence of systemic absorption of toxic levels of drug, and better patient compliance, with only once-weekly insertion of the insert required. **Disadvantages** are that occasionally the inserts are lost from the eye without patient knowledge, there is a transient burst effect of higher drug delivery when new inserts are put in (thus bed-time insertion is preferable), and intolerance or inability to handle the insert in up to 14% of patients.

      The Ocusert P-20 was found to control IOP in patients also controlled by pilocarpine concentrations less than 2%. The Ocusert P-40 generally controlled pressure in patients requiring 2% pilocarpine or stronger for similar IOP reduction.

(3) **Gel.** Pilocarpine HCl has been formulated as a 4% high-viscosity acrylic gel designed to prolong contact time, improve compliance, and reduce adverse side effects because of delivery of a lower total dose. The gel is applied once daily, usually at bedtime. Initial studies indicate that it is effective and well tolerated. It is a useful adjunct to daytime treatment of glaucoma with drops and/or carbonic anhydrase inhibitors. One study reported development of a diffuse subtle corneal granularity in 20% of patients using the gel longer than 2 months and persisting 12 months after the gel was discontinued.

d. **Clinical indications** for pilocarpine include primary open-angle glaucoma, acute and chronic angle-closure glaucoma, certain noninflammatory secondary glaucomas, opening the angle wider for laser trabeculoplasty, tightening the iris longitudinal fibers to optimize laser iridotomy applications, preoperative situations where miosis is desirable, such as corneal transplantation in a phakic eye, and postoperative situations where miosis is desirable, eg, prevention of posterior chamber lens pupillary capture.

e. **Contraindications** include neovascular glaucoma, glaucoma secondary to acute or chronic inflammatory disease such as uveitis, and malignant glaucoma. Miotic therapy is contraindicated in these conditions because of the effect of cholinergics in breakdown of the blood–aqueous barrier, resulting in iritis, ciliary body tightening, and 8–12% shallowing of the anterior chamber. Miotics should be used with caution in patients predisposed to retinal detachment because of drug-induced pull on the peripheral retina as the iris-lens diaphragm is pulled forward. A paradoxical rise in IOP may occur in patients with compromised trabecular meshwork, eg, traumatic angle recession, because of drug-induced decreased uveoscleral flow, an alternative aqueous outflow mechanism of importance in such eyes.

f. **Adverse side effects**

(1) **Ocular.** Cholinergics induce pupillary miosis and ciliary spasm. The miosis may cause a marked decrease in vision, especially if the lens is cataractous. Ciliary spasm may cause deep ocular pain which usually is much worse at the initiation of treatment and becomes tolerable to nonexistent as the eye adapts. Drug-induced myopia often is not correctable with glasses because it fluctuates as each dose wears off or is given. This side effect is more intolerable in younger eyes with greater accommodative power and may necessitate discontinuation of cholinergic treatment. There is a higher inci-

dence of nuclear sclerotic cataract in patients on long-term therapy, but as senile cataract is common in the age group usually using the drugs, development of such opacities is not necessarily due to cholinergic therapy. Pilocarpine also is one of several topical drugs implicated in the development of ocular pemphigoid or conjunctival cicatrization with associated histopathologic and immune changes. There are no human data suggesting teratogenicity during pregnancy, although animal studies have indicated potential syndactyly or abnormal tooth development.

(2) **Systemic** absorption of drug across the nasolacrimal and conjunctival mucous membranes occasionally may result in increased systemic muscarinic activity. This is very rare in the doses given for open-angle glaucoma, but may be seen more frequently in patients receiving multiple doses, as in therapy of acute angle-closure glaucoma. Such muscarinic activity may induce hiccoughs, lacrimation, salivation, nausea, vomiting, diarrhea, tenesmus, bronchospasm, and pulmonary edema. **Therapy of cholinergic poisoning** is parenteral atropine along with appropriate supportive measures.

2. **Carbachol** is the second of the cholinergic agents widely used in glaucoma management (see Table 5-1). It is a synthetic derivative of choline.

a. **Mechanism of action.** Carbachol works both as a direct acetylcholine-like parasympathetic drug and indirectly by displacing acetylcholine from the parasympathetic terminals and by inhibiting cholinesterase. Pharmacologically, this results in contraction of the longitudinal fibers of the ciliary muscle, thus, like pilocarpine, widening the trabecular meshwork spaces and increasing facility of outflow. There is also an intense miotic effect that is unrelated to the IOP reduction. Because of its resistance to cholinesterase, carbachol is longer acting than pilocarpine and, therefore, has a greater effect on the diurnal fluctuation of IOP.

b. **Intraocular penetration.** This synthetic derivative of choline is made from parts of two molecules, acetylcholine and physostigmine. As such, it differs from pilocarpine in reduced bipolarity. This results in poor lipid solubility and, therefore, poor corneal penetration across the epithelial and endothelial layers. To enhance intraocular drug levels, carbachol is prepared with a wetting solution included in the vehicle for topical use. In surgical use the specially formulated drug is administered by direct injection into the anterior chamber.

c. **Preparations.** The two forms of use for carbachol are as a topical agent in therapy of glaucoma and as an intraocular miotic during ocular surgery.

(1) **Topical** carbachol is available in concentrations of 0.75–3.0% under several trade names. It is commonly used 3–4 times daily.

(2) **Intracameral** carbachol (Miostat) is prepared specifically for intraoperative use by instillation into the anterior chamber for the purpose of inducing miosis and controlling postoperative IOP. The preparation used is 0.01% for irrigating the anterior chamber and reforming it as indicated during surgery. It lowers postoperative IOP and is longer lasting than **acetylcholine chloride** (Miochol), which also is used intraoperatively for the rapid induction of miosis, but which has little effect on postoperative IOP.

d. **Clinical indications** for topical carbachol drops are similar to those of pilocarpine: primary open-angle glaucoma, acute primary and chronic angle-closure glaucoma, and certain noninflammatory secondary glaucomas. Because of its longer duration of action, this drug may be better tolerated in younger patients, as there is less fluctuating miosis and myopia. In addition, intraoperative surgical carbachol prevents an acute evaluation of IOP postoperatively in cataract patients and is highly effective intraoperatively in inducing miosis where desired, eg, to prevent dislocation of a posterior chamber IOL or to induce miosis during penetrating keratoplasty to protect the natural or implanted lens.

e. **Adverse side effects and contraindications** are those of all cholinergics and are listed under pilocarpine. **Therapy for overdosage** is parenteral atropine.

B. **Anticholinesterases** may be divided into the short-acting drugs, **physostigmine** and **neostigmine,** and the long-acting drugs, **isofluorophate** and **echothiophate.** The characteristics common to all of these drugs will be discussed in greater detail under echothiophate and, where applicable, referred to under the individual drug descriptions (see Table 5-1).

1. **Echothiophate iodide (phospholine iodide, PI).** PI is one of the most commonly used, very potent, and long-acting miotics.

a. **The mechanism of action** of organophosphorus drugs is through the irreversible binding of both anionic and esteratic sites of cholinesterase to produce an extremely stable phosphorylated enzyme. This allows accumulation of acetycholine at the neural effector junction, thereby extending cholinergic activity for up to 12 hours after a single application. Return of anticholinesterase activity is dependent on synthesis of new enzyme in the eye. Clinically the effect is similar to that of pilocarpine, in that there is contraction of the longitudinal fibers of the ciliary muscle, thus opening the trabecular meshwork spaces to increase aqueous outflow and lower IOP. A secondary effect is miosis, which may be noted as early as 5–10 minutes after topical application and last up to 1 week. The miosis plays no role in reducing IOP in eyes with open-angle glaucoma. The magnitude and duration of drug effect is a dose–response relationship. The maximum drop in pressure after a single application is seen at 24 hours, and the miotic effect and lowering of pressure may last from a few days up to a week. In doses stronger than 0.06%, there is a higher incidence of subjective complaint and local side effects.

b. Intraocular penetration is excellent because of the biphasic nature of the molecule. The drug localizes in the ciliary body, with reduced cholinesterase activity noted within 30 minutes to 2 hours after instillation.

c. Preparations. PI is available in aqueous solution concentrations of 0.03–0.25% for topical use (see Table 5-1). The drug is marketed as a powder and reconstituted at the time of proposed use by mixing an accompanying diluent with the sterile powder. Storage at 4° C (refrigeration) is essential to prevent the aqueous solution of PI from degenerating, with subsequent loss of 20% activity within 1 month at room temperature. The unconstituted powder form of the drug is stable indefinitely. The drop is used topically in the concentration thought to be indicated every 12 hours. It may be given in lower doses once daily or every other day as indicated.

d. Clinical indications for glaucoma therapy are similar to those noted under pilocarpine (see Sec. **II.A.1**) where a stronger agent is desired. The drug may be used more successfully than pilocarpine in young people because its long duration of action avoids the fluctuating myopia that shorter-acting drugs induce in patients with considerable residual accommodative powers.

Accommodative esotropia (crossed strabismus secondary to accommodative overaction) is often responsive to very low doses of PI, 0.03–0.12%, once or twice daily. The mechanism here is the artificial induction of ciliary spasm that blocks the hyperactive covergence reflex by "tricking" the eye and CNS into perceiving maximal accommodation.

e. Adverse side effects and contraindications are common to all cholinesterase drugs. Generally the longer-acting drugs such as PI are prone to more severe local and systemic side effects. The vascular congestive effect and enhanced forward movement of the iris lens diaphragm make use of this drug in iritis or acute angle-closure glaucoma undesirable.

(1) External ocular side effects not infrequently reported include allergic conjunctivitis, contact dermatitis, chronic conjunctival hyperemia, and, rarely, ocular pemphigoid.

(2) **Intraocular** adverse side effects are secondary to drug-induced dilatation of iris blood vessels with breakdown of the blood–aqueous barrier, thus producing an iritis of varying levels of severity. The combination of this iritis with chronic miosis in long-term therapy is not infrequently associated with formation of posterior synechiae to the lens. For this reason, periodic dilatation of the pupil at least 2–3 mm should be attempted, using such agents as Cyclogyl or phenylephrine-tropicamide. Pupillary cysts may be seen with long-term use of PI in as many as 60% of patients. Cysts are prevented by 2.5% phenylephrine drop qd, more common in children under treatment for accommodative esotropia, but also may occur in adults under glaucoma therapy. These cysts are seen less frequently with weaker and shorter-acting agents such as demecarium bromide or physostigmine than with PI. Ciliary body contraction with concomitant relaxation of the lens zonules results in both forward movement and an increased anterior–posterior lens diameter. This both shallows the anterior chamber, making drug use in the presence of already narrow angles of dubious value, and induces artificial myopia, which may require correction by altering the patient's spectacle lenses.

Cataractous changes secondary to long-term drug administration have now been well established. Such lenticular changes begin as small, anterior, subcapsular vacuoles that with continued therapy will evolve into anterior subcapsular and nuclear opacities. Such changes may be noted as early as several months after the initiation of anticholinesterase therapy. This phenomenon appears to be confined to drug treatment in older patients. Except for a single case report of a reversible cataract in a young patient, there is no indication that cataracts occur in children under treatment with anticholinesterase drugs. The mechanism of cataractogenesis is thought to be interference with the normal ionic transport of cholinesterase across the lens capsule. Inhibition of enzyme results in a breakdown of ion transport, resulting in cataract formation.

Retinal detachment, vitreous hemorrhage, vitreous floaters, and frank retinal detachment all have been reported with increased frequency in patients on PI and other cholinesterase therapy. There is no definite cause-and-effect relationship between these drugs and these adverse side effects other than increased incidence. There is evidence, however, that the ciliary muscle spasm results in forward movement of the ora serrata, posterior lens surface, and possibly anterior vitreous face, all of which may lead to increased traction on the peripheral retina and vitreous body, resulting in the vitreoretinal complications noted above.

(3) **Systemic** adverse side effects result from inhibition of at least two types of cholinesterase present in the patient and follow the systemic absorption of the drug across the conjunctiva and nasal mucous membranes into the blood stream. The two key cholinesterases are the **true cholinesterases** present in red blood cells and at the nerve terminals, and the **pseudo-cholinesterases** present in the serum and for which no known function has been ascertained. The serum cholinesterases are the first to be bound by the anticholinesterase drugs, thus leaving the tissue and red blood cell cholinesterases open to attack. The toxic symptoms, both muscarinic and nicotinic, are believed to be due to a decrease in the amount of true cholinesterase, with consequent accumulation of acetylcholine in the neural tissues and red blood cells. The decline in both types of enzymes begins during the first 2 weeks of PI administration, with the maximum depletion occurring within 5–7 weeks. On cessation of the cholinergic drugs, cholinesterase level begins to rise after 7 days.

Clinical manifestation of cholinergic toxicity includes aggravation of bronchial asthma due to bronchial constriction; gastrointestinal side effects of abdominal cramping, diarrhea, and vomiting; adverse effects on blood vessels and cardiac muscles, producing systemic hypertension and bradycardia; and hyperactivity of the secretory glands, resulting in sweating, salivation, and lacrimation. There also may be nicotinic signs secondary to accumulation of acetylcholine at motor nerve endings, resulting in fatiguability, generalized weakness, twitching, and even paralysis.

Prolonged respiratory depression or paralysis may be seen after general anesthesia in patients on PI or other cholinergics. Systemic depletion of pseudocholinesterase results in diminished hydrolysis of succinylcholine, a muscle relaxant used during **general anesthesia.** To avoid such a **complication,** it is recommended that cholinergics such as PI be discontinued for 6 weeks before succinylcholine use.

Therapy of systemic toxicity due to PI or other cholinergics initially is to discontinue the drug(s). For more severe cases, intravenous or intramuscular atropine should be used in repeated doses until muscarinic symptoms have cleared. For peripheral neuromuscular toxicity, pralidoxime chloride (2-PAM), a cholinesterase reactivator, may reverse the toxicity. For severe poisoning in adults, 1 g of 2-PAM diluted in 100 ml NaCl is infused over a 30-minute period or injected IV at a rate not greater than 200 mg/minute after atropine has been given and allowed to exert its effect. Toxicity in children should be managed with IV 2-PAM at doses of 20–40 mg/kg. This drug also may be given orally for mild toxicity. This does not penetrate the cornea or blood–aqueous barrier and, therefore, has little or no effect on counteracting the intraocular effects of these drugs.

Contraindications for the use of PI and other cholinergics are implied in the above discussion, but may be summarized briefly as follows:

- Presence of shallow anterior chamber that may be precipitated into acute angle-closure glaucoma by forward movement of the iris lens diaphragm.
- Glaucoma secondary to uveitis that would be aggravated by drug-induced breakdown of the blood–aqueous barrier with subsequent enhanced inflammation.
- Angle-closure glaucoma secondary to neovascular membrane and peripheral anterior synechiae, all of which are aggravated by use of strong miotics and increase the risk of paradoxical rise in IOP due to interference with uveoscleral outflow by the miotics and in the absence of trabecular meshwork outflow.
- Before use of succinylcholine in general surgery to prevent prolonged respiratory paralysis.
- Before intraocular surgery where intense miosis, contraction of the ciliary body, increased ocular hyperemia, and enhanced postoperative inflammatory reaction are undesirable.

2. **Isoflurophate (diisopropyl fluorophosphate, DFP),** like pholine iodide, is an irreversible inhibitor of cholinesterase. Developed as a toxic agent during World War II, its use has fallen off in favor of newer, more stable drugs.
   a. **The mechanism of action,** onset, duration of action, and pharmacologic effects on the eye are similar to PI.
   b. **Intraocular penetration** is good because of the

high lipid solubility of the drug, which enhances passage across epithelium and endothelium.

c. **Preparations.** DFP is available in an anhydrous vegetable oil or ointment base in concentrations of 0.01–0.1% (see Table 5-1). The drug is rapidly hydrolyzed, necessitating caution to avoid contamination of the bottle with tears or water. Maximum lowering of IOP is achieved with 1 drop once or twice daily.

d. **Clinical indications** are similar to those for pilocarpine and PI. The drug is not used for accommodative esotropia.

e. **Adverse side effects and contraindications** are similar to those of PI.

3. **Demecarium bromide** is a short-acting anticholinesterase synthesized by the linking of two neostigmine molecules.

a. **The mechanism of action** is through binding of acetylcholinesterase. This results in a carbamylated acetylcholinesterase that blocks the hydrolysis of acetylcholine for 3–4 hours. The active enzyme then is regenerated through reaction of the carbamylated enzyme with water. The pharmacologic effects on the eye are similar to those of pilocarpine and PI, with opening of the trabecular meshwork through traction on the longitudinal fibers by ciliary muscle contraction and consequent enhanced outflow facility. Miosis is tight, as with PI, and not related to lowering of IOP. Onset and duration of clinical effect are similar to those of PI.

b. **Intraocular penetration** is good because of the biphasic qualities of the molecule.

c. **Preparations.** The drug is available as an aqueous preparation in concentrations of 0.125–0.25% (see Table 5-1). A single dose results in a marked decrease in IOP persisting for 3–4 days. Miosis is noted in 15–45 minutes and lasts up to 10 days.

d. **The clinical indications** for glaucoma are similar to those for pilocarpine and PI. The drug is not used intraoperatively, postoperatively, or for accommodative esotropia, however.

e. **Adverse side effects and contraindications** are similar to those of all cholinergics such as PI and DFP. Because of its reversible binding of cholinesterase, however, these adverse effects are seen less frequently and are less severe than those of the irreversible drugs.

4. **Physostigmine (eserine)** is, like demecarium bromide, a short-acting anticholinesterase. It is a natural alkaloid long used by the "witch doctors" of West Africa.

a. **The mechanism of action** and **intraocular penetration** are similar to those of demecarium bromide. Both miosis and drop in IOP begin within 30 minutes of application. Maximum IOP-lowering effect is seen at 2 hours; duration of action is 24 hours. The miosis lasts about 12 hours longer.

   b. Preparations. The drug is available as an ointment or as drops in concentrations of 0.25–0.5% (see Table 5-1). The ointment is used once daily at bedtime; the drops may be administered effectively every 6–12 hours.

   c. The clinical indications for glaucoma are similar to those of PI, although the drug is not used in surgical cases or for accommodative esotropia.

   d. Adverse side effects and contraindications are similar to those of PI and all other anticholinesterases. Because the drug is a reversible cholinesterase inhibitor, the adverse effects are less frequent and less severe than those of PI or DFP, irreversible enzyme inhibitors. An unusual adverse side effect seen only with chronic use of physostigmine is depigmentation of the skin of the eyelids in black patients. No other anticholinesterase produces this effect, and it has not been reported in Caucasians or Orientals. The mechanism of action is unknown.

C. **Adrenergic agonists (sympathomimetics).** Three sympathomimetic agents are currently used in the therapy of glaucoma: **epinephrine, dipivefrin,** and **apraclonidine.**

   1. **Epinephrine** is a naturally occurring catecholamine that acts on both the alpha- and beta-receptor sites in the eye.

   a. The mechanism of action is not fully known. Current studies suggest that epinephrine stimulation of the beta-receptors in the eye result in increased cyclic adenosine monophosphate (AMP) production with enhanced aqueous outflow facility. Stimulation of alpha-receptors in the trabecular meshwork also may play a role, as the enhanced aqueous outflow occurs simultaneously with other alpha stimulation effects such as vasoconstriction and pupillary mydriasis. Decreased IOP after epinephrine instillation is also a function of decreased reduction in aqueous humor formation. This is believed to be secondary to drug stimulation of the alpha-receptors in the ciliary body, resulting in decreased blood flow to that structure with consequent decreased production of aqueous. The pharmacologic effects of the drug on the eye are a 10–30% decrease in IOP, which is maximum at 2% concentration. The onset of decreased IOP is within 1 hour of instillation and the maximum effect 2–4 hours later. The duration of the maximal hypotensive effect is 12 hours, with a return to baseline levels at 24 hours, when the higher-dose 1–2% solutions are used. Weaker doses result in a more rapid return to pretreatment IOP levels. Stimulation of the alpha-receptors in the conjunctival blood vessels results in vasoconstriction, which effectively whitens the eye. As this effect wears off, the eye may become abnormally hyperemic until the next drug instillation. Stimulation of the alpha-receptors in the iris results in mydriasis due to activation of the iris dilator muscle. In patients with cataractous lens changes, this mild to moderate mydriasis may be useful in enhancing visual acuity or counteracting the miotic effects of concomitant cholinergic or anticholinesterase drugs.

b. **Intraocular penetration** is good with aqueous levels detectable within 20 minutes of topical instillation of drug.

c. **Preparations.** Epinephrine is marketed as a borate, hydrochloride, or bitartrate salt under several trade names (Table 5-2). There is no significant difference in the clinical efficacy of these preparations in their effect on IOP. The bitartrate preparation contains only about 50% of the labeled concentration as free base drug; 1% epinephrine bitartrate actually has only about 50% drug base in it. This should be taken into account when comparing the bitartrate preparations with the hydrochlorides and borates. Drug concentrations for all three salts range from 0.25–2.0%. They commonly are given every 12–24 hours. Epinephrine is also available in **combination** with the cholinergic agent pilocarpine as 1% epinephrine combined with pilocarpine concentrations of 1–4%. Because the pilocarpine effect is lost within 4–6 hours, combined drugs must be given 4 times daily for optimal effect.

Therapy usually is initiated at a lower drug concentration and changed to a higher concentration if a greater hypotensive effect is deemed necessary for adequate IOP control.

d. **Clinical indications.** Epinephrine is one of the more frequently used drugs in therapy of both primary and secondary noninflammatory and inflammatory open-angle glaucoma. The mild mydriatic effect is particularly useful in enhancing visual acuity in eyes with cataractous lens changes, but the mydriasis necessitates extreme caution when this drug is used in patients with shallowing of the anterior chamber. It is contraindicated in eyes at risk of angle-closure glaucoma, but may be used with miotics in chronic angle-closure glaucoma to decrease aqueous production.

e. **Combination therapy.** Epinephrine is particularly useful in combination with **cholinergics** (see Table 5-2), **anticholinesterases,** and **carbonic anhydrase inhibitors.** The addition of epinephrine to pilocarpine therapy will induce a further drop in IOP of about 13 mm Hg, and triple therapy with pilocarpine, carbonic anhydrase inhibitor, and epinephrine may result in an additional hypotensive effect of up to 21 mm Hg. The combined use of epinephrine and the **beta-blockers** still is controversial, however. There appears to be little additive effect between the two drugs, although this may be a function of individual patients. The combination of beta-blocker and adrenergic agonist should be initiated on a trial basis to ascertain any significant additional efficacy. Because **timolol no longer binds many beta-receptors by 3 hours after application,** optimal epinephrine effect as combination therapy most likely would be achieved by administering this drug 3–4 hours after the instillation of timolol.

f. **Adverse side effects and contraindications.** The mydriatic effect of epinephrine has been mentioned previously as beneficial in patients with lenticular changes and as inducing risk of angle-closure glaucoma in those with shallowing of the anterior chamber. Additional side effects, both topical and systemic, are reviewed below.

(1) **Ocular.** In almost all patients, topical medication results in rebound conjunctival hyperemia, irritation, and stinging. A significant number of patients also complain of eye ache and headache, and some may develop a true allergic conjunctivitis and periocular dermatitis that will resolve only with discontinuation of epinephrine therapy. Some of these patients may, however, safely take dipivefrin without a cross-allergic reaction. Long-term administration of topical epinephrine is associated with black deposits of adrenochrome in the conjunctiva and occasionally in the cornea and nasolacrimal passages. Casts of adrenochrome may block the nasolacrimal ducts. In the cornea, the pigmented deposits may involve virtually all tissue layers, but are most commonly confined to the epithelium and may easily be removed. Conjunctival deposits do not warrant therapy, but adrenochrome casts may have to be removed from the nasolacrimal canals. Epinephrine has also been implicated as one of several topical agents that may induce ocular pemphigoid that is clinically and pathologically similar to the idiopathic disease and that may be arrested by discontinuing the drug. Epinephrine maculopathy is a widely recognized adverse side effect of topical drug in up to 30% of aphakic patients so treated. The cystoid macular edema produced may occur within a few weeks to months after starting therapy and usually is reversible on discontinuing such treatment. This side effect appears to be secondary to the greater uptake of epinephrine by aphakic eyes in comparison with phakic controls. Because the condition does not occur in at least 70% of patients using epinephrine and is reversible on discontinuing the drug, aphakia is not an absolute contraindication to the use

Table 5-2. Medications for glaucoma management: adrenergic agonists, sympathomimetics, combination drugs

Drug commercial names	Mechanism of action	Major clinical indications	Common dosages	Adverse side effects
Adrenergic agonists-sympathomimetics				
Epinephrine: E 1 & 2%, Epitrate, Epifrin, Epinal, Eppy 1N, Glaucon, Murocoll 1 & 2%, Mytrate	Reduced aqueous humor formation (α receptor stimulation in ciliary body). Increased outflow facility (alpha- and beta-receptor in trabecular meshwork)	Primary and secondary open-angle glaucomas. Certain chronic angle closure cases (with miotics) and inflammatory glaucomas	0.25, 0.5, 1.0, and 2.0% qd-q12h	*Ocular:* stinging conjunctival hyperemia, eye ache, headache, allergic conjunctivitis or dermatitis, adrenochrome deposition, mydriasis, ocular pemphigoid, cystoid macular edema *Systemic:* hypertension, angina, tachycardia
Dipivefrin HCl: Propine	As per epinephrine. Prodrug converted to epinephrine. Alpha- and beta-receptor stimulant	As per epinephrine	0.1% drop qd-q12h	*Ocular:* stinging, mydriasis, conjunctival hyperemia, allergic conjunctivitis *Systemic:* as per epinephrine

	Mechanism	Dosage	Indications	Side effects
Apraclonidine: Iopidine	Inhibition of aqueous humor secretion (α-2 stimulant)	1% drop pre and post laser surgery; q12h (see text)	Minimize IOP spikes post laser; ? For chronic glaucomas.	*Ocular:* upper lid retraction, conjunctival blanching, mydriasis, blurred vision, allergic response, subconjunctival hemorrhage. *Systemic:* abdominal pain, nausea, vomiting, diarrhea, bradycardia, vasovagal attack, palpitations, orthostatic hypotension, insomnia, dream disturbance
Combination pilocarpine-epinephrine				
E-pilo (1–6%)	Increased outflow facility and decreased aqueous production (ciliary muscle tension on trabecular meshwork and α and β receptor stimulation)	1% epinephrine with 1, 2, or 4% pilocarpine qd–qid	Primary and secondary noninflammatory open-angle glaucomas. Certain chronic angle closure glaucomas	As per pilocarpine and epinephrine

of epinephrine. If it appears that a patient will benefit from epinephrine therapy, it should be instituted and the clinical course carefully monitored.

(2) **Systemic** adverse side effects. Systemic hypertension, angina, and increased pulse rate may be induced. Patients with cardiovascular disease, diabetes, hyperthyroidism, or cerebrovascular disease should be monitored for adverse side effects, and in patients more severely afflicted by their systemic disease, the use of epinephrine may be contraindicated.

2. **Dipivefrin hydrochloride (dipivalyl epinephrine, DPE, Propine)** is a synthesized prodrug created by the addition of two pivalic acid groups to the epinephrine molecule. This prodrug must undergo biotransformation in the tissues before therapeutic efficacy is achieved. It was synthesized in an attempt to circumvent epinephrine side effects through reduced drug delivery to the eye while retaining maximal hypotensive efficacy.

   a. **The mechanism of action** is similar to that of epinephrine in that this drug is both an alpha- and beta-receptor stimulant. The pharmacologic effect on the eye is both inhibition of aqueous formation by the ciliary body and increased facility of outflow via the trabecular meshwork. The epinephrine effect may be blocked by the administration of the antiprostaglandin agent indomethacin, so it is suggested that both epinephrine and its prodrug DPE also may work by a prostaglandin-mediated mechanism. For this reason it is probably advisable that patients on therapy with either agent minimize or **avoid** use of **prostaglandin inhibitors** such as aspirin, naproxyn, or indomethacin. DPE is metabolized in the eye by the slow removal of the pivalic acid groups by esterases. This results in the release of epinephrine via a metabolic pathway that is slower than that of epinephrine alone. The result is increased bioavailability and longer duration of action of the drug.

   b. **The intraocular penetration** of DPE across the cornea is almost 17 times that of epinephrine. The presence of the pivalic acid groups renders the prodrug more lipophilic, thus enhancing its passage across epithelial and endothelial cell layers. Because of the enhanced passage, a 0.1% solution of DPE induces a lowering of IOP comparable to that induced with 2% topical epinephrine.

   c. **Preparation.** DPE is available as an aqueous solution of 0.1% dipivefrin hydrochloride (see Table 5-2). The drug is commonly used once every 12–24 hours as indicated for control of IOP. DPE is similar to epinephrine in its additive effect when used with cholinergics, anticholinesterases, or carbonic anhydrase inhibitors. A beneficial combination of

DPE with beta-blockers is at best borderline, but may vary from patient to patient. A unilateral trial in comparison with the opposite eye treated with one agent alone may be indicated to establish a significant additional reduction in pressure if the drugs are used in combination. A delay in instillation of DPE for 3–4 hours after the beta-blocker is instilled may, as discussed under epinephrine, enhance any additive effect as the beta-blocker releases from the receptor site.

   d. **Clinical indications** for the use of DPE are similar to those for epinephrine, ie, management of both primary and secondary noninflammatory and inflammatory open-angle glaucoma. Anticipated hypotensive effect is up to 25% below baseline pressure, with even greater effect seen when the drug is used in combination therapy. DPE probably should not be used with the anticholinesterases such as PI, as these latter drugs may inhibit the esterases necessary for the conversion of DPE into epinephrine, thus effectively inactivating the prodrug. Some studies indicate, however, that the combined use of PI and DPE may be beneficial in some patients, and therapeutic trial may be initiated in one eye compared with the opposite eye control in certain patients where indicated.

   e. **Adverse side effects and contraindications** have been minimized with the use of DPE in comparison with those noted with epinephrine use.

      (1) **Topical** DPE may, however, produce the side effects of burning, stinging, rebound conjunctival hyperemia, superficial punctate keratopathy, pupillary mydriasis, and rarely allergic conjunctivitis. There have been no reports of adrenochrome deposits or aphakic maculopathy with the use of DPE. Should such side effects be noted, it may be assumed that the mechanism is similar to that of epinephrine.

      (2) **Systemic** side effects encountered with DPE, although probably less than those seen with epinephrine, may in some patients be comparable to those changes induced by epinephrine with respect to both resting blood pressure and pulse rate.

3. **Apraclonidine** is a synthetic alpha-adrenergic agonist.

   a. **The mechanism of action** is not fully established, but it is known that the drug is a relatively selective alpha-2 stimulant that results in a reduction in IOP through inhibition of aqueous humor formation without effort on outflow. Drug efficacy is seen within 1 hour of instillation, with maximum effect 3–5 hours after application of a single dose.

   b. **Preparation.** The drug is available as an aqueous 1% solution in single-dose 0.25-ml containers (Iopidine; see Table 5-2).

   c. **Clinical indication** is for the control of potential
      increase in IOP commonly seen after **laser surgery**
      such as trabeculoplasty or iridotomy, and possibly
      a variety of **chronic glaucomas.** One drop of apra-
      clonidine is administered in the operative eye 1
      hour before anterior segment laser surgery and a
      second drop in the same eye immediately after com-
      pletion of the procedure. This reduces the incidence
      of post-laser pressure spikes of greater than 10 mm
      Hg to less than 2% of patients treated. As a 40%
      reduction in IOP is noted 3–5 hours after giving
      the drop with effect up to 12 hours, apraclonidine
      has great potential as a q12h drop with efficacy
      comparable to beta blockers, epinephrine, and the
      miotics. Clinical studies are underway.
   d. **Adverse side effects and contraindications**
      (1) **Ocular** adverse effects include upper lid re-
          traction, conjunctival blanching, and pupillary
          mydriasis. Less frequent are burning, discom-
          fort, foreign body sensation, dryness, itching,
          blurred vision, allergic response, and subcon-
          junctival hemorrhage.
      (2) **Systemic** side effects include gstrointestinal
          reactions such as abdominal pain, diarrhea,
          stomach discomfort, nausea, and vomiting. Car-
          diovascular effects include bradycardia, vaso-
          vagal attacks, palpitations, and orthostatic hy-
          potension. Central nervous system reactions
          include insomnia, dream disturbance, irritabil-
          ity, and decreased libido. All of these side effects
          are transient, barring further instillation of the
          drug.
D. **Alpha-adrenergic antagonists (sympatholytics)**
   1. **Thymoxamine** is the only alpha-adrenergic blocker
      currently in clinical use in Europe and Canada. While
      under study in the United States, it is not yet com-
      mercially available.
      a. **The mechanism of action** of this alpha-blocker is
         the competitive antagonism of norepinephrine.
         Topical thymoxamine produces miosis within 15–
         20 minutes, maximum at 45–60 minutes, and last-
         ing up to 2 hours after topical instillation. This
         miosis is the result of isolated inhibition of the
         pupillary dilator muscle without the induction of
         ciliary body contraction. As a result, the drug in-
         duces miosis without any effect on facility of out-
         flow or rate of aqueous formation. There is, there-
         fore, no effect on IOP.
      b. **Preparations.** An aqueous 0.1–0.5% solution of
         thymoxamine is used primarily for diagnostic pur-
         poses, although there may be other potential
         ophthalmic uses (see below, and Table 5-3).
      c. **Clinical indications** are primarily diagnostic. The
         miotic effect opens the anterior chamber angle,
         thus making it possible to differentiate open-angle
         glaucoma with a narrow angle component from true
         angle-closure glaucoma or from true combined-

mechanism glaucoma. It also may be used to determine whether an iridectomy would be sufficient to open an angle wide enough to maintain normal IOP in narrow-angle situations. Additional clinical applications of thymoxamine include reversal of phenylephrine mydriasis, treatment of angle-closure glaucoma, and management of pigmentary dispersion glaucoma. Because of the availability of superior agents, however, the drug is rarely used for these latter indications.

    d. Adverse side effects and contraindications

        (1) Topical thymoxamine induces minimal side effects in the short term, and long-term use has not been investigated. Local effects include mild ptosis, burning, and conjunctival hyperemia.

        (2) Systemic side effects from topical thymoxamine have not been reported, but systemically administered drug may cause vertigo, headache, nausea, diarrhea, hypotension, and facial flushing.

E. Beta-adrenergic antagonists (sympatholytics). Until the 1960s, all the adrenergic blockers were in the alpha category and altered the ability of epinephrine to induce vasoconstriction. Subsequently a new class of sympatholytic was identified that selectively blocked adrenergic action on the smooth bronchial muscles and the myocardium. This group of drugs, known as beta-blockers, were subsequently categorized into beta-1 (cardiac) and beta-2 (smooth muscle). With further investigation it was found that different beta-blockers varied in potency, selectivity for a specific beta-receptor, and nonadrenergic effects such as membrane stabilization. Most beta-blockers such as propranolol possess this membrane-stabilizing effect, which makes them unsuitable for topical use in glaucoma because of the induction of corneal anesthesia. Other early agents such as practolol caused conjunctival cicatrization and severe dry eye with loss of some eyes treated with this agent. Three drugs currently in use topically as glaucoma therapy are **timolol, betaxolol,** and **levobunolol,** all of which share the common beta-blocker molecular structure of an aromatic ring with an alkyl side chain.

    1. Beta-receptor activity. Beta-1 receptors are the primary beta receptors in cardiac tissue. The stimulation of cardiac tissue induces tachycardia, increased inotropism, and increased conduction time. In the lungs the primary beta-receptors are beta-2, and their stimulation induces bronchodilation. Both alpha- and beta-receptors are widely scattered throughout other tissues and regulate such physiologic events as vasodilation in muscle, skeletal, and uterine contraction. The blockade of either receptor by drug action induces the opposite physiologic effect from stimulation of the alpha- or beta-receptor. In the eye the primary receptors appear to be beta-2, and these are primarily in the ciliary processes. There are scattered sparse beta-1 receptors

Table 5-3. Medications for glaucoma management: adrenergic antagonists (sympatholytics)

Drug commercial names	Mechanism of action	Common dosages	Major clinical indications	Adverse side effects
Alpha-adrenergic antagonis (sympatholytic)				
Thymoxamine	Miosis (inhibits pupillary dilator through norepinephrine antagonism)	0.1–0.5% drop	Diagnosis of narrow angle component of combined-mechanism glaucoma, treatment of acute angle closure?, reversal of phenylephrine mydriasis?	*Ocular:* ptosis, burning, hyperemia *Systemic:* vertigo, headache, nausea, vomiting, diarrhea, hypotension, facial flushing
Beta-adrenergic antagonists (beta-blockers, sympatholytics)				
Timolol Timoptic	Decreased aqueous humor production (β-1 and β-2 blockade ciliary muscle)	0.25–0.5% drop qd– q12h	Primary and secondary open-angle glaucomas including inflammatory, angle	*Ocular:* allergic conjunctivitis, orbital pain, blurred vision, ocular myasthenia, diplopia, dry eye, superficial punctate keratitis, corneal erosion,

				corneal anesthesia *Systemic:* bronchospasm aggravating asthma, emphysema, chronic obstructive pulmonary disease, bronchitis
			closure, aphakic, developmental	
Betaxolol (Betoptic, 0.5%) Betoptic S, 0.25%	Decreased aqueous humor production, mechanism not known. Selective β-1 receptor blockade over β-2	0.25–0.5% drop q12h	As per timolol	As per timolol. No corneal anesthesia reported
Levobunolol (Betagan)	Decreased aqueous humor production (β-1 and β-2 blockade). Longer duration of action than other β-blockers	0.5% qd–q12h	As per timolol	As per timolol. No corneal anesthesia reported.

in the eye, but their role in drug action is still speculative. Instillation of a beta-blocker in just one eye often results in a consensual drop in IOP in the untreated, contralateral eye, sometimes nearly equaling that of the eye receiving drug. This is due not just to systemic absorption but, at least in the case of timolol, to actual presence of the drug in the contralateral eye, presumably via the circulatory system.

2. **Preparations** (Table 5-3)

   a. **Timolol** (Timoptic) was the first of the beta-blockers to become commercially available for ophthalmic use.

      (1) **Mechanism of action.** Timolol maleate is a nonspecific beta-1 and beta-2 blocker that induces decreased aqueous humor production without altering facility of aqueous outflow whether given topically or systemically. The relationship between duration of therapeutic effect and drug-binding affinity at the receptor is not understood. It appears that timolol releases from the receptor site as early as 3 hours after topical administration, yet the clinical effect may last up to 2 weeks. This may be the result of a "depot" effect, where there is significant accumulation of drug binding to the iris pigment epithelial melanin. Gradual release of timolol from this depot in the eye would result in prolonged duration of the drug effect. It also may explain the reduced pressure effect on heavily pigmented eyes. While individual responses vary, however, some studies report nearly 50% reduction in aqueous production in glaucomatous eyes. This drug effect is less in dark eyes and in the nearly 25% of patients treated with timolol who are unresponsive to therapy. The mechanism for this refractory primary state is unknown. Some reports suggest that timolol also may induce a slight increase in outflow facility, but it is doubtful that this contributes significantly to its ocular hypotensive effect.

      (2) **The intraocular penetration** of timolol is a direct function of its high lipophilicity. The drug easily passes the various corneal barriers, to appear in the aqueous humor within minutes of topical application, reaching peak levels within 1–2 hours. Aqueous levels have fallen to less than 20% of peak values by 4 hours after administration, but iris levels peak within 15 minutes and remain high for several hours because of melanin binding responsible for the depot effect.

      (3) **Preparations.** Timolol is available in aqueous concentrations of 0.25% and 0.5% to be administered every 12–24 hours (see Table 5-3). With once-daily dosage, it is advisable to monitor

IOP immediately before the next dose to ascertain that there is drug effect at the 24-hour mark. Use of 0.25% every 12 hours may be more effective than 0.5% once daily.

(4) **Clinical indications** for the use of timolol include a wide variety of primary and secondary glaucomas. The drug will lower IOP in both normotensive and glaucomatous patients, including those with primary open-angle glaucoma, secondary open-angle glaucoma, including the inflammatory glaucomas, secondary angle-closure glaucoma after penetrating keratoplasty, aphakic glaucoma, and acute and chronic primary angle-closure glaucoma. The drug also is effective in both developmental glaucoma and secondary glaucoma in children, although these agents are not without special hazards in this age group (see below).

(5) **The combination** of timolol with most other antiglaucoma medications results in a significant additive hypotensive effect. The combination of timolol and miotic agents or carbonic anhydrase inhibitors may decrease the aqueous humor output by more than 50%, significantly more than either agent alone. The combination of timolol with epinephrine, however, is variable and certainly not in the range seen with miotics or carbonic anhydrase inhibitors. The basis of this minimal therapeutic effect in combined epinephrine/timolol therapy is thought to be timolol blockage of the receptors by which epinephrine would normally affect aqueous outflow. This would suggest that optimal effect would be obtained by dosing with epinephrine at least 3 hours after the timolol dose, a time when timolol has begun to release from the beta-receptor sites, thus freeing them for epinephrine action. It also has been postulated that, in eyes in which combined simultaneous therapy with timolol and epinephrine has resulted in some lowering of IOP, the mechanism is epinephrine-induced aqueous reduction through drug action on the alpha-receptors. Timolol's poor additive effect in concert with epinephrine is to be compared with the allegedly good therapeutic efficacy of combined betaxolol–epinephrine therapy.

(6) **Tolerance** to timolol is seen in some patients as manifested by a gradual decrease in IOP control. "Short-term escape" may develop within days of initiating therapy. This form of tachyphylaxis is very rare, however. More common is "long-term drift." This gradual rise in pressure despite continued therapy may develop after many months or years of treatment and may occur as a result of drug modulation

of the ocular receptors themselves. Aqueous suppression near 50% at the end of the first week of timolol therapy may be near 25% suppression after 1 year. This loss of efficacy has not been noted with levobunolol, however, after 1 year of treatment.

(7) **Adverse side effects and contraindications.** Although timolol is relatively well tolerated in comparison with some other antiglaucoma medications, adverse side effects, both topical and systemic, have been associated with ophthalmic application of the drops. It should be remembered that topical drug enters the blood stream through the nasopharyngeal mucosa, thereby avoiding first-pass liver metabolism, and thus is analogous to an intravenous injection rather than to oral administration of a systemic drug.

Ocular adverse side effects are often nonspecific and include allergic conjunctivitis, orbital pain, blurred vision, ocular myasthenia gravis, diplopia, keratoconjunctivitis sicca, superficial punctate keratitis, and, because of its membrane-stabilizing capabilities, corneal anesthesia. Corneal epithelial erosions also have been noted in patients wearing gas-permeable contact lenses shortly after instituting topical timolol therapy. There is some indication in animal studies that the combination of timolol with contact lenses may cause marked alterations in both corneal epithelium and endothelium, although this has not been borne out in human studies of the effects of beta-blockers on the endothelium,

Systemic toxicity of timolol is that of a nonspecific beta-1 and beta-2 blocker and may affect the cardiovascular, respiratory, and central nervous systems. As timolol is 10 times more potent as a beta-blocker than the prototype propranolol, systemic effects may occur with relatively low blood levels of timolol in comparison with therapeutic levels of propranolol. Measurable timolol levels have been found in the blood with 8 minutes of topical administration. Beta-2 blockade in the lungs will increase airway resistance, potentially life-threatening to asthmatic patients or patients with other airway disorders such as emphysema, chronic obstructive pulmonary disease, or bronchitis. Use of the beta-blockers in patients with asthma or allergic bronchitis should be with caution, and the effectiveness of epinephrine in treatment of acute allergic reaction may be inhibited in patients on chronic beta-blocker therapy.

Significant cardiac depression from beta-1 blockade is rare, but heart failure and pulmonary edema have occurred in patients with significant cardiomyopathy. Timolol may also cause atrioventricular dissociation and cardiac arrest in patients with pre-existing partial heart block, particularly those on digitalis, as both drugs depress the AV conduction system. Other cardiac side effects include inhibition of exercise-induced tachycardia resulting in decreased exercise tolerance or lethargy, both indicative of significant systemic absorption of topical drug.

Additional problems include gastrointestinal side effects of nausea, vomiting, and mild diarrhea, and the rare central nervous system side effects of hallucinations, nightmares, insomnia, lassitude, depression, and impotence. When these problems are detected, the first step is discontinuing the drug for 24 hours and then, if indicated, reinstituting it after the patient has been instructed in manual nasolacrimal occlusion and eyelid closure for 1–2 minutes after drug administration. These two steps will decrease systemic absorption of timolol or any other ophthalmic medication.

Children present a special problem in the use of timolol because topical drops given to children in adult dosage may result in very high and toxic blood levels. Apnea spells after topical administration of timolol are more common in young children than in adults, and nursing mothers should be warned that timolol is excreted in breast milk. It may be advisable to discontinue the use of timolol in nursing mothers to avoid undue systemic toxicity in the infant.

b. **Betaxolol (Betoptic** or **Betoptic S)** became commercially available as the second topical betablocker to be released for the treatment of ocular hypertension and glaucoma. Its primary advantage is its relative receptor selectivity. Betaxolol has 100 times more affinity for beta-1 (cardiac) than beta-2 (pulmonary) receptors.

(1) **The mechanism of action** is not established. The ciliary processes have primarily beta-2 receptors, and beta-1 receptors are scattered only sparsely throughout the eye, but betaxolol, a beta-1–selective blocker, induces an ocular hypotensive effect similar to that of nonselective beta-1–beta-2 blockers such as timolol. There is decreased aqueous humor production without an alteration in facility of aqueous outflow. It is postulated that betaxolol may achieve intraocular concentrations sufficiently high to saturate not only the beta-1 but also the beta-2 receptors. It is evident that selectivity for beta-1 receptors is only relative, not absolute. The role of beta-1 blockade in inducing ocular hy-

potension is not established. Although betaxolol is beta-1–selective, it has, in fact, a lower affinity for the beta-1 receptor than does timolol. In systemic dosing, 10 times more betaxolol must reach the beta-1 receptors to exert effects equivalent to those of the nonselective blocker timolol. Betaxolol, like timolol, is metabolized into a predominantly inactive molecule.

(2) **Intraocular penetration** of betaxolol is similar to that of other beta-blockers, being detectable within minutes after application and peaking at 1–2 hours. Betaxolol is 4 times more lipid soluble than timolol and passes the corneal epithelial and endothelial barriers more easily. However, there are 5 times more plasma protein binding and volume of distribution of betaxolol in comparison with timolol, making less drug available for systemic toxicity.

(3) **Preparations.** Betaxolol is available as a 0.5% or 0.25% (equivalent efficacy, less sting) aqueous solution (see Table 5-3). Recommended dosing is once every 12 hours in comparison with timolol and levobunolol, which may be used once every 12–24 hours. Comparative studies between timolol and betaxolol indicate that betaxolol is slightly less potent than timolol and levobunolol. The latter two drugs are comparable in therapeutic efficacy. Betaxolol used as a single agent will lower IOP approximately 30% during the first 6 months. Whether betaxolol is subject to the same "long-term drift" loss of hypotensive effects seen with timolol is yet to be established. **Combination therapy** using betaxolol with other antiglaucoma medications results in significantly additive pressure-lowering effects. These drugs include the miotics, pilocarpine and carbachol, the cholinesterases, the carbonic anhydrase inhibitors, and, unlike timolol, epinephrine. The effect of combined betaxolol–carbonic anhydrase inhibitor therapy is significantly greater than each drug being used alone and slightly less than additive. Studies combining epinephrine (an alpha- and beta-1/beta-2 agonist) with betaxolol, a beta-1 blocker, in comparison with a similar combination of epinephrine with timolol indicated a slightly greater additive effect for the combination of epinephrine and betaxolol. This may have been due to enhanced outflow facility due to stimulation of the beta-2 receptors in the eye. Studies indicate that although betaxolol/epinephrine combination therapy may be significantly more effective than timolol/epinephrine therapy at 1 week's time, this difference is not statistically significant after 4 weeks of therapy. It would appear

clinically that only 20% of patients will have a significant and long-lasting additive pressure-lowering effect from the addition of epinephrine to any topical beta-blocker.

(4) **Clinical indications** for betaxolol therapy are similar to those for all topical beta-adrenergic blockers and include virtually all forms of glaucoma: primary and secondary open-angle and primary and secondary acute and chronic angle-closure (see Timolol).

(5) **Adverse side effects and contraindications.** **Local** adverse effects due to betaxolol therapy include mild to moderate stinging, burning, or irritation, erythema, superficial punctate corneal staining (transient), toxic conjunctivitis, and extremely rare incidence of corneal anesthesia, significantly lower than that noted with timolol. Betaxolol does not have timolol's membrane-stabilizing effects.

Systemic side effects due to absorption of topical drug is similar to all beta-blocker agents with reference to cardiac and central nervous system reactions as listed under timolol. Although it was hoped that pulmonary side effects would be avoided by use of this beta-1–selective agent, increasing clinical evidence indicates that higher doses and greater absorption of betaxolol may induce bronchospasm in some patients. Nonetheless, betaxolol is the **agent of choice** in patients at risk for pulmonary reaction when a beta-blocker is considered a useful potential therapeutic agent. Although betaxolol's cardiac effect is less than timolol's, patients with cardiovascular disease, slow pulse, or heart block should be carefully evaluated before being placed on betaxolol. Acute myocardial infarction within 5 minutes of instilling a single drop of betaxolol has been reported recently.

c. **Levobunolol (Betagan)** is a nonselective (beta-1/beta-2) blocker that appears to have a longer duration of action than other topical beta-blockers.

(1) **The mechanism of action** of levobunolol is ocular hypotension induced through decreased aqueous production in a manner similar both in mechanism and magnitude to that of timolol. The primary effect is blockade of the beta-receptors in the ciliary processes, resulting in decreased aqueous production. Studies carried out for up to 1 year indicate that levobunolol does not have a tendency for long-term drift with loss of effective ocular hypotensive effect.

(2) **Intraocular penetration** is a function of the increased lipophilicity of levobunolol, with aqueous humor levels detectable within minutes of application and peaking at 1–2 hours. The duration of action of the drug is longer than

that of betaxolol and possibly longer than that of timolol. Whether this is a result of depot effect has not yet been ascertained.

(3) **Preparations.** Levobunolol is marketed as a 0.5% aqueous solution for use once every 12–24 hours (see Table 5-3). When once-daily dosing is anticipated, IOP should be measured immediately before the daily dose to ascertain that ocular hypotensive effect at the end of the 24-hour period is satisfactory. Comparative studies indicate that levobunolol is therapeutically as efficacious as timolol, both of which are slightly more effective than betaxolol.

Combination therapy of levobunolol with other antiglaucoma drugs such as miotics, carbonic anhydrase inhibitors, or alpha agonists (epinephrine or dipivefrin) indicate that there is a significant additive effect with the beta-blocker in combination therapy over either drug used alone. The enhanced effect of levobunolol/dipivefrin therapy is comparable to that of combination timolol/dipivefrin therapy. It is proposed that the mechanism of added hypotensive effect is through dipivefrin's further reduction of aqueous production via its alpha agonist activity. It is postulated that the beta-adrenergic-mediated effect on outflow would be blocked by the nonselective blockade of levobunolol. The duration of levobunolol receptor blockade is not known, but may be comparable with or somewhat longer than that of timolol, indicating that administration of the alpha agonist may have optimal effect when given 3–4 hours after the beta-blocker has been instilled.

(4) **Clinical indications** for the use of levobunolol are similar to those for other topical beta blockers and include virtually all forms of glaucoma: primary and secondary open-angle and primary and secondary angle-closure whether acute or chronic (see Timolol).

(5) **Adverse side effects and contraindications** for levobunolol have not yet been fully evaluated because of the relatively short time that the drug has been commercially available. As it is a nonselective alpha- and beta-adrenergic blocker, however, one would anticipate that it has the potential for the same adverse reactions noted with timolol.

F. **Carbonic anhydrase inhibitors (CAI)** in current clinical use for lowering IOP are the sulfonamides: **acetazolamide, methazolamide,** and **dichlorphenamide.**

1. **The mechanisms of action** of the CAI family of drugs are through inhibition of carbonic anhydrase (CA) in the ocular ciliary processes, with consequent reduction

in aqueous humor formation. There is no drug effect on outflow facility or on uveoscleral flow.

CA is an enzyme distributed widely throughout the body. It is the catalyst for the production of carbonic acid from water and carbon dioxide and the buffer for the hydroxyl ion released in oxidation of cytochrome oxidase. The end result is sodium bicarbonate secretion into the posterior chamber, making the aqueous there hypertonic and thus drawing more water into the chamber. CAIs inhibit the transfer of sodium and bicarbonate from plasma in the ciliary processes to the aqueous, thus minimizing diffusion of water into the posterior chamber and reducing aqueous production. Both fluorophotometry and tonographic studies indicate that CAIs inhibit aqueous production by 40–60% when drug dosage sufficient to block 90% of tissue CA activity is given.

The drugs are rapidly absorbed from the gastrointestinal tract, with onset of ocular hypotension within 1 hour, maximal at 4 hours, and return to baseline at about 6 hours, except in the case of sustained-release drug, which may be at least partially effective up to 18 hours after ingestion. The plasma half-life of orally administered aczetazolamide is 5 hours; that of methazolamide, nearly 14 hours. Intravenous administration of acetazolamide will induce an ocular hypotensive effect within minutes of injection and last for 3–6 hours. The clinical effect obtained is directly related in magnitude to the baseline IOP; the higher the initial pressure, the greater the hypotensive effect. Other factors that bear on the efficacy of the CAIs are the degree of drug plasma protein and the concomitant use of other antiglaucoma medications that also work by inhibiting aqueous formation. In the former case the degree of plasma protein binding is inversely proportional to the amount of CAI available to act in the ciliary processes and decrease the production of new aqueous. Acetazolamide is highly protein bound, whereas methazolamide and dichlorphenamide are only minimally bound. As a result, much smaller doses of the latter two drugs are required to achieve therapeutic effects similar to high doses of acetazolamide. If other drugs that block aqueous formation are in use, the effect of CAI will be reduced by the amount of inhibition induced by other agents, eg, beta blockade of the beta-2 receptors in the ciliary processes.

2. **Preparations** (Table 5-4)
   a. **Acetazolamide** (Diamox) is available as 125- and 250-mg tablets to be given 2–4 times daily up to a maximum dose of 100 mg/24 hours. A sustained-release capsule of 500 mg is also available for use once every 12–24 hours. Doses higher than 1000 mg/24 hours do not increase the therapeutic effect, but markedly increase adverse side effects. Parenteral acetazolamide is available as the sodium salt

Table 5-4. Medications for glaucoma management: carbonic anhydrase inhibitors, hyperosmotics

Drug commercial names	Mechanism of action	Common dosages	Major clinical indications	Adverse side effects
Carbonic anhydrase inhibitors				
Acetazolamide: Diamox	Decreased aqueous production (inhibition of carbonic anhydrase in ciliary body processes)	• 250 mg tablet q12h–q6h–8h • 500 mg spansule q12–24h • IV preparation 500 mg/ml	Acute angle closure glaucoma, adjunctive therapy to primary and secondary open and angle closure glaucomas, inflammatory and postoperative glaucomas	*Ocular:* transient myopia *Systemic:* tingling paresthesias, anorexia, nausea, vomiting, lassitude, diuresis, abdominal cramping, renal colic or stone formation, malaise, depression, confusion, coma, decreased libido
Methazolamide: Neptazane	As per acetazolamide	50 mg tablet po q8–12h	As per acetazolamide	As per acetazolamide except minimal effect on renal citrate and therefore minimal chance of renal colic or stone formation

Dichlorphenamide: Daranide	As per acetazolamide	50 mg tablet po q8–12h	As per acetazolamide	As per acetazolamide, except no alkalinization of urine and therefore minimal chance of renal colic or stone formation
Hyperosmotic agents				
Glycerin (oral): Glyrol, Osmoglyn	Movement of water from intraocular structures to circulation due to increased plasma osmolarity	• Per os solutions Glyrol 1–2 ml/kg (3–5 oz/person) Osmoglyn 1.0–1.5 g/kg body weight (4–6 oz/person)	Lowering of IOP in any acute glaucoma or for very high IOP as adjunct to other medications. Preoperative reduction of vitreous volume	Headache, nausea, vomiting, confusion, coma, subdural hematoma, systemic hypertension, congestive heart failure, pulmonary edema, urinary retention, hyperglycemia in diabetics
Glycerin (topical) Ophthalgan	As per oral glycerin	• Topical glycerin	Clearing corneal edema in acute glaucoma	As per oral glycerin
Isosorbide: Ismotic	As per oral glycerin	1.5–3.0 g/kg body weight (1.0–3.0 ml/ lb/patient)	As per oral glycerin	As per oral glycerin
Mannitol: Osmitrol	As per oral glycerin	2 g/kg body weight or 25–50 ml of 20% solution IV	As per oral glycerin	As per oral glycerin

in vials containing 500 mg for intravenous administration. A 2% drop for topical administration q12h is under investigation and appears to induce a drop in IOP of about 20%.

b. **Methazolamide** (Neptazane) is marketed in 50-mg tablets for oral administration every 8–12 hours. The maximum effective dose is 300 mg/24 hours.

c. **Dichlorphenamide** (Daranide) is available as 50-mg tablets for oral administration every 8–12 hours. The maximum effective dose is 200 mg/24 hours.

3. **Clinical indications** for the use of CAIs are as additive therapy for numerous forms of glaucoma not adequately controlled by maximum tolerated topical therapy such as primary and secondary open-angle glaucomas. They are often used as part of primary therapy in acute glaucoma secondary to traumatic hyphema or inflammation, intraoperative and postoperative pressure rises, after laser surgery, and in acute and certain forms of chronic angle-closure glaucoma. Long-term use of CAIs is probably not wise in cases of angle-closure glaucoma where there is not already extensive peripheral anterior synechia (PAS) formation. Such therapy may allow further increase in synechial scarring while maintaining IOP control until the process is so advanced as to cause an irreversible pressure rise. Acute angle-closure patients should undergo iridotomy as soon as some control of the pressure is obtained and the angle opened using CAI and topical agents. CAI therapy then should be discontinued as part of primary therapy. Chronic open-angle glaucoma should be treated with CAIs only when all other maximum tolerated therapy has failed.

4. **Adverse side effects and contraindications**

a. **Ocular** side effects from systemic drug are negligible, other than transient myopia in some patients.

b. **Systemic** toxicity is in large part the result of CAI action on the carbonic anhydrase systems found throughout the body, the systemic acidosis resulting from disturbance of the bicarbonate production, and serum electrolyte depletion. Approximately 50% of patients placed on CAIs will develop sufficiently severe side effects to necessitate discontinuing the drug.

(1) **The most common side effects** are tingling paresthesias in the fingers, anorexia, nausea, and lassitude. Also noted not infrequently are diuresis, abdominal cramping, renal colic and stone formation, malaise, depression, disorientation, and decreased libido. Confusion and even coma have been reported with use of CAIs in patients with hepatic insufficiency.

(2) **Symptoms due to acidosis** may in some cases be alleviated with supplemental sodium bicar-

bonate, and those due to electrolyte imbalance corrected with supplemental sodium and potassium. Electrolyte imbalance is found more frequently in patients on diuretic therapy.

(3) **Cardiac patients,** especially those on digitalis preparations, and **Addisonians,** in whom electrolyte balance is crucial, must be monitored periodically for hypokalemia because of the potentially life-threatening effect. CAIs should be avoided wherever possible in these patients, as they are relatively contraindicated.

(4) **Patients with a history of renal colic or stones** should not be placed on acetazolamide therapy. This drug is actively taken up by the secretory cells of the proximal tubules and excreted almost entirely unchanged in the urine. The effect on renal tubular transport is to make normally acid urine alkaline. This, combined with reduction in citrate concentration, predisposes to calcium carbonate renal stone formation with no change or even a rise in urinary calcium levels. The alternative CAIs put the renal calculus-prone patient at significantly less risk. Dichlorphenamide is cleared by the kidney, but does not induce a pH change from acid to alkaline, thus minimizing the risk of calcium carbonate deposition in the organ. Methazolamide has a minimal action on the kidney and on citrate concentration, thereby obviating the mechanism of stone formation.

(5) **Sickle cell anemia** patients with hyphema probably should not be treated with acetazolamide or other CAIs. These drugs induce an increase in ascorbic acid in the aqueous humor. This, in turn, predisposes to greater sickling in the anterior chamber.

(6) **Idiosyncratic reactions** are rare but similar to those encountered with use of sulfonamides. Immunologic reactions include Stevens-Johnson disease, drug fever, and the maculopapular rash. Hematologic toxicity may be fatal, in the form of agranulocytosis, aplastic anemia, or pancytopenia. CAIs are contraindicated in any patient with a history of any of these reactions. Sulfur allergy is a relative contraindication only.

(7) **Patients with chronic lung disease** should use these drugs with caution and not for extended periods of time unless monitored for aggravation of a pre-existing systemic acidosis.

(8) **Pregnant women** should not take CAIs under any but urgent conditions as these drugs are known teratogens.

G. **Hyperosmotic agents** were originally developed for use as diuretics, but have proved to be excellent short-term ocular hypotensives. A topical form of glycerin is used to clear corneal edema to facilitate gonioscopy and fundus examinations. The drugs of use in ophthalmology are **mannitol, glycerin,** and **isosorbide.**

1. **The mechanism of action** of hyperosmotics is a function of their common characteristics: freely filterable at the renal glomerulus, limited resorption by the renal tubule, pharmacologically inert, and resistant to metabolic alteration. These attributes allow administration of such agents orally or parenterally in sufficiently large quantities to increase the tonicity of the plasma significantly. The unreabsorbed solute (hyperosmotic agent) limits the back diffusion of water from renal tubules to the circulation. The resulting increase in plasma osmolarity widens the gradient between both aqueous and vitreous and the circulating blood. Water moves from the intraocular structures into the iris, ciliary body, and choroidal and retinal vessels, and on out the periocular vessels, resulting in a marked ocular hypotonic effect. For optimal effect, it is essential that the blood–aqueous and blood–vitreous barriers be intact to prevent leakage of hyperosmotic agent across the barrier, thus decreasing the gradient; intraocular inflammation may interfere with this barrier and markedly reduce the potential ocular hypotensive effect of these agents.

2. **Onset of action and the degree of IOP reduction** are in great part a function of route and rate of administration of a therapeutic dose, the presence or absence of intraocular inflammation, and the height of baseline IOP. Intravenous mannitol will cause a significant drop in IOP within 30–60 minutes, reaching maximal decrease of up to 30–40 mm Hg by 2 hours and lasting for about 6 hours. Orally administered glycerin has an onset of action of 10–30 minutes and lasts 4–5 hours, while isosorbide has an onset of 30 minutes, maximal at 1–2 hours, and lasting up to 5 hours. Efficacy is comparable to the parenteral agents, but there is less diuretic action.

3. **Preparations** commercially available are given either topically, orally, or intravenously, depending on the urgency and nature of the situation (see Table 5-4).

   a. **Systemic glycerin (Glyrol, Osmoglyn)** is a derivative of glycerol and, until the advent of isosorbide, was the only oral hyperosmotic agent used in ophthalmology. It does not meet all of the criteria of true hyperosmotic agents in that it is rapidly metabolized and therefore causes relatively little diuresis. Hyperglycemia is produced, however, and contributes to the ocular hypotensive effect. Dosage is 1.0–1.5 g of glycerin/kg body weight. Osmoglyn is a 50% lime-flavored solution for which dosage volume is 2–3 ml/kg body weight or 4–6 oz per individual. Glyrol is a 75% solution for which dosage volume is 1–2 ml/kg body weight or 3–5 oz per individual. Both solutions are better tolerated by the patient if served over cracked ice with a straw and may be given 1–1½ hours preoperatively or every 8–10 hours prn.

b. **Topical glycerin (Ophthalgan)** is a clear, colorless viscous solution. One or two drops are applied to the edematous cornea to induce transient clearing by osmotic withdrawal of water from the cornea, thus allowing a clearer view of the intraocular structures.

c. **Isosorbide (Ismotic)** is a true hyperosmotic diuretic, although the diuresis induced by this orally administered agent is significantly less than that of the parenteral drugs. It is not metabolized and appears in the urine unchanged. Isosorbide is available as a 45% vanilla-mint–flavored solution best served over cracked ice 1–4 times daily prn or 1–1½ hours preoperatively. The ocular hypotensive effect is similar to oral glycerin. Dosage is 1.0–2.0 g/kg body weight (1.5–3.0 ml/lb body weight). A 150-pound patient would take 225 ml isosorbide/dose.

d. **Mannitol** is an IV hyperosmotic available in concentrations of 5–25% in volumes of 50–1000 ml of water. It is the drug of choice when the patient is unable to tolerate or should not take oral medications, eg, nausea, vomiting, or, in some instances, preoperatively. Dosage is 2 g/kg body weight, with the most common administration being 50 ml of 20% solution IV by slow push (approximately 5 min) in patients with stable cardiovascular status. Mannitol should be **warm** (38–39° C) before infusing to redissolve any crystals that may have come out of solution. In patients with systemic hypertension or cardiovascular disease, in whom a sudden increase in plasma volume would be ill advised, either the dose may be lowered or the infusion given over 30–40 minutes, or both. The ocular hypotensive effect is noted in 30 minutes and will last up to 6 hours.

4. **Adverse side effects and contraindications.** Side effects noted with all hyperosmotic agents are a function of induced tissue dehydration. Plasma hyperosmolarity produces cerebral dehydration and may cause headache, nausea, vomiting, confusion, disorientation, and, rarely, coma or even subdural hematoma due to tearing of sagittal veins. Expansion of plasma volume may put an undue strain on a borderline cardiovascular system with a severe rise in systemic blood pressure, congestive heart failure, or pulmonary edema. Patients with prostatic hypertrophy or other causes of urinary retention may require ureteral catheterization. These drugs are contraindicated in oliguria or anuria. All hyperosmotics except glycerol cause diuresis, but only glycerol causes hyperglycemia and glycosuria, which may precipitate a crisis in a brittle diabetic. Isosorbide or mannitol should be used in di-

abetics. Tissue extravasation of mannitol will irritate but not induce tissue damage. True allergic reactions to hyperosmotics are rare.

Information Sources and Suggested Reading (*Antiglaucoma*)

1. Allen, R., Robbin, A., Long, D., Novak, G., Lue, J., and Kaplan, G., A combination of levobunolol and dipivefrin for the treatment of glaucoma. Arch. Ophthalmol. 106:904–906, 1988.
2. Beach, W., Shamsi, S., and Raymond, L., Apraclonidine 1% ophthalmic solution. *Pharmacy News of the Massachusetts Eye and Ear Infirmary* 5(5):3–4, 1988.
3. Betaxolol hydrochloride for ocular hypertension. In *Ocular Therapy Report,* American Health Consultants, Atlanta 1(3):9–12, 1988.
4. Boerner, C., Total punctate keratopathy due to dipivefrin. [Letter], Arch. Ophthalmol. 106:171, 1988.
5. Brown, R., Stewart, R., Lynch, M. et al., ALO 2145 reduces the intraocular pressure elevation after anterior segment laser surgery, Ophthalmol. 95:378–381, 1988.
6. Cairns, J.E. (Ed.), *Glaucoma.* New York: Grune and Stratton, 1986, multiple contributing authors, pp. 453–510 (closed-angle glaucomas—diagnosis and therapy), pp. 511–730 (open-angle glaucomas—diagnosis and therapy), pp. 731–826 (congenital glaucomas—diagnosis and therapy), pp. 827–894 (some secondary glaucomas—diagnosis and therapy).
7. Chamberlain, T., Myocardial infarction after ophthalmic betaxolol. N. Engl. J. Med. 321:1342, 1989.
8. Davies, P.H., and O'Connor, *The Actions and Uses of Ophthalmic Drugs,* 2nd ed. Boston: Butterworths, 1981, pp. 156–175 (miotics).
9. Development of topical carbonic anhydrase inhibitors. In *Ocular Therapy Report,* American Health Consultants, Atlanta 2(6):21–24, 1989.
10. Ellis, P., *Ocular Therapeutics and Pharmacology,* 7th ed. St. Louis: C.V. Mosby, 1985, pp. 60–79, 162–186, 296–297, 305–307 (antiglaucoma agents, therapy of glaucomas).
11. Epstein, D.L., *Chandler and Grant's Glaucoma,* 3rd ed. Philadelphia: Lea & Febiger, 1986, pp. 129–411 (diagnosis and treatment of adult glaucomas), pp. 469–528 (diagnosis and treatment of childhood glaucoma).
13. Fiore, P., Jacobs, I., and Goldberg, D., Drug-induced pemphigoid: a spectrum of diseases. Arch. Ophthalmol. 105: 1660–1664, 1987.
14. Fiore, P., and Cinotti, A., Systemic effects of intraocular epinephrine during cataract surgery. Ann. Ophthalmol. 20:23–25, 1988.
15. Fraunfelder, F., and Roy, F.H. (Eds.), *Current Ocular Therapy 2,* 2nd ed. Philadelphia: W.B. Saunders, 1990, multiple contributing authors, pp. 461–580 (accommodative esotropia, spasm), pp. 539–579 (the glaucomas).
16. Gilman, A.G., Goodman, L.S., Rall, T., and Murad, F. (Eds.), *The Pharmacological Basis of Therapeutics,* 7th ed. New

York: Macmillan, 1985, pp. 100–110 (cholinergic agonists, Taylor, P.), pp. 110–130 (anticholinesterase agents, Taylor, P.), pp. 145–181 (sympathomimetics, Weiner, N.), pp. 181–214 (adrenergic blocking agents, Weiner, N.).

17. Givens, K., and Lee, D., Topical beta blockers, part 1: clinical pharmacology. In Starita, J. (Ed.), *Clinical Signs in Ophthalmology.* St. Louis: C.V. Mosby, 1988, pp. 2–15.

18. Greenridge, K., Angle closure glaucoma. In Starita, R. (Ed.), *Clinical Signs in Ophthalmology.* St. Louis: C.V. Mosby, 1988, pp. 2–15.

19. Gressel, M., Parrish, R., II., and Folberg, R., 5-Fluorouracil and glaucoma filtering surgery: animal model. Ophthalmology 91:378–383, 1984.

20. Havener, W.H., *Ocular Pharmacology,* 5th ed. St. Louis: C.V. Mosby, 1983, pp. 261–417 (autonomic drugs), 539–564 (osmotic agents), pp. 575–597 (secretory inhibitors).

21. Heuer, D., Parrish, R. II., Gressel, M., Hodapp, E., Palmberg, P., and Anderson, D., 5-Fluorouracil and glaucoma filtering surgery. II: pilot study. Ophthalmology 91:384–394, 1984.

22. Kolker, A., and Heatherington, J., Jr., *Becker-Shaffer's Diagnosis and Therapy of the Glaucomas,* 5th ed. St. Louis: C.V. Mosby, 1983, pp. 187–363 (diagnosis and therapy), pp. 373–415 (medical therapy).

23. Kooner, K., and Zimmerman, T., Antiglaucoma therapy during pregnancy—part II. Ann. Ophthalmol. 20:208–211, 1988.

24. Levobunolol Study Group, Levobunolol: A four-year study. Ophthalmology 96:642–645, 1989.

25. Lichter, P., Musch, D., Medzihradsky, F., and Standardi, C., Intraocular pressure effects of carbonic anhydrase inhibitors in primary open-angle glaucoma. Am. J. Ophthalmol. 107:11–17, 1989.

26. Lynch, M., Whitson, J., Brown, R., Nguyen, H., and Drake, M., Topical beta blocker therapy and central nervous system side effects. Arch. Ophthalmol. 106:908–912, 1988.

27. Pavan-Langston, D., and Epstein, D., Glaucoma. In Pavan-Langston, D. (Ed.), *Manual of Ocular Diagnosis and Therapeutics,* 3rd ed. Boston: Little, Brown, 1990.

28. Ritch, R., Shields, M.B., and Krupin, T. (Eds.), *The Glaucomas.* St. Louis: C.V. Mosby, 1989, multiple contributing authors, pp. 515–556 (pharmacologic agents), pp. 761–788 (congenital glaucoma), pp. 789–824 (open-angle glaucomas), pp. 825–868 (primary angle-closure glaucomas), pp. 869–1348 (the secondary glaucomas: developmental disorders, associated ocular disease, systemic disease, drugs, inflammation and trauma, ocular surgery).

29. Robin, A., Pollack, I., and deFaller, J., Effects of topical ALO 2145 (p-aminoclonidine) on acute intraocular pressure rise after argon laser iridotomy. Arch. Ophthalmol. 105:1208–1211, 1987.

30. Rumelt, M., Blindness from misuse of over-the-counter eye medications. Ann. Ophthalmol. 20:26–30, 1988.

31. Samples, J., Use of topical beta-adrenergic antagonists for the contemporary therapy of glaucoma. Contemp. Ophthalmol. Forum 5(4):139–143, 1987.

32. Sears, M.L. (Ed.), *Pharmacology of the Eye.* Vol. 69, Handbook of Experimental Pharmacology. New York: Springer-

Verlag, 1984, pp. 149–180 (cholinergics, Kaufman, P., Weidman, T., Robinson, J.), pp. 193–233 (autonomic nervous system: adrenergic agonists, Sears, M.L.), pp. 249–272 (autonomic nervous system: adrenergic antagonists, Lotti, V., LeDouarec, J., Stone, C.), pp. 279–303 (carbonic anhydrase inhibitors, Friedland, B., Maren, T.).

33. Shihab, Z., Antiglaucoma therapy. In Lamberts, D., and Potter, D. (Eds.), *Clinical Ophthalmic Pharmacology.* Boston: Little Brown, 1987, pp 193–256.

34. Stock, J., Sulfonamide hypersensitivity and acetazolamide, Arch. Ophthalmol., 108:634, 1990.

35. Systemic side effects of ophthalmic beta-adrenergic blocking agents. In *Ocular Therapy Report,* American Health Consultants, Atlanta 1(4)13–16, 1988.

36. West, D., Lischwe, T., Thompson, V., and Ide, C., Comparative efficacy of the beta blockers for prevention of increased IOP after cataract extraction. Am. J. Ophthalmol. 106:168–173, 1988.

37. Wood, T., Effect of (intraoperative) carbachol on postoperative intraocular pressure. J. Cataract Refract. Surg. 14:654–656, 1988.

6

Antiparasitic Drugs

With increased ease of travel and iatrogenic and disease-induced immunosuppression, ocular parasitic disease never previously seen by many doctors may now be encountered anywhere. Most parasitic disease is systemic, but certain organisms such as *Toxoplasma* and *Onchocerca* involve the eye as a primary site, and others such as *Taenia* and *Toxocara* frequently have ocular involvement. Numerous parasites may cause ocular complications requiring chemotherapy or surgical intervention and certainly hygienic and nutritional measures to prevent reinfection (Table 6-1). As only minimal immunity is conferred by parasitic disease, even adequately treated patients are fully susceptible to multiple exogenous reinfections. Protozoal infections tend to persist despite treatment, although the patient may be made asymptomatic. Helminthic infections are considered adequately treated even if only the egg production is stopped and the adult worms survive. The latter do not multiply in the human host. Attempts to completely eradicate either protozoal or helminthic infection may result in the use of intolerably toxic drug doses with no particular advantage to the patient. It often is preferable to use a less toxic second-choice drug rather than a more toxic drug of first choice because of the numerous side effects of many antiparasitic agents. Similarly, two courses of treatment with a less toxic drug of first choice that has failed the first time may be preferable to switching to a more toxic alternative agent for the second line of therapy. The decision may even correctly be made to withhold therapy if the illness is less severe than the anticipated drug-induced side effects.

The antiparasitic drugs discussed below are not all approved by the United States Food and Drug Administration, but many may be obtained, if so indicated below, from the Centers for Disease Control (CDC) in Atlanta, Georgia. Others may be obtained from the manufacturer on a clinical investigational basis. See Tables 6-1 and 6-2.

A. **Antimony compounds** are best tolerated parenterally, are very irritating to the GI tract, and have a low therapeutic index. Patients treated with them should be monitored for heavy-metal poisoning.
1. **Clinical indication** for the trivalent compound, **antimony potassium or sodium tartrate** (tartar emetic), is for therapy of trematode infestations, being effective against all **Schistosoma** species, *S. haematobium, S. japonicum, S. mansoni,* and *S. mekongi.* It is a second-line drug of choice but more readily available commercially, as the drug of first choice, praziquantel, is still considered investigational by the FDA. Antimony sodium tartrate is equally therapeutically effective and believed to be somewhat less toxic than the potassium formulation, but must be used with the

continued on page 148

Table 6-1. Ocular parasitic diseases: Anti-helminthics

Parasite	Ocular lesions	Geographic distribution	Laboratory tests	Therapy*	Source
Ascaris lumbricoides (roundworm, ascariasis)	Rare intraocular worm	Worldwide	Eggs in stool, complement fixation larva in ocular granuloma or histopathology	Mebendazole, or pyrantel pamoate	Janssen Pfizer
Echinococcus granulosus (hydatid cyst, echinococcosis, tapeworm)	Orbital cyst (common), intraocular cyst (rare)	Sheep-raising areas	Skin test, indirect hemagglutination or immunofluorescent serology, X ray, CT scan	Praziquantel	Miles
Loa loa (loaiasis, eyeworm, Calabar swelling)	Subcutaneous or subconjunctival nodule, periorbital swelling and pain	Africa, South America	Blood smear, tissue biopsy	Diethylcarbamazine	Lederle
Onchocerca volvulus (river blindness, onchocerciasis)	Uveitis, keratitis, secondary glaucoma, optic atrophy and neuritis, skin and eye nodules, chorioretinitis	Africa, Central and South America	Skin snip, nodule biopsy	Ivermectin or diethylcarbamazine followed by suramin	Merck Lederle Bayer (Germany)
Schistosoma haematobium (bilharzia, schistosomiasis)	Dacryoadenitis, conjunctival and orbital granulomas	Africa, Middle East	Eggs in urine, lesion biopsy, CT scan	Praziquantel, niridazole	Miles CDC

Organism	Ocular manifestation	Distribution	Diagnosis	Treatment	Supplier
Schistosoma japonicum (bilharzia, schistosomiasis)	Orbital granuloma (rare)	China, Japan, Philippines	Eggs in urine, lesion biopsy, CT scan	Praziquantel, antimony potassium tartrate	Miles CDC
Taenia saginata (beef tapeworm)	Orbital granuloma (rare)	Worldwide	Eggs in segments in stool, scotch tape swab rectum	Praziquantel, niclosamide	Miles Miles
Taenia solium (cysticercosis, pork tapeworm)	Intraocular granuloma	Worldwide	Skin test, X ray for calcified cysts	Praziquantel, niridazole	Miles Miles
Chelazia callipeda or *californiensis*	Conjunctivitis, extraocular muscle paresis, orbital granuloma	Central America	Biopsy lesion for worm	Surgical excision	
Toxocara cari, cati (toxocariasis)	Panuveitis, endophthalmitis, posterior and peripheral retinal granuloma	Worldwide	ELISA on aqueous, vitreous, serum for antibodies	Diethylcarbamazine, thiabendazole, or mebendazole	Lederle Merck Janssen
Trichinella spiralis (trichinosis)	Lid and periorbital edema, extraocular muscle paresis and pain	Worldwide	Serology, skin biopsy	Thiabendazole and steroids	Merck Many
Wuchereria bancrofti, brugia, malayi (filariasis, elephantiasis)	Orbital lymphedema, periorbital swelling	*W. bancrofti* and *W. brugia*—tropical areas *W. malayi*—Japan	Nocturnal blood smear	Diethylcarbamazine	Lederle

CDC, Centers for Disease Control, Atlanta, GA.
* Dosages given in text.

Table 6-2. Ocular parasitic diseases: protozoal

Parasite	Ocular lesions	Geographic distribution	Laboratory tests	Therapy*	Source
Acanthamoeba	Indolent, painful corneal ulcer and infiltrates, iridocyclitis	Worldwide	Culture on *E. coli*, calciflor white stain	Topical pentamidine and neomycin; ? ketoconazole	May & Baker (England) See Antibiotics chapter Janssen
Entamoeba histolytica (amebiasis)	Cutaneous amebiasis of lids	Worldwide	Cysts and trophozoites in stool or lesion biopsy	Iodoguinol Paromomycin Tetracyclines	Glenwood Corp., others Parke-Davis Many
Giardia lamblia	Retinal vasculitis	Worldwide	Cysts and trophozoites in stool	Metronidazole	Searle
Leishmania tropica (Oriental sore, Aleppo boil)	Lid ulcer	Middle East, Asia Minor, Central and South America	Scrapings of skin lesions	Antimony sodium gluconate	Burroughs-Wellcome

Leishmania braziliensis (forest jaws, espundia, mucocutaneous leishmaniasis)	Lid ulcer	Yucatan, Mexico, South America	Scrapings of skin lesions	Antimony sodium gluconate	Burroughs-Wellcome
Pneumocystis carinii	Retinal infarcts (cotton wool spots) in AIDS patients	Worldwide	Bronchial washings, sputum cultures	Pentamidine isothionate Pyrimethamine	Lypho-Med Burroughs-Wellcome
Toxoplasma gondii (toxoplasmosis)	Chorioretinitis, papillitis, retinal vasculitis, uveitis, secondary glaucoma	Worldwide	Serology: immunofluorescent antibody, indirect hemagglutination, ELISA, fluoroimmunoassay (FIAX), immunoperoxidase assay	Pyrimethamine + trisulfapyrimidine or sulfadiazine; spiramycin, steroids, laser, cryotherapy	Burroughs-Wellcome Poulenc, Canada

* Dosages given in text.

same precautions. The pentavalent antimony compound, **sodium stibogluconate,** is the drug of choice in therapy of visceral, cutaneous, and mucocutaneous **leishmaniasis.**

2. **Dosage**

   a. **Antimony potassium tartrate** is available in sterile crystalline form or as a 0.5% solution in ampules. Its action against schistosome phosphofructokinase is about 100 times that against mammalian cells, thus enhancing its therapeutic index. Therapy is begun with a slow IV injection of 8 ml of the 0.5% solution. Drug is administered on alternate days, increasing dosage by 4 ml up to a maximum of 28 ml/day. The usual maximum total dose is 360 ml. Excretion is slow and via the kidneys, with only 30% of drug recoverable at 1 week and detectable drug levels in the urine persisting at 100 days. This slow release of trivalent compound is thought to be a function of the rapid uptake of injected drug by the erythrocytes, with consequent low plasma levels and hemoglobin malfunction.

   b. **Sodium stibogluconate (sodium antimony gluconate, Pentostam)** is available from the CDC as a solution for IM or IV administration. The solution contains 330 mg/ml of drug, which is the equivalent of 10% or 100 mg/ml of pentavalent antimony. The drug is easily degraded by light and should be protected from it. Therapy is 20 mg/kg/day by IV or IM injection of up to 800 mg/day for 20 days. A severely debilitated patient should receive the drug only on alternate days. Children tolerate the same doses of pentavalent drug as adults. Because sodium stibogluconate is not taken up by erythrocytes, plasma levels are much higher and renal clearance much faster than for the trivalent compound. About 50% of the drug is recovered in the urine by 24 hours.

3. **Adverse side effects** are similar for both trivalent and pentavalent compounds, but significantly less frequent for the latter because of its rapid clearance. **Ocular** side effects are listed in Part II of this book (see Table 15-4). **Systemically,** too rapid injection may result in coughing, vomiting, arm and chest pain, and syncope. Anaphylactic reaction becomes a risk by the sixth or seventh injection. During the course of therapy, slowly reversible electrocardiographic changes or a total arrythmia may occur, and joint, muscle, or back pain, bradycardia, or hypotension may require cessation of therapy. Pneumonia is commonly seen with trivalent drug but not with pentavalent, and hepatitis is rare but may occur with either. Miscellaneous side effects include headache, dizziness, fatigue, rash, apnea, dyspnea, nausea, anorexia, diarrhea, abdominal pain, constipation, excessive salivation, metallic taste

in the mouth, fever, herpetic dermatitis, and conjunctival hyperemia. Antimony potassium tartrate is contraindicated in the presence of renal, hepatic, cardiac, or pulmonary disease unrelated to the parasitic disease.

B. **Clindamycin** is a lincomycin derivative discussed in greater detail in the chapter on Antibiotics.

1. **Clinical indication** in parasitic disease is in therapy of both acute and latent *Toxoplasma gondii* as an effective drug of second choice. The drug may induce rapid healing of active chorioretinitis and, because of its activity against the encysted forms, may in some cases prevent recurrences. This efficacy may be in part a function of iris and choroidal concentration of bioactive drug by uveal melanin binding followed by slow drug release.

2. **Dosage** is 15–50 mg by subconjunctival injection every other day and/or 300 mg po qid for 3–4 weeks. High drug concentrations are found in the uveal tract experimentally 6 hours after subconjunctival injection and remain relatively high at 24 hours when serum levels have decreased. There may be synergistic action between clindamycin and the drugs of first choice for toxoplasmosis, pyrimethamine, and trisulfapyrimidines.

3. **Adverse side effects** are discussed in greater detail in the chapter on Antibiotics and in Part II of this book. In general, this drug should be used with caution in patients with renal or liver disease. The drug also may block the action of erythromycin and enhance neuromuscular blocking agents. Diarrhea is a common side effect (8%), and a potentially fatal pseudomembranous colitis may develop infrequently.

C. **Diethylcarbamazine (Hetrazan, Banocide, Notezine)** is a piperazine derivative in wide use for the past 30 years.

1. **Clinical indications** for use include therapy of filarial infestation: **onchocerciasis** (*Onchocerca volvulus*) as a drug of second choice, and **loaiasis** (*Wuchereria bancrofti, W. brugia,* or *W. malayi, Mansonella ozzardi,* and *Loa loa*) as drug of first choice. It is also a drug of first choice in treating **toxocariasis.**

2. **Dosage.** The drug is easily absorbed from the GI tract with peak concentrations in 3 hours and total elimination from the body in 24 hours. The initial dose should not exceed 0.5 mg/kg po when treating ocular disease. This dose is given once on day 1 and bid on day 2, increased to 1 mg/kg tid on day 3, and to 2 mg/kg tid by day 5 for a total of 21 days. The regimen is the same for onchocerciasis, loaiasis, and toxocariasis. In the case of *Onchocerca,* therapy will kill microfilariae in the skin but not in nodules. The drug causes redistribution of microfilariae in the body and exposes parasitic surface antigens. The consequent augmented host immune response results in death of the young

organisms. As the adult worms are not killed, short drug treatment courses may be necessary every few months to prevent replacement of the microfilarial population. Another recommended regimen is an initial course of diethylcarbamazine followed by a short course of the macrofilaricidal drug, suramin.

3. **Adverse side effects,** either ocular or systemic, are not common.

   a. **Ocular side effects** include a keratopathy characterized by punctate fluffy opacities in the cornea. Histopathologic study reveals dead microfilariae with associated inflammatory changes. Also noted are transient retinal pigment epithelial disturbance, papillitis, increased retinal vascular permeability, and white spots beneath the internal limiting membrane. These posterior segment changes are associated with high levels of circulating immune complexes, particularly C-lg complement sequence. Additional ocular effects are listed in Table 15-4 in Part II of this book.

   b. **Systemic side effects** include severe allergic reactions in response to the release of foreign antigen from dead microfilariae (Mazzotti reaction). Treatment with systemic corticosteroids is often required. Other side effects are nausea, vomiting, diarrhea, and, less frequently, headache, vertigo, dermatitis, lymphadenopathy, and encephalopathy.

D. **Ivermectin (Mectizan, Ivomec)** is a hydrogenated analog of the macrocyclic lactone avermectin B. It is considered an investigational drug by the FDA, but is available from the manufacturer.

   1. **Clinical indications** for this broad antiparasitic agent is as the drug of choice for *Onchocerca volvulus* infestation (filariasis) and possibly *Ancyclostoma duodenale* (hookworm), although mebendazole is the drug of first choice for the latter disease. In onchocerciasis, the drug acts against microfilariae either as an agonist of the neurotransmitter γ-aminobutyric acid (GABA) or by prolonging its release from inhibitory nerve endings.

   2. **Dosage** varies, depending on whether there is ocular involvement. In the absence of ocular involvement, the adult and pediatric dose is 150 mg/kg po once and repeated every 6–12 months to reduce rapidly and keep reduced the microfilarial load and prevent microfilarial migration. If there is ocular involvement, the dose is 200 mg/kg po once with periodic repetition. This higher dose is as effective as diethylcarbamazine in decreasing the number of microfilariae, with fewer adverse ophthalmic reactions.

   3. **Adverse side effects** include transient generalized pruritus, dizziness, and weakness. No cardiovascular, hematologic, biochemical, or drug-induced ocular abnormalities have been reported. A major advantage of ivermectin over diethylcarbamazine is the absence of the Mazzotti systemic and ocular allergic reaction to released microfilarial antigens.

E. Mebendazole (Vermox, Mebutar, Neniasole, Pantel-min, Sirben, Mebandecin, Vermirax) is a benzimida-zole structurally and therapeutically related to thiaben-dazole.

1. **Clinical indications** for mebendazole are broad and include *Ascaris lumbricoides* (roundworm), *Enterobius vermicularis* (pinworm), *Trichuris trichura* (whip-worm), *Gnathostoma spinigerum,* and *Toxocara* spp.

2. **Dosage** varies with the nature of the infestation. The drug is available as 100-mg tablets (Vermox in the United States and Canada) and given as follows. For roundworm and whipworm, mebendazole is the drug of first choice and given as 100 mg bid po for 3 days to adults and to children over 2 years of age. For pinworm it is equal to pyrantel pamoate, the alternative drug, and dosage is 100 mg po once and repeated in 2 weeks. Toxocariasis is treated with 200–400 mg/day for 5 days.

3. **Adverse side effects** are extremely rare, probably because of poor absorption, although heavily infested patients may have transient abdominal pain and diar-rhea.

F. Minocycline is a semisynthetic tetracycline discussed in greater detail in the chapter on Antibiotics.

1. **Clinical indication** for minocycline in therapy of par-asitic disease is as a second-line adjunctive drug with sulfadiazine in therapy of retinal *Toxoplasma gondii.* It is not FDA approved for this use.

2. **Dosage** is 100 mg po bid for 2–4 weeks with sulfadi-azine.

3. **Adverse side effects systemically** include vestibular toxicity symptoms of ataxia, dizziness, nausea, and vomiting, which clear within a day or two of discontin-uing treatment. Allergic reactions are uncommon. **Ocular** side effects are listed in Part II of this book.

G. Niridazole (Ambilhar) is a nitrothiazole derivative available from the CDC as an experimental drug.

1. **Clinical indications** include use as an alternative drug in therapy of schistosomiasis and possibly as an effective agent against adult *Onchocerca volvulus.* The drug appears to work by inhibiting glucose-6-phos-phate dehydrogenase in the adult worm.

2. **Dosage.** The drug is available in 100- and 500-mg tablets. Usual therapy is 25 mg/kg po daily in 2 divided doses, as the drug is rapidly metabolized in the liver. Maximum dose is 1.5 g daily; duration of therapy is 5–10 days. As *Schistosoma japonicum* response may be variable, treatment dosage is longer at 15 mg/kg in 2 divided doses daily for 24 days or 3 10-day courses with 30 days between courses.

3. **Adverse side effects** are not commonly seen. Central nervous system toxicity is the most important reaction and may present as mood change, confusion, or con-vulsion. Other effects are anorexia, nausea, vomiting, diarrhea, headache, insomnia, somnolence, T-wave changes on ECG, tachycardia, and urticarial rash. Pa-

tients with glucose-6-phosphate dehydrogenase deficiency frequently develop hemolytic anemia and therefore should not take this drug. It also is contraindicated in malnutrition, severe anemia, and severe concomitant infectious disease such as hookworm and tuberculosis. The drug should be used with caution in patients with nonparasitic liver, renal, cardiac, or neurologic disease.

H. Pentamidine isethionate (Lomidine) is a diamide derivative available from the CDC.

1. **Clinical indications** for use of this drug include *Trypanosoma gambiense, T. rhodesiense* (African sleeping sickness), but not *T. cruzi* (Chagas' disease, South American trypanosomiasis), *Leishmania donovani* (kala azar, visceral leishmaniasis), and *Pneumocystis carinii,* the opportunistic infection common in AIDS. It is the drug of second choice for the infestations in which it is indicated. The drug is thought to work by binding to trypanosomal mitochondrial DNA.

2. **Dosage** varies with the nature of the infestation, and the IM route is preferred. For African trypanosomiasis and pneumocystic infections, dosage is 4 mg/kg IM daily for 10 days (trypanosomiasis) or 14 days (*Pneumocystis*). Pentamidine inhalers are used for pneumocystis prophylaxis in AIDS patients but 2% still see ocular *P. carinii* choroiditis. As the drug does not cross the blood–brain barrier, it is ineffective in *T. rhodesiense* infection with CNS involvement, which may be quite early with this species. Therapy of visceral leishmaniasis (*L. donovani*) is 2–4 mg/kg daily for 12–15 doses, followed by a second course after 1–2 weeks.

3. **Adverse side effects** include immediate shortness of breath, systemic hypotension, tachycardia, dizziness, headache, syncope, and vomiting. It should be used with caution in patients with hepatic or renal disease or diabetes.

I. Propamidine isethionate (Brolene) is an aromatic diamidine structurally related to pentamidine and hydroxystilbamadine. The drug is sold over the counter as a drop (propamidine isethionate) or ointment (dibromopropamidine) in England, but is available only as an investigational drug through Janssen Corporation in the United States.

1. **Clinical indication** for propamidine is in therapy of *Acanthamoeba* amoebic keratitis. In the search for effective therapy for this very resistant and progressive corneal disease, studies on numerous drugs have indicated that only the aromatic diamidines like propamidine, the antibiotic aminoglycosides (neomycin, paromomycin), and the antifungal imidazoles (miconazole, clotrimazole, ketoconazole) have some efficacy in tolerable doses as topical agents. Polymyxin B also may have some efficacy.

2. **Dosage.** Although no drug or combination of drugs has yet been found to be consistently effective and

penetrating keratoplasty may be required, the combination of topical **propamidine** and **neomycin** appears to be reasonably good treatment. Initial therapy is 1% propamidine isethionate drop followed 5 minutes later by a drop of neomycin sulfate-polymyxin B sulfate-gramicidin (Neosporin or similar ophthalmic solution) every 15 minutes to 1 hour while the patient is awake and dibromopropamidine and neomycin sulfate-polymyxin B sulfate-bacitracin zinc ointment (Neosporin or similar ophthalmic ointment) every 2 hours during the hours of sleep for the first week. The medication then is slowly tapered (eg, q2h by day and q4h by night for 2–4 weeks) to a long-term maintenance dose of 1 drop of each medication qid to bid for a year or longer, depending on the clinical response. This regimen should be followed even if penetrating keratoplasty has been performed.

3. **Concurrent topical steroid** use is controversial. If the patient is already taking steroids, dosage should be tapered to the lowest dose tolerable to the patient, and stopped completely as soon as possible.

4. **Additive therapy to propamidine.** Oral **ketoconazole** may be added in severe infections (see chapter on Antifungals). **Clotrimazole** has been used as a 2% suspension 4–8 times in artificial tears or in an ointment base with effective results. **Miconazole** is not well tolerated topically and is unstable in solution.

5. **Adverse side effects** of topical propamidine include reversible chemical conjunctivitis, punctate keratitis, and an unusual keratopathy characterized by clear intraepithelial microcysts that tend to be linear in arrangement. They disappear with tapering of medication. Neomycin toxicity may be similar to that of propamidine, with the exception of this cystic keratopathy.

J. **Physostigmine (Eserine)** is an anticholinesterase discussed also in the chapter on Glaucoma.

1. **Clinical indication** for use of this drug in parasitic disease is in therapy of **phthiriasis (lice)** of the eyebrows and lashes. The drug affects neural transmission in the louse but not the nits (eggs).

2. **Dosage** is liberal application of the 0.25% ointment bid to tid for several weeks. This will assure the killing not only of the parent lice but also of the progeny that hatch from the eggs 8–10 days after being laid.

3. **Adverse side affects** are not encountered when the ointment is confined to brows and lashes. If some medication contacts the eye, the side effects may include reversible conjunctival hyperemia, ciliary spasm, myopia, miosis, paralysis of accommodation, superficial keratitis, and possibly other effects on lens, pupil, and retina, as listed in the chapter on Glaucoma.

K. **Praziquantel (Biltricide)** is a pyrazinoisoquinoline derivative with broad activity.

1. **Clinical indications** for use are as the drug of first

choice in therapy of liver flukes (*Fasciola* spp., *Clonorchis* spp.), against all four *Schistosoma* species (*S. haematobium, S. japonicum, S. mansoni, S. mekongi*), and for larval and adult cestodes (tapeworms: *Diphyllobothrium* spp., *Taenia* spp., *Hymenolepsis* spp., and *Cysticercus* spp.).

2. **Dosage** is 20 mg/kg po tid for 1 day in both adult and childhood schistosomiasis and for liver flukes. For tapeworm infestation, treatment is 25 mg/kg po once, with the exception of *Cysticercus,* which requires 50 mg/kg/day in 3 divided doses for 14 days.

3. **Adverse side effects** frequently include headache, malaise, and dizziness, with occasional sedation, abdominal discomfort, fever, sweating, nausea, fatigue, eosinophilia, and, rarely, a pruritic rash.

L. **Pyrimethamine (Daraprim)** is a 2,4-diaminopyrimidine structurally similar to folic acid.

1. **Clinical indication** is as part of the drug combination of first choice, pyrimethamine plus trisulfapyrimidine or sulfadiazine, in treatment of systemic and ocular **toxoplasmosis** (*Toxoplasma gondii*). The drug binds more to the parasitic cell than to the mammalian cell and enters by nonionic diffusion. It acts by substrate inhibition to block dihydrofolate reductase, an enzyme essential to tetrahydrofolate production and subsequent synthesis of purines and pyrimidines for DNA and RNA.

2. **Dosage** of pyrimethamine is 25 mg/day po for adults, or 2 mg/kg/day for 3 days and then 1 mg/kg/day po in children for 3–4 weeks. A loading dose triple that of maintenance may be given for the first 2 days. The drug is available as 25 mg scored tablets or as an elixir. The drug is slow in onset of action and ineffective in nondividing organisms. Dosage of concurrent trisulfapyrimidine or sulfadiazine is 4–6 g/day in 2–3 divided doses for adults and 100–200 mg/kg/day in children for 4 weeks.

3. **Adverse side effects** result from the prolonged use of the medication, including bone marrow suppression with leukopenia, pancytopenia, thrombopenia, agranulocytosis, and a megaloblastic anemia similar to that seen in folic acid deficiency. To combat these effects, 3 mg of **folinic acid** (leucovorin) should be given po or IM biw. Patients should drink copious amounts of fluid and keep their urine alkalinized by taking 1 teaspoonful of sodium bicarbonate tid. A complete blood count and platelet count should be done once or twice weekly even if patients are taking folinic acid, as adverse hematologic effects are not entirely blocked by this drug. Other toxic effects seen in pyrimethamine therapy include nausea, vomiting, and, rarely, rash or shock. The drug may be teratogenic and therefore used with caution in pregnancy.

4. **Concurrent therapy.** Topical **corticosteroids** and **cycloplegics** may be used for the anterior uveitis that may be seen when posterior segment lesions are active.

Periocular injections should **not** be used, however, as they induce prolonged local immunosuppression in the area of active toxoplasmic disease. A 1–2-week course, but not longer, of systemic prednisone at a dosage of 30–40 mg po bid may be given to minimize inflammatory damage encroaching on the optic nerve and macula or for significant vitritis. **Photocoagulation** and **cryotherapy** have been used successfully to destroy encysted parasites and to wall off existing chorioretinal scars to prevent the spread of new lesions from the old ones.

M. **Spiramycin (Rovamycin)** is a macrolide antibiotic derived from *Streptomyces ambofaciens.*
   1. **Clinical indication** for spiramycin in parasitic disease is as a second-line drug for therapy of *Toxoplasma gondii.* It is less effective than combined pyrimethamine and sulfadiazine, but a reasonable alternative regimen should toxicity prevent use of the former agents. The drug acts by binding the 50s ribosome unit, inhibiting peptide chain translocation and, therefore, protein synthesis in the parasites.
   2. **Dosage** in adult patients is 500 mg po qid, and for children 50–100 mg/day in 2–4 divided doses for 3–4 weeks. The drug is well absorbed from the GI tract and slowly inactivated, with only 5–15% recovered in the urine. Adjunctive therapy of ocular toxoplasmosis is discussed under Pyrimethamine.
   3. **Adverse side effects** of spiramycin include nausea, pseudomembranous colitis, diarrhea, and, rarely, peripheral paresthesias and skin rash.

N. **Suramin (Antrypol)** is a polycyclic trypan dye available from the CDC as a sterile powder. Foreign commercial names include Germanin, Bayer 205, Moranyl, Forneau, Naphuride, Naganol, and Belganyl.
   1. **Clinical indication** for use is as the drug of first choice for African (but not South American) **trypanosomiasis** and for *Onchocerca volvulus.* The mode of action is not known, but may be related to intracellular membrane damage.
   2. **Dosage.** The sterile powder is made up in sterile water for injection as a 10% solution immediately before use. It is potentially highly toxic. In therapy of **trypanosomiasis,** adult dosage is a 100–200 mg test dose slowly IV and then 0.5–1.0 g IV on days 1, 3, 7, 14, and 21, with weekly doses thereafter for 5 weeks. For children the dose is 20 mg/kg on days 1, 3, 7, 14, and 21 with weekly doses thereafter for 5 weeks. In therapy of **onchocerciasis,** the drug is an effective macro- and microfilaricide. Indications for treatment in sight-threatening disease are the finding on clinical exam of (1) 20 or more microfilariae (Mf) in the anterior chamber or 50 Mf in the cornea, (2) severe uveitis, (3) early sclerosing keratitis, (4) 15 Mf in an outer canthal skin biopsy, (5) 100 Mf in the skin elsewhere, (6) head nodules, (7) reduced visual acuity, or (8) visual field loss.

3. **Alternative suramin therapy.** Although ivermectin is the drug of first choice, a recommended, very effective alternative is a course of diethylcarbamazine to kill the microfilariae followed by a course of suramin to kill both remaining micro- and macro (adult)-filariae. The recommended treatment regimen for an average 60-kg patient is: days 1–2, dexamethasone 4 mg/day po; days 3–4, diethylcarbamazine (DEC) 50 mg po; days 5–10, DEC 100 mg po bid. Week 4, suramin 0.2 g IV. Week 5, suramin 0.4 g IV, increasing each weekly dose by 0.2 g through week 8 (1.0 g IV), then 0.8 g IV week 9, and nodulectomy of all palpable nodules week 10.

4. **Adverse side effects systemically** may be seen even after small dosages of suramin and are worse in malnourished patients. Immediate side effects are nausea and anaphylactic shock. Photophobia and peripheral neuritis may develop in 24 hours, and albuminuria is common late in treatment. Rarely, agranulocytosis and hemolytic anemia may occur. The drug is sufficiently toxic that it should be given only under close supervision. **Ocular toxicity** of suramin includes a vortex keratopathy, corneal epithelial and subepithelial opacities, and similar deposits in conjunctiva and lens epithelium. These deposits are membranous lamellar inclusion bodies, similar to other drug-induced lysosomal lipid-storage diseases. Iritis, subconjunctival and retinal hemorrhages, optic atrophy, and urticaria also have been noted.

O. **Thiabendazole (Mintezol)** is an imidazole derivative.

1. **Clinical indications** for use are in therapy of nematodes, in **toxocariasis** (visceral larva migrans, *Toxocara cati,* and *T. cani*) and in **trichinosis** (*Trichinella spiralis*). Its mode of action is not known, but may be related to fumarate reductase inhibition in helminths and to its anti-inflammatory, antipyretic, and analgesic effects.

2. **Dosage** in adults and children is 25 mg/kg daily up to a maximum of 3 g/day for 2–4 weeks (nematodes) and for 5 days (toxocariasis, trichinosis). In therapy of trichinosis and toxocariasis, systemic corticosteroids, such as prednisone 40 mg/day po for 3 weeks, also are given to minimize inflammatory side effects in reaction to death of the parasites.

3. **Adverse side effects** of thiabendazole are frequently seen **systemically** as CNS toxicity characterized by dizziness, headache, and drowsiness. Other effects include anorexia, nausea, vomiting, diarrhea, and pruritus. Rarely seen are tinnitus, numbness, hyperglycemia, enuresis, systemic hypotension, leukopenia, crystalluria, and hepatotoxicity. **Ocular** side effects are blurred vision, red-green color vision defect, yellow-tinged vision, visual hallucinations, angioneurotic edema, keratoconjunctivitis sicca, and retinal hemorrhages. See Table 15-4 in Part II of this book.

Information Sources and Suggested Reading (*Antiparasitics*)

1. Burd, E., Antiparasitic agents. In Tabbara, K.F., and Hyndiuk, R.A. (Eds.), *Infections of the Eye.* Boston: Little, Brown, 1986, pp. 275–291.
2. Drugs for parasitic infections. The Medical Letter on Drugs and Therapeutics. The Medical Letter, New Rochelle, NY 30(759):15–22, 1988.
3. Fraunfelder, F., and Roy, F.H. (Eds.), *Current Ocular Therapy* 3rd ed. Philadelphia: W.B. Saunders, 1990, multiple contributing authors, pp. 98–124 (parasitic disease).
4. *Handbook of Antimicrobial Therapy.* New Rochelle, NY: The Medical Letter, 1989, pp. 110–129 (antiparasitic agents).
5. Havener, W., *Antihelminthics, Ocular Pharmacology,* 5th ed. St. Louis, C.V. Mosby, 1983, pp. 220–222.
6. Holland, E., Stein, C., Palestine, A., et al., Suramin keratopathy. Am. J. Ophthalmol. 106:216–220, 1988.
7. Johns, K., Head, S., and O'Day, D., Corneal toxicity of propamidine (Brolene). Arch. Ophthalmol. 106:68–70, 1988.
8. Ludwig, I., and Meisler, D., Acanthamoeba keratitis. In Tabbara, K.F., and Hyndiuk, R.A. (Eds.), *Infections of the Eye.* Boston: Little, Brown, 1986, pp. 665–678.
9. Matoba, A., Pare, P., Lee, T., and Osato, M., Effects of freezing and antibiotics on the viability of acanthamoeba cysts. Arch. Ophthalmol. 107:439–440, 1989.
10. Moore, M.B., Parasitic infections. In Kaufman, H., McDonald, M., Barron, B., and Waltman, S. (Eds.), *The Cornea.* New York: Churchill Livingstone, 1988, pp. 271–279.
11. Nussenblatt, R.B., and Palestine, A.G., *Uveitis: Fundamentals in Clinical Practice.* Chicago: Yearbook Medical Publ., 1989, pp. 325, 336–354 (toxoplasmosis), pp. 355–362 (toxocariasis).
12. Schuman, J., Weinberg, R., Ferry, A., and Guerry, R.K., Toxoplasmic scleritis. Ophthalmology 95:1399–1403, 1988.
13. Smolin, G., and Thoft, R.A. (Eds.), *The Cornea.* 2nd ed. Boston: Little, Brown, 1987, pp. 177–178 (parasitic microbiology, Okumoto, M.), pp. 225–227 (parasitic disease, Forster, R.).
14. Tabbara, K.F., and Hyndiuk, R.A. (Eds.), *Infections of the Eye.* Boston: Little, Brown, 1986, pp. 635–652 (toxoplasmosis, Tabbara, K.), pp. 665–678 (acanthamoeba keratitis, Ludwig, I., Meisler, D.)
15. Tabbara, K.F., Other parasitic infections. In Tabbara, K.F., and Hyndiuk, R.A. (Eds.), *Infections of the Eye.* Boston: Little, Brown, 1986, pp. 679–695.
16. Taylor, H., and Dax, E., Ocular onchocerciasis. In Tabbara, K.F., and Hyndiuk, R.A. (Eds.), *Infections of the Eye.* Boston: Little, Brown, 1986, pp. 653–664.
17. Webster, L. Jr., Chemotherapy of parasitic diseases. In Gilman, A.G., Goodman, L.L., Rall, T., and Murad, F. (Eds.), *The Pharmacological Basis of Therapeutics,* 7th ed. New York: Macmillan, 1985, pp. 1004–1065.

7

Antiviral Drugs

There are currently seven antiviral drugs of major interest for therapy of ocular disease in the United States: **idoxuridine** (IDU), **vidarabine** (Ara A), **trifluridine** (F_3T), **acyclovir** (ACV), **ganciclovir** (DHPG), **azidothymidine** (AZT), and **foscarnet** (PFA). IDU, F_3T, and Ara A are commercially available for topical therapy of herpes simplex viral (HSV) keratitis. Ara A and ACV are also used systemically in treatment of herpetic encephalitis, mucocutaneous herpes, and neonatal herpes. Topical ACV is therapeutically effective for HSV keratitis and systemic ACV for genital herpes, herpes zoster ophthalmicus (HZO), and possibly HSV keratouveitis, but is not yet FDA approved for either of the latter two uses. DHPG is efficacious in cytomegalovirus (CMV) retinitis and is FDA approved for this use. It is possibly effective against Epstein–Barr virus (EBV). AZT is FDA approved for use in acquired immune deficiency syndrome (AIDS). Two other antivirals, **bromovinyldeoxyuridine** (BVDU) and **ethyldeoxyuridine** (EDU), are used in ocular HSV and HZO (BVDU only) in Europe, but are not available in the United States. **Interferon** drops have been studied in this country and found to be somewhat effective in HSV keratitis, but are not available for use pending further study. BVDU, EDU, and interferon will not be discussed further in this book.

I. **Viral Infection and the Basis of Antiviral Toxicity and Failure**
   A. **Viral life cycle.** With the exception of the AIDS virus (human immunodeficiency virus, HIV-RNA virion), and adenovirus (DNA virion) the major ocular viral infections are caused by the herpesviruses and, unlike adenoviruses, are generally amenable to antiviral therapy. The viral DNA core is encapsulated in a protein coat and, in certain cases, by an outer lipoprotein envelope. After viral entry into the host cell by a phagocytic mechanism, the DNA protective coats are digested by the cell, and the viral DNA (vDNA) enters the cell nucleus. The vDNA then transcribes messenger RNA and initiates the genetic cascade that results in production of virus-specific proteins such as thymidine kinase and DNA polymerase. The former is essential for initial phosphorylation of purine and pyrimidine bases for their ultimate incorporation into new vDNA and the latter for the incorporation of the triphosphorylated bases into vDNA. Viral DNA cores synthesized in the cell nucleus migrate to the cytoplasm to be coated by the protein capsid, and are subsequently released from the cell by lysis.
   B. **The site of viral infection** influences drug efficacy and toxicity. Superficial epithelial infections are easily managed with therapeutic titers using topical drugs, whereas deeper tissues such as the corneal stroma or intraocular disease can be managed only, if at all, by systemic therapy. Therapeutic efficacy of either administration route is dependent on drug solubility, absorption, and toxicity.

C. **Basis of antiviral toxicity.** Because viruses are obligate intracellular parasites and because all current agents of importance in ocular therapy act at an intracellular level, the potential for toxic side effects is great. Current chemotherapy is based primarily on disruption of viral DNA synthesis. The mechanisms of action of all antivirals discussed here are not known, but those that are known are dependent on drug activation by viral or host enzymatic phosphorylation. Toxicity is a function of host enzymes also activating drug in uninfected cells; the more specific the drug activation by viral enzymes only, the less host toxicity is produced by the drug.

D. **Treatment failure** usually may be attributed to one or more of six factors:
   1. **Poor patient compliance.**
   2. **Premature discontinuation** of therapy.
   3. **Inadequate drug potency.**
   4. **Viral resistance,** primary or secondary to drug exposure.
   5. **Drug intolerance** due to toxicity or allergy.
   6. **Incorrect diagnosis,** eg, sterile ulcer or punctate keratitis of dry eye.

II. **Specific Antiviral Agents**
   A. **Idoxuridine** (IDU, 5-iodo-2′-deoxyuridine, Stoxil, Herplex), the oldest of the antiviral agents, is a halogenated pyrimidine that resembles the DNA base, thymidine.
      1. **Spectrum of activity.** IDU's therapeutic effect is limited to the large DNA viruses herpes simplex (HSV) types 1 and 2, varicella (chicken pox, varicella zoster virus [VZV]), and vaccinia. There is also in vitro activity against herpes zoster (VZV) and cytomegalovirus (CMV), but this has no useful clinical application.
      2. **Mechanism of action.** Drug entry is via thymidine transport in normal cells and diffusion across leaky membranes in infected cells. IDU competes with cellular thymidine for phosphorylation by thymidine kinase (TK). As a triphosphate, it is preferentially incorporated into viral and, to a certain extent, into host cellular DNA (thus host toxicity). This DNA is fragile, and abnormal viral and host proteins result from faulty transcription. IDU also interferes with the activity of viral TK and DNA polymerase by feedback inhibition, thereby again interfering with viral and some host DNA synthesis.
      3. **Routes of administration and dosage.** Because of its toxicity, IDU is used only topically as a 0.1% drop every 1–2 hours by day and every 2–3 hours at night, 0.5% ointment 5 times daily or drops q1–2h by day and ointment HS for 2 weeks in acute infectious keratitis, or at lower doses as prophylaxis with concurrent steroid therapy (See specific viral infections). There is no indication for systemic, subconjunctival, or intravitreal administration.
      4. **Ocular penetration and metabolism.** IDU is minimally soluble in water (0.1%) and penetrates the cornea very poorly, limiting its efficacy to epithelial dis-

ease. The drug is rapidly metabolized in serum or tissue to an inactive compound, iodouracil. In herpetic corneal ulcers not complicated by concomitant use of steroids for viral immune disease, IDU is as efficacious (85–90%) as Ara A, F_3T, and ACV (90–95%). In the face of steroid therapy, however, this drug falls to 70–80% efficacy compared with the others, which retain their therapeutic effect despite use of steroids.

5. **Adverse side effects**

   a. **Topical IDU** toxicity is not uncommon and includes short-term, reversible tissue changes due to interference with uninfected host cell DNA metabolism. These include superficial punctate keratitis (SPK), follicular conjunctivitis, lid margin thickening and keratinization, punctal occlusion, and ptosis. Long-term therapy may result in permanent conjunctival cicatrization, permanent punctal occlusion, and corneal scarring. A true **delayed hypersensitivity** reaction to IDU also may develop and is like any other local drug reaction: marked itching, puffy lid edema, redness, induration, and leathery dermatitis. This reaction resolves within 2–3 days of stopping the medication. Topical IDU is **teratogenic** in animals. No human data is available, but cautious use is advised in pregnant women.

   b. With the advent of less toxic antivirals, **systemic** IDU therapy is too toxic to justify its use.

   c. **Wound healing.** Topical IDU does not interfere with the rate of corneal epithelial wound healing, but does cause mild to moderate toxic intracellular edema. There also is significant interference with stromal wound healing, a factor of importance in thinning or recently transplanted corneas.

B. **Vidarabine** (Ara A; 9-β-D-arabinofuranosyl-adenine, Viral A) is a purine analog of the DNA base adenosine.

   1. **Spectrum of activity.** Vidarabine is clinically active against the DNA viruses herpes simplex types 1 and 2, herpes zoster, and vaccinia. It is more efficacious than IDU and slightly less effective than trifluridine when concomitant steroids are being used in the eye, with 80–90% of eyes healing by 14 days of treatment.

   2. **Mechanism of action.** The drug enters uninfected cells via the purine transport system and by diffusion across the membranes of viral infected cells. It is phosphorylated to the active triphosphate state in the cytoplasm by cellular enzymes. Absence of Ara A dependence on viral enzymes is of clinical importance. This drug is effective in certain infections in which viral resistance to more specific antivirals such as acyclovir and ganciclovir has developed via loss of the viral enzyme production necessary for drug phosphorylation. The active vidarabine triphosphate inhibits several viral and cellular enzymes, particularly viral DNA polymerase. Small amounts also are incorporated into

viral and cellular DNA, resulting in DNA chain termination.

3. **Routes of administration and dosage**

   a. **Topical.** The most common use of this drug is as a 3% ointment given 5 times daily for 14–21 days in therapy of infectious herpes simplex epithelial keratitis. It may also be used 2–3 times daily for several weeks as prophylaxis against recurrent corneal infection if immunosuppressive drugs are in use or in the presence of herpetic lid or periocular lesions. There is no efficacy against stromal herpes, which is primarily an immune reaction to viral antigen, and no proven effect in infectious herpes zoster epithelial keratitis.

   b. **Systemic.** Because of its relative lack of toxicity, vidarabine is a very useful systemic agent in treatment of herpes simplex encephalitis. The intravenous suspension is available as 200 mg/ml. Dosage of 15 mg/kg/day IV for 10 days reduces mortality from 70 to 28%. Intravenous vidarabine also is therapeutically effective in acute herpes zoster infections, including ophthalmicus, at dosage of 10 mg/kg/day for 5 days, particularly if begun within 6 days of onset of the rash and in patients under 40 years of age. With the advent of acyclovir, systemic vidarabine is now more useful as an alternative drug for treatment of acyclovir- or ganciclovir-resistant herpes simplex infections of the immunosuppressed.

   c. **There is no oral form** of vidarabine, and **intravitreal use** has **not** been **reported.**

4. **Ocular penetration and metabolism.** Although it is relatively insoluble (0.1%), topical 3% vidarabine ointment does penetrate the cornea to achieve virucidal concentrations of 6 μg/ml 2 hours after application. The drug is rapidly metabolized to hypoxanthine arabinoside, which possesses about 20% of the antiviral potency of the parent compound. It is excreted in the urine.

5. **Adverse side effects**

   a. **Topical** drug reactions are less frequent than those seen with IDU, because there is less interference with host cell metabolism. Toxic effects noted are largely reversible and include punctate keratitis, follicular conjunctivitis, and punctal occlusion. Prolonged treatment may, rarely, result in irreversible punctal occlusion, cicatricial conjunctivitis, and corneal scarring. Patients also may develop a true delayed hypersensitivity reaction, characterized by itching, redness, and lid and facial edema, all of which resolve on discontinuation of the drug. There is no cross-allergenicity between vidarabine and IDU or trifluridine.

   b. **Intravenous** vidarabine at doses of 5–15 mg/kg/day may produce nausea and diarrhea in a small percentage of patients. At doses of 15–20 mg/kg/day, many patients will develop gastrointestinal symptoms, bone marrow depression, and central nervous system toxicity, as manifested by tremor, dizziness, hallucinations, ataxia, confusion, and encephalopathy.

c. **Wound healing.** Vidarabine ointment has no adverse effect on rate of corneal epithelial wound healing, although there is mild cellular toxicity. However, stromal healing is significantly slowed. This factor should be considered in patients with active corneal thinning or in penetrating keratoplasty where interference with stromal healing is undesirable.

C. **Trifluridine (F_3T, TFT, Viroptic, trifluorothymidine)** is a thymidine analog similar in structure to IDU but halogenated with three fluoride atoms at the 5-methyl group of the pyrimidine base.

1. **Spectrum of activity.** This drug effectively inhibits several DNA viruses, including herpes simplex virus (HSV) types 1 and 2, vaccinia, adenovirus, and cytomegalovirus in vitro. However, its use is confined exclusively to topical therapy of HSV keratitis.

2. **Mechanism of action.** The drug enters the uninfected cell by the thymidine transport system and the infected cell by diffusion across the cell membrane. In its triphosphate nucleotide form, F_3T is a potent inhibitor of both viral and cellular thymidilate synthetases and thymidine kinase, enzymes essential to phosphorylation of nucleic acid bases before incorporation into the chain. The key antiviral event is probably the inhibition of viral DNA polymerase and incorporation of drug into viral DNA to produce defective virus. Drug action is not totally selective for viral products; some host cell toxicity and death occur at therapeutic levels and increase markedly at higher levels. Viruses deficient in thymidine kinase activity demonstrate increased resistance to F_3T, but in many cases the cellular TK enzyme will phosphorylate the drug to achieve clinical efficacy.

3. **Routes of administration and dosage**

a. **Topical F_3T** is given as a 1% drop to the HSV-infected eye 9 times daily for 14 days or 4–5 times daily as prophylaxis against infection over several weeks to months in high-risk patients. The drug is significantly more effective than IDU, especially with concurrent topical steroid use and probably more effective than Ara A in the presence of steroid use. Both F_3T and Ara A have healing rates in the 90–95% range. Absence of healing by 5–7 days may indicate toxicity or viral resistance. A viral culture or enzyme-linked immunosorbent assay (ELISA) test (Herpchek, DuPont) should be taken and therapy switched to IDU or Ara A.

b. **Systemic F_3T** is of no use in herpetic disease because of its marked cellular toxicity and its rapid metabolism into inactive byproducts. **Intravitreal** use has not been reported, but drug toxicity would dictate against this route.

4. **Ocular penetration and metabolism.** F_3T crosses the cornea with minimal catabolism to achieve therapeutically effective aqueous titers ranging from 5–50 μmol/liter, depending on the epithelial integrity. Its superior solubility (1%) makes F_3T preferable to IDU and Ara A in this regard. The drug is actively metabolized to trifluorothymine and deoxyribose by cellular enzymes, and it is very unstable at a pH greater than 7.6. These factors, coupled with toxicity, make F_3T of no use systemically.

5. **Adverse side effects**
   a. **Topical** F_3T is the most toxic of the ocular agents used, followed by IDU, Ara A, and acyclovir in descending order. Clinically, short-term, reversible adverse effects of F_3T include follicular conjunctivitis, superficial punctate keratitis, punctal occlusion, thickening and keratinization of the lid margins, meibomian gland pouting, and ptosis. Prolonged treatment may result in irreversible punctal occlusion and conjunctival and corneal scarring. Patients may also develop a true delayed-type hypersensitivity with itching, redness, puffy edema and dermatitis of the lids and face, and chemosis. Unlike IDU, topical F_3T has not been shown to be teratogenic in animals, but any antimetabolite should be used with **caution in pregnancy.**
   b. **Systemic** and **intravitreal** F_3T are not used clinically because of marked cell toxicity.
   c. **Wound healing** in the cornea is not affected with reference to the rate of epithelial closure, but the cells show more cytotoxicity than is seen with other antivirals. Similarly, stromal wound healing is impaired and should be taken into account in patients with thinned corneas or in recent postoperative situations.

D. **Acyclovir** [9-(2-hydroxyethoxymethyl) guanine, Zovirax, ACV] is the first of the second-generation antivirals, being selective in action and therefore significantly less toxic than IDU, Ara A, and F_3T. The drug is a purine analog similar to Ara A but with the deoxyribose ring broken open (acyclic nucleoside), a feature that conveys specificity of action.

1. **Spectrum of activity.** ACV is an extremely potent inhibitor in vitro of HSV types 1 and 2, and of varicella/zoster virus (VZV). There is minimal activity against the other herpesviruses, cytomegalovirus (CMV), and Epstein–Barr virus (EBV). Clinically, the drug is used primarily for HSV and VZV infections.

2. **Mechanism of action and resistance.** ACV penetrates both infected and uninfected cells. It is converted to its monophosphate form, however, only in the infected cells and only by viral, not cellular, thymidine kinase gene-specified deoxypyrimidine kinase. Subse-

quent phosphorylation to the active triphosphate state is by host-derived guanidylate kinase. ACV-triphosphate is the active antiviral. It is a highly effective inhibitor of viral DNA polymerase and, to some extent, incorporated into viral DNA as a chain terminator. The drug is essentially inactive in normal tissues.

Resistance to ACV is achieved through a single base mutation by the virus such that it lacks the genes for thymidine kinase and/or DNA polymerase. HSV and VZV resistant to ACV are still susceptible to Ara A, IDU, and F_3T because of their ability to use cellular enzymes for activation. Because of the ease of mutation and the selection of naturally existing resistant virus, ACV should be used judiciously and only in situations where it has been shown to be clinically effective.

3. **Routes of administration and dosage**
   a. **Topical** ACV is used as a 3% ophthalmic ointment 5 times daily for 14 days in therapy of infectious HSV keratitis. It appears to be as effective as Ara A and F_3T, even with concurrent steroid use. The ophthalmic drug is licensed for use in the United Kingdom, where it is also used for zoster keratitis, and in several other countries as well. It is not FDA approved for use in the eye in the United States. The ointment is available for ophthalmic use, however, on a compassionate plea basis from the manufacturer. A 5% ointment for genital herpes is FDA approved, but is too toxic for use in the eye because of the carrier vehicle.
   b. **Oral** ACV is available as 200-mg tablets for therapy of genital herpes. In the eye it is used primarily in treatment of acute herpes zoster ophthalmicus (HZO) at doses of 600–800 mg po 5 times daily for 10 days, preferably starting within 72 hours of onset of the rash. There is some controversial evidence that herpes simplex keratouveitis may respond favorably to 200 mg po 5 times daily, but the risks of the long-term treatment currently required may outweigh potential benefit. The drug is not FDA approved for either of the above uses. It is FDA approved for long-term use to prevent recurrent genital herpes with dosage of 400 mg po BID. Recurrence on prophylactic therapy is treated with 200 mg po 5 times daily for 5 days and then return to prophylaxis levels. There is a single report of a possible slow response of Epstein–Barr iritis responding over 5 months to oral ACV in doses used for zoster in combination with topical 3% ACV ointment qid and systemic steroids, the patient having failed to respond to steroids alone.
   c. **Intravenous** ACV has been particularly useful in therapy of herpes simplex and herpes zoster immunocompetent and immunocompromised patients with progressive cutaneous, CNS, or visceral dissemination of disease. The IV drug has also been highly effective in resolving zoster retinitis and

acute retinal necrosis (ARN), a disease usually due to zoster and occasionally to herpes simplex. Dosage is 5–10 mg/kg or 500 mg/m² IV q8h for 5–7 days (not FDA approved for this use).

   d. **Intravitreal** infusion of 10 and 40 μg/ml ACV has been reported in treatment of ARN coupled with vitrectomy and scleral buckle with resolution of disease and return of vision.

4. **Ocular penetration and metabolism.** ACV as a 3% ointment penetrates the intact corneal surface easily to achieve virucidal titers in the aqueous as unmetabolized drug (7.5 μmol/liter). Only 25% of **oral** ACV is absorbed from the GI tract, but this is sufficient to achieve virucidal serum levels. Because of minimal toxicity, very high serum levels (10 μg/ml) are achieved with **IV** administration. The ocular penetration after these routes of dosing is not known, but CSF concentrations are about 50% of serum levels. Seventy percent of the drug is excreted via the urinary system as unmetabolized ACV, the remainder as inactive carboxymethoxymethylguanine.

5. **Adverse side effects**
   a. **Topical** ACV has almost no adverse side effects, with only occasional punctate keratitis and conjunctivitis noted. One case of punctal occlusion was reported, but may have been due to the basic disease, zoster ophthalmicus.

   b. **Oral** ACV may produce nausea on a dose-dependent basis that, after adjustment, allows the patient to continue therapy. Rarely noted are headache, diarrhea, anorexia, leg pain, and rash. There is no significant bone marrow, liver, or neurotoxicity or teratogenicity. A potential toxic side effect is drug crystallization in the lower renal nephrons resulting in renal dysfunction reversible on drug discontinuation.

   c. **IV** ACV may produce a local phlebitis, nausea, vomiting, diaphoresis, and hypotension. At doses of 500 mg/m² or greater, renal toxicity, rash, headache, and hematuria may be noted. Mild bone marrow suppression and neuropsychiatric changes have been reported, but may have been due to concurrent drugs or disease. CBCs and creatinine levels should be checked every few weeks on chronic therapy.

   d. **Wound-healing** studies in the cornea indicate that ACV is the most benign antiviral of all. Topical ACV did not interfere with the rate and quality of epithelial healing and stromal wound healing. This latter factor makes it a drug of choice in corneal thinning situations where an antiviral is required.

E. **Ganciclovir [DHPG, Cytovene, 9-(1,3-dihydroxy-2-propoxymethyl) guanine].** This purine analog is a close relative of ACV, differing only in the addition of a 3'-methoxyl group to the acyclic side chain. It has the advantages over ACV of greater and more effective antiviral spectrum and higher solubility. The drug is now FDA approved for therapy of CMV retinitis.

1. **Spectrum of activity.** DHPG has excellent activity against herpes simplex virus types 1 and 2, herpes varicella zoster virus, and cytomegalovirus. It has good activity against Epstein–Barr virus. Currently its clinical use is for ocular and systemic CMV infections.

2. **Mechanism of action and resistance.** CMV does not encode for virus-specified thymidine kinase in infected cells and, therefore, fails to activate ACV. DHPG, however, is phosphorylated in CMV-infected cells by an unknown mechanism to its active form. This drug form inhibits CMV DNA polymerase with 30-fold greater efficacy than does ACV.

   Resistance of HSV and VZV to ganciclovir is through single base mutations in the DNA chain that result in changes in either the virus-encoded thymidine kinase or DNA polymerase genes. In the case of CMV, resistant strains have been reported, but the mechanisms have not yet been elucidated. Resistant virus may arise either by random mutation after multiple courses of drug therapy, or the drug may select out resistant viruses already present in the host.

3. **Routes of administration and dosage**
   a. **No oral** preparation is available for clinical use but GI-stable forms are under study.
   b. **Intravenous** DHPG is used for therapy of CMV retinitis, particularly in immunosuppressed patients. Dosage ranges from 5 mg/kg body weight bid for 3–4 weeks to 2.5 mg/kg q8h for 10 days and then maintenance dosage of 5 mg/kg/day 5 days weekly for several weeks. Recurrence of retinitis is treated with the initial high dose and maintenance given 7 days a week for several weeks.
   c. **Intravitreal** DHPG is used in patients myelosuppressed or hepatotoxic on systemic DHPG. It successfully suppresses CMV retinitis at dosages of 200–300 μg/0.1 ml. Induction therapy is 200 μgm/0.1 ml q2–3d for 6 doses and then once weekly maintenance during office visits. This may be repeated at least 56 times with no apparent increase in toxicity and may be coupled with systemic AZT therapy.

4. **Ocular penetration and metabolism.** Little is known of the ocular pharmacokinetics of DHPG. Although the drug is effective in therapy of CMV retinitis, gastrointestinal infection, and hepatitis, and variably effective in pneumonitis, it has not been effective in CMV encephalitis. This suggests limited blood–brain barrier penetration, although ocular effects indicate that therapeutic drug levels do enter the eye. After IV administration at doses of 15 mg/kg/day in three divided doses, peak serum concentrations at 2 hours were highly virucidal at 25 μmol/liter; 78% of the drug was excreted in the urine in unaltered state.

5. **Adverse side effects.** DHPG is minimally toxic, but

does have a greater suppressive effect on the bone marrow than does ACV at doses higher than 7.5 mg/kg/day in humans. Other side effects reported in animals include testicular atrophy, hepatotoxicity, diarrhea, vomiting, and obstructive nephropathy. CBCs and liver chemistries should be checked weekly to monthly.

F. **3-Azidothymidine (AZT, zidovudine, Retrovir)** is one of the few promising drugs in the therapy of AIDS. It is FDA approved for therapy of symptomatic and asymptomatic infection.

   1. **Spectrum of activity.** AZT inhibits the infectivity of the AIDS virus, the HIV (human immunodeficiency virus), both in vitro and in human studies. Recent evidence indicates that the virus breaks through after a period of improvement. This may be due to development of resistance or to overwhelming of the drug by a large viral burden.

   2. **Mechanism of action.** AZT is a nucleoside analog of thymidine that is activated by conversion to the triphosphate state. The activated drug appears to work by inhibition of the HIV reverse transcriptase by competing with cellular triphosphates for the substrates essential to formation of proviral DNA by the reverse transcriptase. There also is evidence that AZT is a nucleic acid chain terminator in the synthesis of proviral DNA.

   3. **Routes of administration and dosage.** For asymptomatic HIV infection, AZT is given as a 100 mg pill po every 4 hours while awake. For symptomatic HIV infection, starting dose for adults is 200 mg po q4h (1200 mg/d) for 1 m, then 100 mg po q4h (600 mg/d).

   4. **Ocular penetration and metabolism.** Little is known about the ocular pharmacodynamics of AZT. Successful therapy of AIDS-related neurologic abnormalities and iritis indicate that the drug crosses the blood–brain and blood–eye barriers in therapeutic levels.

   5. **Adverse side effects.** AZT may induce significant bone marrow suppression, with resulting leukopenia and anemia. CBCs should be checked weekly to monthly. Other reported adverse reactions include headache, asthenia, diarrhea, abdominal pain, fever, and grand mal seizures. The drug also may interact adversely with concurrent acyclovir to produce almost overwhelming fatigue reversible on discontinuing either drug. It should not be used with IV DHPG because both are myelosuppressives.

G. **Foscarnet (PFA, phosphonoformate),** like phosphonoacetic acid (PAA), is a unique antiviral agent that does not require metabolic activation.

   1. **Spectrum of activity.** PFA is effective against viruses possessing genes that encode for DNA polymerase. These include HSV types 1 and 2, VZV, CMV, EBV, hepatitis B, vaccinia, and possibly AIDS virus. The drug is used on a study basis as therapy of CMV reti-

nitis and of viruses resistant to acyclovir, particularly HSV types 1 and 2. Resistant strains of HSV and CMV are emerging more frequently among AIDS patients.

2. **Mechanism of action.** The drug works by binding to the pyrophosphate exchange site of the viral DNA polymerase. PFA also binds to the viral polymerase with 10–30 times the affinity it has for cellular DNA polymerase, thus reducing its toxicity.

3. **Route of administration and dosage.** PFA is given IV in dosage of 50–60 mg/kg body weight tid for about 2–3 weeks with longer-term maintenance given once daily.

4. **Ocular penetration and metabolism.** No data are available on ocular penetration, but initial studies indicate efficacy similar to that of ganciclovir in therapy of CMV retinitis in AIDS patients, suggesting that it crosses the blood–eye barrier in therapeutic levels.

5. **Adverse side effects.** PFA is not myelosuppressive, but is nephrotoxic and should be used with caution in patients with renal failure.

III. Clinical Management of Ocular Viral Disease

A. **Herpes simplex virus (HSV)** infection of the eyes is almost invariably due to type 1 HSV, except in congenital disease, where type 2 is more frequent. Both viruses have similar drug susceptibilities. Ocular HSV is managed according to its diagnostic category. Not infrequently, patients may have two or more forms of disease, infectious and immune, at the same time. In these cases therapies must be adjusted and combined.

1. **Infectious epithelial herpes** is primary (first infection) or recurrent (established antibodies and cellular immunity from previous exposure).

a. **Clinically,** infectious epithelial herpes is characterized by the variable presence of clear to crusting umbilicated lid vesicles, conjunctival tearing and hyperemia, and branching dendritic, dendrogeographic, or irregular, map-shaped corneal ulcers. Primary disease tends to have much more extensive periocular involvement than does recurrent disease, and, if the cornea is also infected, atypical diffusely scattered dendrites. The stroma or deeper tissues may or may not be involved in concurrent immune reaction.

b. **Diagnosis** is usually based on clinical impression, but may be supported by the office diagnostic test, Herpchek (DuPont), or by sending the patient for tissue culture studies in a major medical center. Serial serologic tests 1 month apart showing a rise in HSV antibody from <1:8 to >1:16 indicates primary disease. Serial titers are unreliable in the diagnosis of recurrent HSV.

c. **Therapy** is gentle debridement of the ulcer to remove excess antigen using a sterile, soft-tip applicator. Antiviral drops or ointment (Table 7-1) are begun the same day and continued for 2–3 weeks. See specific antivirals (Part II) for details of resistance or toxicity. If the cornea is not ulcerated but lids or conjunctiva are infected, drug dosage may be lowered to **prophylactic** levels of IDU 6–8 times/day, F_3T qud, or IDU or Ara A ointment tid for 2 weeks.

2. **Trophic post-HSV ulcer** is a sterile epithelial defect that looks much like an infected geographic ulcer. It is, in fact, the result of previous viral damage to the basement membrane, thus causing a mechanical healing problem.

   a. **Clinically,** trophic post-HSV ulcer may be recognized by its indolent, often ovoid shape, thickened gray edges, and tendency to heal and break in cycles.

   b. **Diagnosis** is based on clinical suspicion of a persistent ulcer in a patient adequately treated with antivirals and having the above clinical pattern. Viral cultures and Herpchek are negative.

   c. **Therapy** includes application of a high-water-content therapeutic soft contact lens (SCL), such as the Sauflon flat (9.0 BC, 14.5 diameter) or plano Permalens (9.0 BC, 15.0 diameter) until healthy epithelium has healed across the ulcer base, usually 1–3 months. Antibiotic drops bid are advisable along with artificial tears qid for lubrication. If melting and cornea thinning ensue, sealing the ulcer with cyanoacrylate tissue adhesive (Nexacryl) and the use of SCL and artificial tears may prevent corneal perforation. Use of tissue adhesive in corneal ulcers is currently under study in anticipation of FDA review. Antivirals are not indicated except as prophylaxis if steroids are in use for stromal disease.

3. **Limbal vasculitis** is thought to be a local immune Arthus immediate-type hypersensitivity reaction.

   a. **Clinically** limbal vasculitis is recognized by focal or extensive limbal hyperemia and edema, which can become quite intense.

   b. **Diagnosis** is by clinical appearance.

   c. **Therapy** ranges from nothing if the disease is mild to ⅛% prednisolone qid with gradual taper for more marked cases. In patients prone to infectious virus recurrences or those receiving higher steroid dosages, prophylactic antiviral therapy (see **1.c** above) should be used until a ⅛% prednisolone therapy level of once or twice daily is reached.

4. **Stromal immune disease** may present in three forms, alone or in combination: (1) white, necrotic **interstitial keratitis (IK),** often with deep neovascularization, (2) Wessley **immune rings,** partial or complete, and (3) **disciform edema,** which may be focal or diffuse and with or without keratic precipitates (KPs, lymphocytes) clinging to the affected endothelium.

   a. **Clinically IK** and the rings are thought to be immediate hypersensitivity reactions and disciform to be delayed hypersensitivity. All are recognized by

Table 7-1. Antiviral agents

Drug	Class	Spectrum of activity in vitro	Therapeutic use	Dosage	FDA approved
Idoxuridine (IDU, Stoxil, Herplex)	Pyrimidine nucleoside	HSV-1, HSV-2, VZV, CMV, vaccinia	HSV-1 and HSV-2 keratitis	0.1% q1h by day, q2h at night, 2–3 wks	Yes
				0.5% ointment 5 times/day, 2–3 wks	Yes
				Prophylaxis: reduce dose daily by 40–50%	—
Vidarabine (Ara A, Vira A)	Purine nucleoside	HSV-1, HSV-2, VZV, CMV, vaccinia	HSV-1 and HSV-2 keratitis and encephalitis, varicella keratitis	5% ointment 5 times/day, 2–3 wks (ocular)	Yes
				15 mg/kg/d, IV, 7–10d (encephalitis)	Yes
Trifluorothymidine (TFT, F₃T, Viroptic)	Pyrimidine nucleoside	HSV-1, HSV-2, VZV, CMV	HSV-1 and HSV-2 keratitis	1% drop 9 times/day, 2–3 wks	Yes
Acyclovir (Zovirax)	Purine acyclic sugar	HSV-1, HSV-2, VZV, EBV, CMV	HSV-1 and HSV-2 keratitis, VZV ophthalmicus, ? EBV + CMV borderline efficacy, iritis, retinitis	3% ointment 5 times/day, 2–3 wks (keratitis)	No
				800 mg 5 times/day, 10d (VZV ophthal.)	Pending review

Acute retinal necrosis (ARN)	500 mg/m², IV q8h, 7d (ARN, VZV retinitis)	No
Mucosal, skin, HSV-1 and HSV-2 in immunocompromised, primary and recurrent genital HSV	5 mg/kg, IV, q8h, 5–10d (HSV retinitis)	No
	5 mg/kg, IV, over 1h, q8h, 5–7d (skin, mucosa of immunocompromised, severe primary genital HSV)	Yes
	5% ointment, 6 times/day, 2 wks (primary genital HSV—*not* ocular form)	Yes
	400 mg po BID, 1–3 yrs (prophylaxis recurrent genital HSV) 200 mg po 5 times/day, 5d then 400 mg po BID, 1–3 yrs (breakthrough genital HSV)	Yes

Table 7-1. (continued)

Drug	Class	Spectrum of activity in vitro	Therapeutic use	Dosage	FDA approved
Ganciclovir (DHPG, Cytovene)	Purine acyclic sugar	HSV-1, HSV-2, VZV, EBV, CMV	CMV retinitis, and disseminated disease	2.5 mg/kg, IV, q8h, 10d, then 5 mg/kg/d, 5d/wk maintenance or 7d/wk if recurrent 200–300 µg/0.1 ml, intravitreal, ×2–3 injections (CMV retinitis)	Yes
Azidothymidine (AZT, Retrovir)	Purine nucleoside	HIV (HTLV-III, AIDS virus)	HIV infection (HIV uveitis)	Symptomatic: 200 mg po q4h, 1 m, then 100 mg po q4h. Asymptomatic: 100 mg po q4h indefinitely	Under FDA IND Yes (No)
Phosphonoformate (PFA, Foscarnet)	Phosphonoacids	HSV-1, HSV-2, CMV, EBV, hepatitis B, vaccinia	CMV retinitis	60 mg/kg, IV, tid, 2–3 wks, then 60 mg qd 5d/wk maintenance	Under FDA IND

HSV, herpes simplex virus; VZV, varicella-zoster virus; CMV, cytomegalovirus; EBV, Epstein–Barr virus. IND, investigational new drug.

the above clinical descriptions and may be associated with epithelial ulcers or iritis.

b. Diagnosis is based on clinical appearance.

c. Therapy is nothing or artificial tears for mild cases. Moderate to severe disease that threatens the visual axis, develops progressive neovascularization, or occurs in patients previously treated with steroids is managed with continued topical steroid drops. The dose range is ⅛% prednisolone daily up to 0.1% dexamethasone 6–8 times daily for a short time in more severe reactions. Taper of steroid therapy is gradual, dropping the dose no more than 50% at a time. Antiviral prophylaxis is used as noted in **1.c** (see also Table 7-1). Daily antibiotics are advisable at higher steroid doses.

5. Herpetic iritis is a diffuse lymphocytic infiltrate of the iris stroma. Infectious virus may play a role in this disease as well.

a. Clinically there is deep aching, tearing, limbal hyperemia, cells and flare in the anterior chamber, and a miotic pupil. The cornea may have active disease, either immune or infectious.

b. Diagnosis is based on clinical exam.

c. Therapy is cycloplegia only for mild disease or topical steroids as in stromal disease for more severe forms along with cycloplegia. If the cornea is ulcerated, topical therapy should be minimized and systemic steroid such as prednisone 50–80 mg po in two divided doses after meals and tapered over 7–10 days. Antiviral prophylaxis is advisable for higher-dose steroid levels or in patients known to have infectious recurrences. The potential value of systemic ACV 200 mg po qd in HSV keratouveitis is currently under multicenter study. No data is available as yet.

6. Combined infectious epithelial and stromal immune disease is managed by initially treating with full antiviral therapy and little or no topical steroid for 1–2 days before increasing steroids to the level necessary to control the immune reaction. Full antiviral therapy is given for 2–3 weeks before discontinuing or dropping back to prophylactic levels, depending on steroid dose (see Part II A 1c and 3c).

7. Combined trophic ulcer and stromal immune disease is treated by application of a continuous-wear therapeutic soft contact lens, artificial tears qid, antibiotic drops bid, and, if needed to increase lens tolerance, cycloplegia bid. Topical steroids such as ⅛ prednisolone bid to 0.1% dexamethasone bid may be introduced at the same time to control stromal disease. Because of a risk of corneal thinning, taper of the steroids as rapidly as possible to the lowest dose that will control the immune reaction is recommended. In the presence of active thinning, 1% medroxyprogesterone (Provera) may be a safer steroid, as it does not interfere with collagen synthesis, but its potency is somewhat less than ⅛% prednisolone. Cyanoacrylate tissue adhesive (Nexacryl) also may be indicated in active melting (see **2.c** above). To minimize interference with stromal healing, antiviral therapy is either not used or kept at prophylactic levels.

B. **Herpes zoster/varicella virus** (VZV) infections are caused by the same organism, the chicken pox virus.

1. **Varicella or chicken pox** is the primary infection with this virus.

a. **Clinically,** in the eye the virus may produce vesiculopapular lesions on the lids and conjunctiva, classically at the limbus. Focal scarring may occur. The infectious keratitis may be punctate or dendritic, and an immune reaction in the stroma similar to the disciform reaction of herpes may occur weeks to months after the original infection.

b. **Diagnosis** of infectious disease may be made on clinical findings and confirmed, if necessary, by viral tissue culture or by scrapings for Giemsa stain (pink intranuclear inclusion bodies denote either HZV or VZV infection, but not which one).

c. **Therapy** of the infectious form of ocular disease is full-dose topical vidarabine (see Table 7-1) for 2 weeks. Stromal immune disease is managed with mild topical steroids. Antivirals are not indicated in immune keratitis.

2. **Herpes zoster ophthalmicus (HZO)** is the recurrent form of chicken pox and is precipitated by a depressed white cell-mediated immune response whether through aging, AIDS, blood dyscrasia, or iatrogenic immunosuppression of organ transplant recipients— all increasing factors in our society.

a. **Clinically,** HZO may begin with headache, malaise, fever, chills, and neuralgia. This is followed within 2–3 days by edema, erythema, and the eruption of often multiple crops of vesicles in the affected dermatome, the first division of cranial nerve VII. The lesions do not cross the midline and may map out the dermatome accurately, often leaving behind telltale pitted scars after the vesicles have resolved 2–3 weeks after onset. Because the virus may spread through the orbit to involve many nerves inside and outside the eye, complications are many. They include cicatricial lid retraction, paralytic ptosis, conjunctivitis, scleritis, keratitis (dendritic and sterile trophic ulcers, and interstitial, immune ring, and disciform stromal immune disease), iridocyclitis, retinitis (hemorrhagic vasculitis), acute retinal necrosis (ARN), optic neuritis, retrobulbar neuritis, Argyll-Robertson pupil, secondary glaucoma, 3rd, 4th, or 6th nerve palsies, and sympathetic ophthalmia. Corneal anesthesia is much denser in HZO than in comparable herpes simplex keratitis.

b. **Diagnosis** is based on clinical observation and may be confirmed by viral tissue culture on human-derived cells usually available in major medical centers. Smears with Giemsa may show intranuclear inclusions, indicating VZV or HZV infection. Serial serologic tests 1 month apart may show a diagnostic two-fold rise in titer against zoster.

c. **Therapy** is systemic and topical and may be summarized as follows:

(1) For all but the mildest disease of skin and eye, **acyclovir** (Zovirax) 200 mg 3–4 tablets po 5 times daily for 10 days, preferably starting within 72 hours of onset of disease in immunocompetent patients. For immunocompromised patients 800 mg po 5 times daily for 10 days or, for these patients or those with even the mildest retinitis or ARN: intravenous acyclovir 500 mg/m^2 body surface area is given q8h over 1 hour infusion for 7–10 days (acyclovir is not yet FDA approved for the above indications). Systemic ACV has been shown to stop viral replication, hasten recovery, and minimize acute and late corneal or uveal disease, but not to affect post-herpetic neuralgia.

(2) Mild or no pain or ocular involvement: **warm compresses** to keep involved skin clean and minimize scarring.

(3) For moderate to severe corneal disciform disease with intact epithelium (IK and immune rings are minimally responsive) or for iritis: **topical steroids** ($\frac{1}{8}$% prednisolone 2–4 times daily up to 0.1% dexamethasone in the same frequency, as warranted by disease). Taper over several weeks.

(4) **Antiviral** ointment or drops are **optional** unless there is any question that herpes simplex may be mimicking HZO. Some British studies indicate that 3% acyclovir ointment 5 times a day for 2–3 weeks has highly favorable effects on zoster keratouveitis provided steroids are not used.

(5) Topical **antibiotics** should be used once or twice daily if there is an open ulcer or steroids are in use.

(6) **Cycloplegics** as needed for iritis.

(7) **Artificial tears** and ointment for unstable tear film or exposure keratopathy.

(8) Nonnarcotic or narcotic **analgesics** daily for 7–10 days for significant or increasing neuralgia. If there is no resolution of pain at this time and the patient is immunocompetent, consider instituting **systemic steroids.** Dosage commonly given is prednisone 20 mg po tid–qid for 7 days, then 15 mg po bid for 7 days, then 15 mg po daily for 7 days before stopping. All other medications as above are continued as indicated. Monitor the patient carefully for dissemination; consult with in-

ternist or dermatologist. Use only with great caution (or not at all) in immunocompromised patients (such as in AIDS) and with an internist directly involved. Systemic steroids are the only drug shown in some studies to prevent or minimize post-herpetic neuralgia, but this point is still controversial.

(9) For chronic exposure or corneal thinning with ulceration, **therapeutic soft contact lenses, cyanoacrylate tissue adhesive** (not yet FDA approved for the eye), **partial tarsorrhaphy, conjunctival flap,** or (rarely) **corneal transplant with partial tarsorrhaphy** if perforation occurs or threatens. See Herpes simplex trophic ulcers.

(10) For chronic **post-herpetic neuralgia,** nonnarcotic **analgesics;** 90% will resolve spontaneously over 9–12 months. **Antidepressants** such as amitriptyline or imipramine 50 mg TID or QID po are highly effective in all longterm pain. For severe persistent incapacitating neuralgia not controlled medically, consider **trigeminal block or ablation** as a last resort.

C. **Cytomegalovirus (CMV)** is a herpesvirus transmitted in 2–3% of all live births. Ocular manifestations are chorioretinitis and optic atrophy and are a sign of systemic infection whether congenital or adult-onset.

1. **Clinical** findings differ in the two groups.

a. **Congenital CMV** infection of the eye may be peripheral or in the posterior pole and range from just a few patchy peripheral retinal infiltrates or vasculitis to total bilateral retinal necrosis. Lesions frequently mimic congenital toxoplasmosis and resolve to leave heavily pigmented and atrophic chorioretinal scars.

b. **Adult-acquired CMV** infection may result from reactivated congenital infection or occur as a new infection via fomites, sexual contact, or contaminated blood. More than 80% of the young adult population is CMV positive on serologic testing. Immunosuppression is the key triggering factor to disease. The rapidly spreading AIDS epidemic and increasing numbers of organ transplants in this age group are making this normally latent CMV infection clinically active in thousands of patients. Clinical appearance of the eye varies with location and may be the presenting disease in immunosuppressed patients or an asymptomatic finding in early AIDS or in ARC (AIDS-related complex). Typically the posterior pole is involved, with dense, patchy, white retinal necrosis most frequently along the vascular arcades and often with intraretinal hemorrhaging. These areas of active retinitis are invariably preceded by cotton-wool spots (microinfarctions due to deposition of AIDS immune complexes), which damage vascular endothelium, allowing CMV access to the retina. Peripheral CMV of the retina is a more granular, white retinitis that is less intense and may or may not have associated hemorrhages. CMV retinitis of AIDS often may be distinguished from that of patients immunosuppressed from other causes. Untreated AIDS patients have a vitritis due to intact granular cell function, whereas the other groups tend to have quiet vitreous due to panleukopenia.

2. **Diagnosis** is based on clinical appearance and on isolation of CMV from urine, white cell buffy coat, and/or saliva.

3. **Therapy** is generally unsatisfactory in the long run, but effective for weeks or months given as systemic ganciclovir (DHPG) and/or intravitreal DHPG or, in resistant cases, with systemic foscarnet (PFA). DHPG (Cytovene) is FDA approved for ocular use.

   a. **Ganciclovir** is given initially as 2.5 mg/kg IV q8h for 10 days and then changed to maintenance dosage of 5 mg/kg/day 5 days weekly indefinitely or until the basic immunosuppression can be resolved. Recurrent disease is treated with restarting the initial dose and giving maintenance therapy 7 days/week.

   b. **Intravitreal ganciclovir** is being used in increasing numbers of IV DHPG-toxic patients, and with very encouraging results. Indications are either host myelosuppression forcing discontinuation of systemic ganciclovir for CMV retinitis or progressive retinitis despite maximum tolerable doses of IV drug. Intravitreal dose is 200–300 μg in 0.1 ml, which may be repeated multiple (>56) times as necessary, with no discernible local or systemic drug toxicity. An acute rise in intraocular pressure from the increased vitreous volume may necessitate anterior chamber paracentesis with a 25-gauge needle and syringe for decompression if optic disc circulation is compromised more than 2–3 minutes or IOP remains at >40 more than 30 minutes.

   c. **Foscarnet (FPA)** is an experimental drug reported to be therapeutically effective in both HSV and CMV infections. It is effective in viral strains resistant to acyclovir or ganciclovir. Dosage is 60 mg/kg body weight tid for 2–3 weeks before starting maintenance dose once daily; optimal dosage is yet to be ascertained.

D. **Epstein-Barr virus (EBV)** is also a herpesvirus, the etiologic agent of infectious mononucleosis and probably African Burkitt's lymphoma and nasopharyngeal carcinoma.

   1. **Clinically** in the eye the virus may cause a follicular conjunctivitis, epithelial punctate or microdendritic keratitis, or immune anterior stromal pleomorphic, nummular, or ring-shaped deposits. The uveal tract may be involved in acute or chronic iritis or pancho-

rioretinitis. Neurologic lesions include optic neuritis, papilledema, convergence insufficiency, and extraocular muscle paresis.

2. **Diagnosis** is by heterophile or Monostat serologic testing for EBV antibodies at diagnostic titers.

3. **Therapy** of EBV ocular disease is still ill defined. External disease and neurologic manifestations usually self-resolve. Uveitis may or may not respond well to topical and/or systemic steroids, but should be tried if disease severity warrants. One case report of successful therapy of EBV panuveitis resistant to steroids involved 10 months of combined oral acyclovir 600 mg po 5 times daily, with no success until topical 3% acyclovir ointment qid was added in combination with topical and systemic steroids. Over the ensuing 5 months, the eye disease totally resolved.

E. **Acquired immune deficiency syndrome (AIDS)** is caused by the human immunodeficiency virus (HIV). It is a transmissible viral infection of the cellular immune system characterized by multiple, recurring, opportunistic infections with or without neoplasms or neuropsychiatric disorders. Ocular opportunistic infection may be the presenting illness.

1. **Clinically** the ocular findings in AIDS and ARC (AIDS-related complex) include punctate or geographic ulcerative keratitis, follicular conjunctivitis, Kaposi's sarcoma, iritis, glaucoma, retinal cotton-wool spots (white, fluffy, nerve fiber layer microinfarctions), retinal hemorrhages, Roth's spots, microaneurysms, ischemic maculopathy, retinal periphlebitis, and papilledema. Although the HIV itself appears capable of producing any of the above, probably through deposition of immune complexes in the vessels and by direct viral invasion, multiple opportunistic ocular infections also may be superimposed. These include herpes simplex virus, varicella zoster, CMV, cryptococcus, toxoplasma, *Candida,* and *Mycobacterium avium-intracellulare* choroidal granulomas. Herpes zoster ophthalmicus or CMV retinitis in a previously healthy, relatively young person is AIDS until proven otherwise.

2. **Diagnosis** is made by culture of the virus from tears, conjunctiva, corneal epithelium, or blood. Serologic testing for HIV antibody and assessment of the ratio of T-helper to T-suppressor lymphocytes.

3. **Therapy** is unsatisfactory in terms of cure, but palliative treatment is now available in the form of azidothymidine (AZT, zidovudine). For symptomatic infection 200 mg po q4h for 1m, then 100 mg po q4h. For asymptomatic AIDS, 100 mg po q4h as long as tolerated or effective. The drug inhibits viral replication, prolongs survival, and improves the quality of life in AIDS patients. CMV retinitis may respond well to AZT therapy alone by increasing immunocompetence. One steroid-recalcitrant iridocyclitis in a patient growing HIV from the aqueous humor responded well to AZT 100

mg po qid for 10 days and then 200 mg po q4h for an additional 2 weeks. There have recently been reports, however, of HIV breakthrough during AZT treatment of AIDS due possibly to emergence of resistant virus. Other antivirals of use in opportunistic viral infection in AIDS include acyclovir for herpes simplex and zoster and ganciclovir for CMV. AZT and acyclovir may interact adversely. See specific drugs in this chapter.

F. **Adenovirus** infection of the eyes is a self-limited DNA viral disease.

   1. **Clinically** it is characterized acutely by moderate to severe ocular discomfort, preauricular adenopathy, lid edema, hyperemic follicular conjunctivitis, occasional iritis, and often a punctate keratitis, which may leave behind classic round anterior stromal immune deposits. There may be sore throat and fever to 104° F. The acute disease resolves in 10–14 days and the corneal deposits over several weeks to months.

   2. **Diagnosis** is by clinical appearance and confirmed by viral isolation on tissue culture, where available. Scrapings show monocytes, but no epithelial inclusion bodies.

   3. **Therapy** is largely reassuring the patient that the illness will self-resolve. Antivirals have been of no therapeutic use, and mild steroids (1/8% prednisolone 2–3 times/day for 1–2 weeks) will relieve acute symptoms and corneal infiltrates, but the latter will recur when steroids are withdrawn.

Information Sources and Suggested Reading (*Antivirals*)

1. Bach, M., Possible drug interaction during therapy with azidothymidine and acyclovir for AIDS. [Letter]. N. Engl. J. Med. 316:547, 1987.

2. Chatis, P., Miller, C., Schrager, L., and Crumpacker, C., Successful treatment with Foscarnet of an acyclovir-resistant mucocutaneous infection with herpes simplex virus in a patient with AIDS. N. Engl. J. Med. 320:297–300, 1989.

3. Ehrlich, K., Mills, J., Chatis, P., et al., Acyclovir-resistant herpes simplex virus infections in patients with AIDS. N. Engl. J. Med. 320:293–296, 1989.

4. Ellis, P., *Ocular Therapeutics and Pharmacology*, 7th ed. St. Louis: C.V. Mosby, 1985, pp. 291–293 (antiviral agents).

5. Erice, A., Chou, S., Biron, K.K., Stanat, S.C., Balfour, H.H., Jr., and Jordan, M.C., Progressive disease due to ganciclovir-resistant cytomegalovirus in immmomocompromised patients. N. Engl. J. Med. 320:289–293, 1989.

6. Farrell, P., Heinemann, M.-H., Roberts, C., Polsky, B., Gold, J., and Mamelok, A., Responsive human immunodeficiency virus-associated uveitis to zidovudine. Am. J. Ophthalmol. 106:7–10, 1988.

7. Fischer, P., and Prusoff, W., Chemotherapy of ocular viral infections and tumors. In Sears, M.L. (Ed.), *Pharmacology of*

the Eye. Vol. 69, Handbook of Experimental Pharmacology. New York: Springer-Verlag, 1984, pp. 553–584.

8. Fraunfelder, F., and Roy, F.H. (Eds.), *Current Ocular Therapy 3,* 3rd ed. Philadelphia: W.B. Saunders, 1990, multiple contributing authors, pp. 72–97 (viral infections).

9. Harris, P., and Caceres, C., Azidothymidine in the treatment of AIDS. [Letter]. N. Engl. J. Med. 318:250, 1988.

10. Havener, W.H., Antiviral drugs. *Ocular Pharmacology,* 5th ed. St. Louis: C.V. Mosby, 1983, pp. 244–260 (antiviral drugs).

11. Heineman, M.-H., Long-term intravitreal ganciclovir therapy for cytomegalovirus retinopathy. Arch. Ophthalmol. 107:1767–1772, 1989.

12. Hermans, P., and Cockerill, F., III., Symposium on antimicrobial agents—part IV: antiviral agents. Mayo Clin. Proc. 58:217–222, 1983.

13. Hymes, K., Greene, J., and Karpatkin, S., Effect of azidothymidine on HIV-related thrombocytopenia. [Letter]. N. Engl. J. Med. 318:516–517, 1988.

14. Kaufman, H.E., and Rayfield, M., Viral conjunctivitis and keratitis. In Kaufman, H.E., McDonald, M., Barron, B., and Waltman, S. (Eds.), *The Cornea.* New York: Churchill Livingstone, 1988, pp. 299–332.

15. Kini, M., Retina and vitreous. In Pavan-Langston, D. (Ed.), *Manual of Ocular Diagnosis and Therapeutics.* Boston: Little, Brown, 1990, pp. 139–161.

16. Kleinert, R., Corticosteroid use in ocular infectious disease. In Tabbara, K.F., and Hyndiuk, R.A. (Eds.), *Infections of the Eye.* Boston: Little, Brown, 1986, pp. 293–302.

17. Lass, J., Antivirals. In Lamberts, D.W., and Potter, D.E. (Eds.), *Clinical Ophthalmic Pharmacology.* Boston: Little, Brown, 1987, pp. 107–156.

18. Liesegang, T., Ocular herpes simplex infection: pathogenesis and current therapy. Mayo Clin. Proc. 63:1092–1105, 1988.

19. Leopold, I.H., Anti-infective agents. In Sears, M.L. (Ed.), *Pharmacology of the Eye.* Vol. 69, Handbook of Experimental Pharmacology. New York: Springer-Verlag, 1984, pp. 441–443 (antivirals).

20. Max, M., Schafer, S., Culnane, M., et al., Amitriptylene but not lorazepam relieves postherpatic neuralgia. Neurology 38:1427–1432, 1988.

21. Nussenblatt, R.B., and Palestine, A.G., *Uveitis: Fundamentals in Clinical Practice.* Chicago: Yearbook Medical Publ., 1989, pp. 407–415 (acute retinal necrosis), pp. 416–430 (viral uveitis).

22. Pavan-Langston, D., and Dunkel, E., Principles of antiviral chemotherapy. In Duane, T.D., *Biochemical Foundations of Ophthalmology.* Philadelphia: Harper & Row, 1986, Vol. 2: Chap. 100.

23. Pavan-Langston, D., Herpetic infections. In Smolin, G., and Thoft, R.A. (Eds.), *The Cornea,* 2nd ed. Boston: Little, Brown, 1987, pp. 240–266.

24. Pavan-Langston, D., Uveal tract. In Pavan-Langston, D. (Ed.), *Manual of Ocular Diagnosis and Therapy,* 3rd ed. Boston: Little, Brown, 1990, pp. 163–200.

25. Pavan-Langston, D., and Foulks, G., Cornea and external

disease, in *Manual of Ocular Diagnosis and Therapy,* 3rd ed. Boston: Little, Brown, 1990, pp. 65–117.

26. Pavan-Langston, D., Ocular viral diseases. In Galasso, G., Merigan, T., and Whitley, R. (Eds.), *Antiviral Agents and Viral Diseases of Man,* 3rd ed. New York: Raven Press, 1990, pp. 207–245.

27. Pepose, J., Newman, C., Bach, M., et al., Pathologic features of cytomegalovirus retinopathy after treatment with antiviral agent ganciclovir. Ophthalmology 94:414–424, 1987.

28. Pizzo, P., Eddy, J., Falloon, J., et al., Effect of continuous intravenous infusion of zidovudine (AZT) in children with symptomatic HIV infection. N. Engl. J. Med. 319:889–896, 1988.

29. Pollard, R., Egbert, P., Gallagher, J., and Merigan, T., Cytomegalovirus retinitis in immunosuppressed hosts: adenine arabinoside. Ann. Intern. Med. 93:655–664, 1980.

30. Samet, J., and Nero, A., Failure of zidovudine to maintain remission in patients with AIDS. [Letter]. N. Engl. J. Med. 320:594–595, 1989.

31. Sande, M., and Mandell, G., Antifungal and antiviral agents. In Gilman, A.G., Goodman, L.S., Rall, T., and Murad, F. (Eds.), *The Pharmacological Basis of Therapeutics,* 7th ed. New York: Macmillan, 1985, pp. 1219–1239.

32. Satterthwaite, J., Tollison, C.D., Kriegel, M., Use of tricyclic antidepressants for the treatment of intractable pain. Compr. Ther. 16(4):10–15, 1990.

33. Schwab, I. Oral acyclovir in the management of herpes simplex ocular infections. Ophthalmology 95:423–430, 1988.

34. Smolin, G., and Thoft, R.A. (Eds.), *The Cornea.* Boston: Little, Brown, 1986, pp. 156–168 (viral microbiology, Oh, J.), pp. 240–265 (herpes simplex and zoster, Pavan-Langston, D.), pp. 266–284 (adenovirus, misc. viruses, Vastine, D.).

35. Survival in AIDS patients receiving zidovudine. Hosp. Ther. 2:14, 1989.

36. Tabbara, K.F., and Hyndiuk, R.A. (Eds.), *Infections of the Eye.* Boston: Little, Brown, 1986, multiple contributing authors, pp. 93–106 (diagnostic virology), pp. 257–274 (antiviral agents), pp. 343–368 (herpes simplex keratitis), pp. 369–386 (varicella-zoster), pp. 387–412 (nonherpetic viral keratitis), pp. 437–460 (conjunctivitis), pp. 487–498 (viral retinitis), pp. 625–634 (AIDS).

37. Ussery, F., Gibson, S., Conklin, R., Piot, D., Stool, E., Conklin, A., Intravitreal ganciclovir in treatment of AIDS-associated cytomegalovirus retinitis. Ophthalmol. 95:640–648, 1988.

38. Yarchoan, R., Mitsuya, H., Myers, C., and Broder, S., Clinical pharmacology of 3′-azido-2′-3′-dideoxythymidine (zidovudine) and related dideoxynucleosides. N. Engl. J. Med. 321:726–738, 1989.

8

Corticosteroids, Immunosuppressive Agents, and Nonsteroidal Anti-inflammatory Drugs (NSAIDs)

I. **The immune/inflammatory system (IIS)** is a complex cellular and cell-product circuitry that functions, for the most part, in a manner beneficial to the host by warding off infectious or other foreign and potentially harmful antigens. To develop a rational therapeutic approach to IIS disease in the eye, as with any other site in the body, it is essential to understand the nature and function of the various components of the immune/inflammatory reaction before discussing the drugs that affect them and their use in various ocular diseases. The IIS response is primarily a function of the leukocyte system, which provides the cells and mediators responsible for the inflammatory immune reaction. Involved cell lines include macrophage/monocytes, polymorphonuclear leukocytes, or polymorphonuclear neutrophils (PMNs) (neutrophils, eosinophils, basophils), lymphocytes (T and B cells), mast cells, and indigenous ocular immune cells. Of these cell types, those considered primarily **immune** in nature are the mononuclear phagocytes, lymphocytes, resident ocular cells, and eosinophils. Those classified as **inflammatory** are neutrophils, basophils, and mast cells. Many reactions are mixed, and all cell types will be reviewed briefly here.

   A. **The general order of events in the inflammatory reaction** includes the foreign or antigenic stimulus for initiation of the reaction. A chemoattractant for cells is produced to induce **IIS** cell migration into the involved area, where chemical mediators are released from these cells. This induces amplification of the reaction through additional cell recruitment and activation and further mediator release until, ultimately, the antigen is inactivated or destroyed, usually with at least some host tissue damage.

   B. **Mononuclear phagocytic cells** are bone marrow derived and include **monocytes,** which are circulating intravascular phagocytic cells, **macrophages,** which are monocytes that have migrated from the circulation to the tissues because of maturation or chemotaxis, and two derivatives of the tissue macrophage, **epithelioid cells,** and their fusion product seen in chronic inflammation, **multinucleated giant cells.** Macrophages perform at least three major functions in the IIS:

      1. **Destruction** of microbes or diseased tissue, in part by release of hydrogen peroxide, with subsequent **engulfment** of the microbe or tissue. The macrophage may also serve as a repository for inactive but live organisms such as in chorioretinal toxoplasmosis.

      2. **Activation** of the immune system occurs with macrophage internalizing, processing, and presenting of

antigen to T cells, and macrophage production of interleukin-1, both of which activate helper T lymphocytes and other T cell subsets.

3. **Secretion of enzymes** ensues. These include numerous proteases, collagenase, elastase, hydrolases, prostaglandins, PMN chemotactic factor, DNase, cathepsin D, acid phosphatase and ribonuclease, lipase, hyaluronidase, proteoglycanases, lysozyme, catalase, esterases, arylsulfatase, and plasminogen activator. The degradation products resulting from reactions induced by the above mediators are **chemotactic** and enhance the immune response still further.

C. **Lymphocytes** are broadly categorized as T cells (thymus-dependent), which are derived from the thymus and other lymphoid tissue systems, and B cells (bursa-equivalent), which have their origin in the bone marrow.

1. **T cells** are found largely in the systemic circulation. There are numerous subsets of T cells, whose many functions include cellular lifelong immunologic memory or anamnestic capacity once sensitized to an antigen, assistance in B cell antibody production, and enhancement of cell-mediated reactions by immune cell recruitment or suppression of immune reaction by blocking various immune cell functions. Helper T cells (OKT4) comprise about 60–80% of all T cells and aid in B cell response and cell-mediated immunity. Suppressor or cytotoxic T cells (OKT8) constitute about 20–30% of T cell totals, suppress B cell activity, are one of the predominant cell types in **corneal transplantation rejection,** and are probably important in other ocular disease states. Intercellular communication is mediated largely by cytokines (lymphokines and monokines), hormone-like proteins produced by lymphocytes and macrophages. Depending on the protein produced, the immune response will be suppressed or augmented. One of the most important of these is **interleukin-2,** a lymphokine that stimulates lymphocyte growth and enhances certain immune responses.

2. **B cells** mature into **plasma cells,** secretors of the five major classes of **antibodies,** or immunoglobulins, IgA, IgG, IgM, IgD, and IgE, and thus are the effector cells in humoral immunity. **IgG** makes up about 75% of the body's immunoglobulins. Plasma cells producing IgG are found mainly in the spleen and lymph nodes. Because the IgG molecule is small, it readily crosses the placental, blood–brain, and blood–eye barriers. **IgM** is a large molecule that, because of its size, stays mainly within the circulatory system. As it is expressed very early on the B cell surface, **IgM** antibody response indicates a **newly acquired infection.** The major role of IgG and IgM is to aid immune effector cells such as T cells or macrophages by enhancing the interaction between the cells and the complement system. Antibody-coated antigen is susceptible to the action of the immune cells. **IgA** is the major extravascular anti-

body; plasma cells secreting it are found in the gut, respiratory tract, tonsils, salivary glands, and lacrimal glands. IgA is a very important component of the ocular surface defense system and appears to work by binding with infectious agents to inactivate them and by impeding absorption of toxins and allergens. **IgE** is a short-lived antibody bound by mast cells and basophil surface receptors and as such is a major mediator in anaphylaxis and allergic reactions. It is intimately involved in certain ocular surface diseases, but apparently not in intraocular inflammation. **IgD** is found only in minute quantities in the body simultaneously with IgM on B cells before stimulation. It appears to be a B cell membrane receptor for antigen.

D. **Indigenous ocular immune cells** include the corneal **Langerhans cells** and **retinal pigment epithelial** (RPE) cells, which function much like macrophages, and the retinal **Müller cells,** which may have marked effects on the ocular immune system. Both RPE and Müller cells may affect fibrocyte growth and division and participate actively in ocular inflammatory/immune disease.

E. **Mast cells** play an integral part in type I hypersensitivity reactions, but are inflammatory rather than true immune-class cells. They are discussed in greater detail in Chapter 2 on Antiallergy Drugs. In brief, they release histamine to cause smooth muscle contraction and increased small vessel permeability, serotonin to cause vasoconstriction, prostaglandins to induce many reactions including vasoconstriction and vasodilation, leukotrienes, which are chemotactic for neutrophils and basophils, and which increase vascular permeability, and chemotactic factor of anaphylaxis to attract eosinophils and neutrophils. Mast cells are found in abundance in the periocular area, in the choroid, and in several other areas of the eye.

F. **Polymorphonuclear leukocytes**

1. **Neutrophils** migrate in response to the chemotactic factors: bacterial endotoxin, cell-membrane–bound antibody, and the C5A component of the complement pathway. The enzyme-containing cytoplasmic lysosomes discharge a wide variety of enzymes and other mediators of the inflammatory reaction that result in destruction of foreign materials, and, unfortunately, of host tissues as well. Enzymes released include collagenase, lysozyme, lactoferrin, myeloperoxidase hydrolases, proteinases (cathepsins), elastase, and proteoglycases. Hydrogen peroxide, hyperchloric acid, and hydroxyl radicals also are produced and result in marked intracellular and membrane cytotoxicity. Massive enhancement of the inflammatory reaction results from a third component of neutrophil function, the generation and release of prostaglandin and leukotriene mediators.

2. **Eosinophils** contain an abundance of the same enzymes released by neutrophils, with the exception of lysozymes. Eosinophils also contain a number of anti-

inflammatory enzymes, such as histaminase, arylsulfatase, and kininase. Eosinophils are attracted to an IIS reaction by the release of mast cell mediators. Once at the inflammatory focus, they play an immunomodulatory role while in the presence of activated **basophils** and mast cells. The anti-inflammatory products of eosinophils neutralize mast cell histamine and slow-reacting substance of anaphylaxis (SRA), and prostaglandins released by eosinophils inhibit basophil function. These cells also are phagocytic in their capability to engulf mast cell granules and are highly responsive to parasitic invasion, binding tightly to the organisms through surface receptors and then releasing peroxidase to kill the invaders.

G. **The complement system** comprises a series of sequentially activating proteolytic enzymes that aid antibody function in the immune system. The complement cascade may be initiated by C1 interaction with membrane-bound antibodies or by an alternative pathway not requiring antibody but direct contact with bacterial cell walls. The end result of the sequence C1 through C9 (with multiple C enzymes within each step) is the generation of chemotactic protein fragments. Various fragments induce mast cell degranulation, smooth muscle contraction, neutrophil phagocytosis, and promotion of cell lysis. The complement system thus is involved in numerous aspects of the inflammatory reaction.

II. **Classification of Immune Hypersensitivity Reactions** is one of the keys to understanding the mechanisms of many ocular diseases, thereby assisting in the selection of therapeutic agents. The inflammatory response may involve more than one type of hypersensitivity reaction.

A. **Type I** reaction is antibody mediated and, in particular, involves IgE binding to mast cells and basophils, resulting in degranulation. Ocular allergic reactions such as perennial or seasonal allergic conjunctivitis (hayfever conjunctivitis) are type I reactions.

B. **Type II** reaction is mediated by cytotoxic antibodies that bind to the target tissue receptors. The association of T cells in some diseases implies that some type II reactions may be antibody dependent, cell-mediated cytotoxic reactions. This appears to be exemplified by ocular pemphigoid, in which the apparent mechanism is attachment of cytotoxic antibodies to the basement membrane of the mucosal surface in association with T cell infiltration.

C. **Type III** reaction is antigen-antibody-complement (immune complex)–mediated with production of chemotactic factors that attract cells that cause tissue damage. The Arthus reaction of herpetic vasculitis, Behçet's disease, and phacoanaphylaxis appear mediated in great part by type III reaction.

D. **Type IV** hypersensitivity is a cell-mediated immune reaction driven solely by T cells and not involving antibodies. Delayed hypersensitivity such as seen in PPD skin testing, sarcoid granulomatous responses, herpetic disciform keratitis, and sympathetic ophthalmia are all classified as type IV responses.

III. **Establishing the Basis for Medical Therapy.** The object of therapy for undue host IIS disease is to prevent or minimize permanent tissue damage without impairing elimination of the inciting antigen. It is not within the scope of this book to discuss fully patient evaluation and diagnostic testing, but a brief list of factors to be considered before undertaking drug therapy is noted below.

A. **Clinical history**
   1. **Onset.** When, where, how, initial or recurrent, unilateral or bilateral.
   2. **Signs and symptoms.** Pain, itching, burning, foreign body sensation, redness, discharge, visual changes, floaters.
   3. **Demography.** Age, sex, race, ethnic heritage, travel, family history, sexual history, allergen exposure (pets, hair spray, make-up).
   4. **General medical condition** and known allergies and atopy (hay fever, eczema).
   5. **Drug therapy.** Current and previous, response.
   6. **Other systemic signs and symptoms.** Headache, deafness, paresthesias, weakness, mental alterations, skin changes, oral and skin ulcers, lacrimal and salivary gland swelling, arthritis, cough, shortness of breath, diarrhea.

B. **Ocular examination**
   1. **Vision.** Uncorrected or best corrected, pinhole.
   2. **Extraocular muscle function** and confrontation fields.
   3. **Lids and periocular skin** redness, swelling, dermatitis, rash, ulcers, atrophy, vitiligo, retraction, ptosis, follicles, papillae, membranes.
   4. **Conjunctiva and sclera.** Discharge, hyperemia (focal, diffuse, deep, superficial), nodules, forniceal shortening, symblepharon, scleral thinning.
   5. **Cornea.** Ulcers, scars, infiltrates, neovascularization, edema, keratic precipitates.
   6. **Anterior chamber (AC), pupil, iris, and lens.** AC cells and flare, fibrin, hypopyon, hyphema, synechiae, miosis, rubeosis, iris nodules, Marcus Gunn pupil (optic nerve assessment), cataract.
   7. **Vitreous, retina, and choroid.** Cells or haze, hemorrhages, infiltrates, vasculitis, neovascularization, old scars, macular edema, cotton wool spots (infarcts), retinal edema, choroid lesions with or without retinal involvement, peripheral retinal lesions.
   8. **Optic disc.** Hyperemia, papillitis, papilledema, atrophy, cupping, neovascularization.
   9. **Intraocular pressure**

C. **Diagnostic testing** can be excessively expensive and time-consuming and reveal little unless the physician has some idea of what he or she seeks to confirm or deny. In many cases such as seasonal allergic conjunctivitis or herpetic dendritic keratitis, the diagnosis usually may be made on history and exam alone. In other cases, such as some of the uveitides, the evaluation may be much more involved.

IV. **Initiating Therapy.** A presumptive or definitive diagnosis having been made, the physician then may initiate anti-inflammatory therapy, coupled where indicated with other drugs specifically oriented to killing and eliminating the offending antigen, eg, replicating microbes. Before starting anti-inflammatory therapy, the following factors should be assessed or recommendations noted:

   A. Begin therapy only if potential **benefits** are felt to **outweigh** potential **risks,** eg, blind eyes do not warrant aggressive therapy.

   B. Consider the patient's **age** and **life expectancy.**

   C. Is the **patient reliable** in terms of compliance with the prescribed medicine, or should alternative arrangements for receiving therapy be made, eg, visiting nurse, friend, injections in office rather than pills at home.

   D. Try to **avoid long-term systemic drugs** in patients with unilateral ocular disease unless concurrent systemic disease warrants it, eg, juvenile rheumatoid arthritis.

   E. **Avoid systemic therapy** in **children** if at all possible, as immunosuppressive agents have lifelong effects on growth and development. Local subconjunctival, sub-tenon, or retrobulbar injection and topical therapy should suffice. Exceptions, again, are concurrent systemic disease that demands systemic therapy.

   F. **Diabetes and systemic hypertension** may be aggravated by corticosteroids and renal disease; systemic hypertension may be aggravated by cyclosporine.

   G. **Discuss** the disease, prognosis, and drug **side effects** with the patient, making sure that the situation is understood by the patient or person(s) responsible for the patient. Signed **informed consent** is advisable when undertaking long-term systemic therapy with corticosteroids and certainly with immunosuppressive agents.

V. **Corticosteroids (steroids)** have been the foundation of therapy for ocular immune/inflammatory disease since the early 1950s. The naturally occurring steroid hormones are produced by the adrenal cortex. Physicians more commonly use synthetic steroids today because of their more selective immunosuppressive action and reduction in some of the less desirable side effects such as salt retention. Drugs of ocular therapeutic use are topical and systemic preparations of prednisolone, dexamethasone, fluorometholone, medrysone, medroxyprogesterone, prednisone, and triamcinolone.

   A. **Mechanism of action.** Steroids are thought to act by controlling the rate of protein synthesis. The drug is met at the susceptible host cell surface by an appropriate receptor, complexes with it, and then migrates to the nucleus. There the drug affects DNA transcription and increases mRNA production that codes for enzymes that synthesize specific proteins. **Glucocorticoid receptors** are present not only on all cells of the immune system but, in the eye, are found in the **iris, ciliary body,** and adjacent **corneoscleral tissue.**

   B. **Metabolism.** Steroids are effectively absorbed into the body from local application of drug to mucous membranes and skin as well as from oral administration and systemic injection. The drugs are metabolized in the liver (70%) and kidney to an inactive substance. Most of the metabolite is excreted in the urine within 72 hours.

C. **Steroid effects on the IIS** are both **anti-inflammatory** and **immunosuppressive.** The anti-inflammatory effects are nonspecific in terms of the disease process, reacting to almost any stimulus. The immunosuppressive effects vary among cell types. Basically, these drugs do not achieve their effect via cytotoxicity (lysis) but by affecting function and distribution of virtually all cellular components of the immune system. Steroid effects are protean and include:

1. **Suppression of lymphocyte proliferation** and **sequestration** of large numbers of T cells, particularly the T helper subset, out of the intravascular circulation and into bone marrow within 4–6 days of dosing. This greatly diminishes recruitment of immunoreactive cells to the inflammatory focus. **B cells are far less steroid-sensitive than T cells.** Antibody production therefore is minimally affected, while cell-mediated immunity is quite suppressed. Very high doses of steroids may, however, reduce levels of serum immunoglobulin and complement.

2. **Increased neutrophil release** from the marrow into the circulation within 4–6 hours of dosing, increased neutrophil production, decreased neutrophil adherence to the vascular endothelium with consequent reduced migration to the inflammatory reaction.

3. **Eosinopenia** and **monocytopenia.**

4. **Inhibition of macrophage migration** across the vascular endothelium to the inflammatory site with consequent decreased macrophage processing of particulate antigen for presentation to the T lymphocytes, without which cell-mediated immunity is depressed.

5. **Inhibition of degranulation** of neutrophils, macrophages, mast cells, and basophils through lysosomal membrane stabilization with consequent blocked release of inflammatory mediators such as histamine, SRA, and other chemotactic factors.

6. **Decreased capillary permeability** and suppressed vasodilation resulting in less protein and fluid leakage and inflammatory cell passage out into the tissues.

7. **Inhibition of prostaglandin synthesis** by decreased arachidonic acid production.

8. **Depressed monocytic/macrophage bactericidal activity.**

9. **Suppressed lymphokine** action, eg, macrophage migration and aggregating factors.

D. **Clinical indications.** The relative anti-inflammatory potency of various corticosteroids is shown in Table 8-1 and clinical uses in Table 8-2.

1. **Topical corticosteroids** are used in the treatment of alkali burns, allergic keratoconjunctivitis, anterior uveitis, bacterial keratitis (marginal and central), cor-

Table 8-1. Relative dose potency of commonly used corticosteroids

Drug	Equivalent anti-inflammatory dose (mg)	Relative anti-inflammatory potency
Cortisone	25	0.8
Hydrocortisone	20	1.0
Prednisolone	5	4.0
Prednisone	5	4.0
Methylprednisolone	4	5.0
Triamcinolone	4	5.0
Dexamethasone	0.75	26.0
Betamethasone	0.60	33.0

neal transplant rejection, episcleritis, immune viral (herpes simplex, zoster, adenovirus), interstitial keratitis, phlyctenulosis, postoperative inflammation, and scleritis.

2. **Combined topical** and **systemic** steroids usually are used in the treatment of autoimmune disease (rheumatoid arthritis, polyarteritis, lupus), anterior uveitis, bacterial or sterile endophthalmitis, Mooren's ulcers, ocular cicatricial pemphigoid, scleritis, and sympathetic ophthalmia (?).

3. **Systemic** and/or **periocular** steroids are used (usually with topical steroids) in dysthyroid ophthalmopathy, some cases of optic neuritis, posterior uveitis, and temporal arteritis.

4. **Intravitreal** steroids may be used, at the discretion of the physician, in certain endophthalmitis patients under appropriate anti-infective therapy. See Endophthalmitis in Chapter 3 on Antibiotics.

5. **Infection.** Any **infectious component** of an ocular inflammatory condition must, of course, be appropriately treated with specific agents. Steroids cannot be used alone in these cases without enhanced spread of the invading organism.

6. **Variable responses.** Certain ocular immune/inflammatory conditions will not respond to steroid therapy and require the use of immunosuppressive cytotoxic agents. Other conditions will respond to steroids and then be kept under control with nonsteroidal anti-inflammatory drugs without need for continued steroid therapy. Section **IX.B** and Table 8-2 address the general therapeutic approach to many of these clinical entities.

E. **Topical steroid preparations and dosages** commonly used in ocular inflammatory disease *in order of decreasing potency*; see Table 8-3 and Section V for doses in specific clinical situations.

continued on page 194

Table 8-2. Anti-inflammatory/immunosuppressive drugs used in specific ocular diseases

Disease	Topical steroid	Periocular steroid	Systemic steroid	Cyclosporine A[a]	Cytotoxic[a] Antimetabolites	Cytotoxic[a] Alkylating agents	Sulfone[a]	Immune-related adjuvant
Alkali or acid burn	+ (<10 days)	—	—	—	—	—	—	—
Allergic keratoconjunctivitis, atopy, vernal	+	—	—	—	—	—	—	Cromolyn[c]
Anterior uveitis and/or cyclitis (idiopathic, recurring)	+	+	+	+	+	+	—	Bromocriptine[a]
Bacterial keratitis Marginal Central	+	—	—	—	—	—	—	—
Bacterial or sterile endophthalmitis	+	Intravitreal?	+	+	—	—	—	—
Behçet's disease	—	—	±	+	—	+	—	Colchicine[a] Plasmapheresis
Birdshot retinochoroidopathy	—	+	+	+	—	—	—	—

Bullous pemphigoid, pemphigus vulgaris	–	–	+	+	+	+	+	Plasmapheresis
Corneal transplant rejection	+	–	–	+	–	–	–	–
Crohn's disease	–	–	+	+	–	–	–	–
Dermatitis herpetiformis[b]	–	–	–	–	–	–	+	–
Dysthyroid ophthalmopathy	–	–	+	–	–	–	–	–
Eales' disease	–	–	–	–	±	±	–	–
Episcleritis	+	–	–	–	–	–	–	–
Graft-versus-host	–	–	–	+	–	–	–	Bromocriptine[a]
Herpetic iritis (H. simplex, zoster)	+	–	+	–	–	–	–	–
Immune viral keratitis (herpes simplex, zoster, adenovirus)	+	–	–	–	–	–	–	–
Lupus erythematosus	+	–	+	–	+	+	–	Plasmapheresis
Mooren's ulcer	+	–	+	+	+	+	–	–
Ocular cicatricial pemphigoid	–	–	+	±	+	+	+	–
Optic neuritis	–	+	+	–	–	–	–	–

Table 8-2. (continued)

Disease	Topical steroid	Periocular steroid	Systemic steroid	Cyclosporine A[a]	Cytotoxic[a] Antimetabolites	Cytotoxic[a] Alkylating agents	Sulfone[a]	Immune-related adjuvant
Pars planitis, intermediate uveitis	+	+	+	+	−	−	−	−
Phlyctenulosis	+	−	−	−	−	−	−	−
Polyarteritis nodosa	−	−	+	−	+	−	−	−
Posterior endogenous uveitis								
Unilateral	−	+	+	−	−	−	−	−
Bilateral	−	+	+	+	+	+	−	−
Postoperative inflammation	+	+	+	−	−	−	−	−
Progressive systemic sclerosis (scleroderma)	−	−	+	−	−	−	−	−
Relapsing polychondritis	−	−	+	−	−	−	+	−
Scleritis	+	−	+	−	+	+	−	−

Serpiginous choroidopathy	—	—	+	±	—	—	—	—
Rheumatoid arthritis	+	+	+	—	+	±	—	—
Sarcoid	+	+	+	+	±	±	—	—
Stevens-Johnson disease (erythema multiforme)	+	—	±	—	—	—	—	—
Sympathetic ophthalmia	+	+	+	+	+	+	—	—
Syphilitic interstitial keratouveitis	+	+	+	—	—	—	—	—
Temporal arteritis	—	—	+	—	+	—	—	—
Ulcerative colitis	—	—	+	—	+	—	—	—
Vogt-Koyanaga-Harada disease	—	—	+	+	±	±	—	Plasmapheresis
Wegener's granulomatosis	—	—	±	—	+	—	—	—

^a Not FDA approved for treatment of ocular disease.

a Not FDA approved for treatment of ocular disease.
b Plasmapheresis used to lower circulating immune complexes.
c See chapter on Antiallergy drugs.

1. **Dexamethasone phosphate** 0.1% solution, 0.05% ointment, or 0.1% suspension daily to q1h, depending on the disease state. This drug is the most potent of all topical ocular steroids with regard to immunosuppressive and anti-inflammatory effect, as well as potential adverse reactions.

2. **Prednisolone acetate** 0.12, 0.25, or 1.0% suspension, prednisolone sodium phosphate 0.12–1.0% solution, and prednisolone phosphate 0.5% solution or 0.25% ointment daily or less to q1–2h, depending on the clinical condition. Although corneal penetration of the acetate and phosphate forms differs, no clinical differences have been noted in efficacy between the two. Efficacy is a function of concentration and frequency of dosing. Prednisolone in higher doses is one of the most potent ocular steroids in terms of both efficacy and potential side effects. It is used for significant external and anterior segment intraocular inflammation.

3. **Hydrocortisone** acetate 2.5% suspension, 1.5% ophthalmic ointment, and 0.2% solution daily to tid for mild to moderate external ocular inflammatory or allergic disease. There is minimal intraocular inflammatory effect, but steroid glaucoma risk is greater than with fluoromethalone or hydroxymedrysone.

4. **Fluoromethalone** 0.1–1% suspension or 0.1% ointment daily to tid for milder superficial ocular inflammation and allergy. Because of lower potency and less intraocular penetration than all other steroids except medrysone, there is less tendency for development of steroid glaucoma. IOP elevation has been reported in some susceptible individuals.

5. **Medroxyprogesterone** 1% solution is not available commercially as an eye drop. It is FDA approved for parenteral administration. The eye drop is used in some ulcerative inflammatory external ocular diseases because it appears to interfere significantly less with collagen synthesis and wound healing than do other steroids. Its relative potency is somewhat less than 0.12% prednisolone, and dosage is daily to qid. The eye drop is made by the hospital pharmacy from the parenteral solution.

6. **Medrysone** 1.0% solution is a low-potency, superficial-acting steroid used in mild external ocular inflammation daily to qid. It is probably the safest of all steroids in terms of adverse ocular effects, but also of lower efficacy.

7. **Combination corticosteroid-antibiotic** preparations are available for hydrocortisone, prednisolone, and dexamethasone. These are reviewed in Table 3-4 in the chapter on Antibiotics.

F. **Systemic (oral or injected) corticosteroids** should be taken with food or antacid. Those steroids commonly used in ocular inflammatory/immune disease **in order of decreasing potency** include:

1. **Dexamethasone** sodium phosphate for **injection** 4, 10, or 24 mg/ml IM, IV, subconjunctival, intralesional,

or dexamethasone acetate suspension for IM or subconjunctival injection (not intravenous or intralesional) 8 or 16 mg/ml are the most potent of all steroids used for retrobulbar, subconjunctival/subtenon, or chalazion injection. The drug is 25 times more effective as an anti-inflammatory agent than is hydrocortisone. The usual injected dose is 4–8 mg via the retrobulbar or subtenon route and 0.1–0.2 ml (0.8–1.6 mg) for intralesional injection.

Dexamethasone is also available in **tablet** form in doses of 0.25, 0.5, 0.75, 1.5, 4, and 6 mg. At equipotent anti-inflammatory doses, dexamethasone almost totally lacks the sodium-retaining, potassium-losing properties of hydrocortisone. Initial dosage may range from 0.75 mg for milder disease to 9 mg po daily for the most severe inflammatory reactions. Food or antacid should be given with po steroids.

2. **Prednisone tablets** come in 1, 2.5, 5, 10, 20, 25, and 50 mg doses and as an oral solution of 5 mg/5 ml or 10 mg/10 ml. It is the most common oral steroid used in managing ocular disease and should always be taken with food, milk, or antacid. Dosages may range from 2.5 mg every other morning to 80–100 mg daily in 2 divided doses for short periods.

3. **Triamcinolone tablets** are available in doses of 1, 2, 4, and 8 mg and the **syrup** as 2 mg/5 ml. It also is marketed as **dermal** (nonophthalmic) 0.025, 0.5, and 1% cream and ointment and for IM **injection** 40 mg/ml (diacetate or acetonide). The drug has about 5 times the potency of hydrocortisone and some advantage over hydrocortisone and dexamethasone in that it is virtually devoid of mineralocorticoid activity in therapeutic doses. Triamcinolone, therefore, causes little or no sodium retention or potassium loss. Initial doses vary from 4–48 mg daily, depending on the clinical condition. Like any other orally administered steroid, it should be taken with food or antacid.

4. **Prednisolone tablets** are available in a 5-mg dose. It has 4 times the anti-inflammatory potency of hydrocortisone and is used in ophthalmic disease far more frequently as the topical preparation **(drops or ointment)** than as an oral medication. Common dose range is 5 mg every other morning to 50 mg daily in divided doses, depending on the clinical disease.

5. **Hydrocortisone tablets** come in strengths of 10 and 20 mg and in the **injectable** form (IM, IV, or subconj.) as 50, 100, 250, and up to 1000 mg/ml. The common injectable dose for subconjunctival use is 50 or 100 mg/ml. Systemic hydrocortisone is commonly used in therapy of such systemic diseases as ankylosing spondylitis, and systemic lupus erythematosus, to name a few among many. All of these diseases may have concurrent ocular inflammatory reactions that will respond to the hydrocortisone treatment of the systemic diseases. The drug also may be used in purely ophthalmic inflammatory disease. Initial doses may range from

Table 8-3. Corticosteroid preparations

Generic and (commercial) names	Oral (PO)	Injectable route (I)	Ophthalmic (O) or dermal (D)
Cortisol, hydrocortisone (Cortef, Hydrocortone, others)	5–20 mg tab	25, 50 mg/ml suspension IM	0.125–2.5% (D)
Cortisol, hydrocortisone sodium phosphate (Hydrocortone Phosphate, others)	—	50 mg/ml IV, IM	—
Cortisol, hydrocortisone sodium succinate (A-hydroCort, Solu-Cortef: I, O)	—	100–1000 mg (powder) IV, IM	Injectable solution 50 mg/ml subconj. (O)
Dexamethasone sodium (Decadron)	0.25–6.0 mg tab 0.5 mg/5 ml elixir 0.5 mg/0.5 ml solution	—	—
Dexamethasone $NaPO_4$ or acetate (Decadron PO, Dexasone, Hexadrol: PO, I); (AK-Dex, Baldex, Decadron, Dexotic, I-Methasone solution and ointment, Maxidex susp.: O)	0.25–6 mg	4–24 mg/ml IV ($NaPO_4$) IM (acetate)	0.1% (D); 0.05, 0.1% (O); Injectable solution subconj., intralesion (O) (see text for formulation)
Fluorometholone (FML, Fluor-Op-)	—	—	0.1, 1.0% (O)
Medrysone (HMS)	—	—	1.0% (O)
Methylprednisolone (Medrol)	2–32 mg tab	—	—

Methylprednisolone acetate (Depo-Medrol, Medrol-Acetate, others: I)*	—	20–80 mg/ml suspension IM	0.25, 1% (D); Injectable intralesion (O), subconj. (O)
Methylprednisolone Na$^+$ succinate (A-Methapred, Solu-Medrol: I)	—	40–1000 mg (powder) IV, IM	Injectable solution subconj. (O)
Medroxyprogesterone (Provera)	2.5, 10 mg	100–400 mg/ml IM	1% solution (O)
Prednisolone (Delta-Cortef, others: PO)	1, 5 mg	—	—
Prednisolone acetate: I (AK-tate, Pred Mild, Pred-Forte, Econopred, Econopred Plus, I-Pred, Predulose: O)	—	25–100 mg/ml suspension IM	0.12–1.0% suspension (O)
Prednisolone NaPO$_4$: I (Inflamase, Inflamase Forte, B-H Prednisolone, AK-Pred: O)	—	20 mg/ml IM, IV	0.12, 1.0% solution (O)
Prednisolone PO$_4$ (Hydeltrasol, Hydeltrasol ointment, Metreton)	—	—	0.5% solution (O); 0.25% ointment (O)
Prednisone (Deltasone, others)	1–50 mg	—	—
Triamcinolone diacetate (Aristocort, Kenacort: PO, I)	1–16 mg	40 mg/ml IM	25 mg/ml intralesion
Triamcinolone acetonide (Kenalog, others: I, D)	—	40 mg/ml suspension IM	0.025–0.5% (D)

* Depot form.

20–240 mg or more daily, depending on disease severity. Food or antacid should be taken concurrently.

6. **Methylprednisolone** is available for **IM, IV, intralesional** (eg, chalazion), or **subconjunctival** injection as the sodium succinate form in doses of 40 mg/ml, 125 mg/2 ml, and higher, up to 2 g/30 ml. Subconjunctival dose is commonly 40 mg/ml. A **depot** form of methylprednisolone is available as the acetate in doses of 20, 40, and 60 mg/ml. In ophthalmic practice its use is largely restricted to subconjunctival and retrobulbar injections where prolonged (about 10 days) release of a relatively potent steroid is desired locally while minimizing (but not eliminating) systemic absorption. The most common dose is 40 mg/ml. Relative potency is 4 times that of hydrocortisone.

G. **Adverse side effects** of corticosteroids may be localized to the eye or be systemic, regardless of administration route. Topical or locally injected steroid will, of course, have fewer systemic side effects than orally or parenterally administered drug, but higher doses and prolongation of treatment increase the chances of both local and systemic adverse reactions. Occlusion of the nasolacrimal canal with finger compression over the medial canthal area for about 3 minutes will reduce systemic absorption of topical drugs by decreasing drug accessibility to nasal mucous membrane and the GI tract.

1. **Ocular side effects** are in some cases idiopathic and in others drug dose- and/or duration-related.

   a. **Secondary open-angle glaucoma (steroid glaucoma)** may develop in about one third of the population after 4 weeks of daily topical 0.1% dexamethasone drops, 5% of this group having an IOP rise of 16 mm Hg or greater. IOP returns to normal in about 2 weeks after discontinuing medication. Medrysone and fluoromet halone have far less tendency to raise IOP than do prednisolone and dexamethasone, but all may induce glaucoma in sufficiently sensitive individuals. Severe intractable glaucoma may occur after periocular steroid injection. If a depot form was used, surgical removal of the residual drug, often a difficult procedure, may be necessary.

   b. **Posterior subcapsular cataracts** have been associated with both topical and systemic corticosteroids. This side effect appears to be idiopathic, as there is no correlation in either children or adults between development of the cataracts and age, total dose, or duration of treatment. In some children the cataract may regress after therapy is discontinued or markedly lowered. Studies indicate that patients receiving less than 10 mg/day of prednisone equivalent or treated with steroids for less than 1 year were unlikely to develop cataractous changes.

   c. **Microbial infections** may be enhanced by corticosteroid therapy. Topical steroids should be used in eyes actively infected with herpes simplex virus (dendritic or geographic ulcerative keratitis) only with antiviral prophylaxis and only if a corneal stromal immune reaction or iritis warrants their use. Bacterial infections should be adequately treated with appropriate antibiotics before introduction of any steroidal therapy, particularly if *Pseudomonas* was the invading organism. Quiescent trachoma has also been activated by topical steroid, and anterior uveitis exacerbation has been noted in patients with a positive treponemal antibody absorption test. There appears to be no place for use of steroids in fungal infections of the external or internal eye because of the marked risk of augmenting infections that are at best difficult to treat. Similarly, systemic steroids are contraindicated in toxoplasma retinitis that is not under appropriate antimicrobial therapy and also in AIDS patients with opportunistic ocular infection of any type.

d. **Wound healing** is significantly interfered with by all topical steroids, with the probable exception of medroxyprogesterone. These drugs interfere with collagen synthesis and should be used with caution and at minimal required dose in the presence of scleral or corneal ulceration and thinning. Drug effect on rate of postoperative healing should not be forgotten in terms of protecting the eye from even minor trauma.

e. **Ptosis** and mild **mydriasis** often are seen with topical steroids.

f. **Pseudotumor cerebri** has been precipitated in children by too-abrupt withdrawal of systemic steroid, and exophthalmos may result from prolonged systemic therapy.

2. **Periocular steroid** injections, particularly when given repeatedly, may be associated with several potential complications in addition to glaucoma. These include globe perforation, proptosis, atrophy and fibrosis of the extraocular muscles, allergic reactions to the drug vehicle, enhanced scleral or corneal ulcer melting, and central retinal artery occlusion.

3. **Systemic side effects** of corticosteroids are greater with parenteral or oral drug and minimized but not eliminated with topical agents or periocular injection. These side effects include:

a. **Immune response suppression** with enhanced susceptibility to bacterial, viral, fungal, and other infections.

b. **Cushing's syndrome** characterized by moon facies, buffalo hump, purpura, acne, hirsutism, muscle atrophy, and pathologic fractures.

c. **Gastrointestinal:** gastric or duodenal peptic ulcers, gastric hemorrhage, intestinal perforation, and pancreatitis.

    d. **Cardiovascular** side effects of hypertension and congestive failure secondary to renal sodium and water retention and potassium loss.

    e. **Metabolic** precipitation of hyperglycemia and ketoacidosis in diabetics, hyperosmolar nonketotic coma, centripetal obesity, and hyperlipidemia.

    f. **Central nervous system** reactions of psychotic break, hallucinations, and pseudotumor cerebri.

    g. **Endocrine system** effects of growth failure, secondary amenorrhea, hypothalamic-pituitary-adrenal axis suppression, and Addisonian crisis with too-rapid steroid taper.

    h. **Impaired wound healing** and **subcutaneous tissue atrophy.**

H. **Principles of corticosteroid therapeutic regimen:** maximize efficacy and minimize adverse side effects.

    1. **Topical corticosteroids.** The strength and frequency of dosage deemed necessary to bring the inflammatory process under control is initiated, and then slow taper is begun when improvement is noted. For a moderate allergic conjunctivitis ⅛% prednisolone qid may suffice with tapering begun in 1–2 weeks. A severe, fibrinous, noninfectious anterior uveitis may require hourly 0.1% dexamethasone during the waking hours, eg, 6:00 A.M.–11:00 P.M., with steroid-antibiotic ointment such as dexamethasone-neomycin qh for several days. Steroid drops, however, are generally more potent than their ointment counterpart. A significant number of treatment failures are due to underdosing, and the more chronic the disease, the longer it will take to bring it under control. Patients should be told ahead of time the nature, prognosis, and probable length of time treatment will be necessary. They also should be told to **shake any steroid suspension** before use to avoid inadequate drug concentration, and instructed in nasolacrimal digital compression to minimize nasal mucosal drug absorption and swallowing of ocular medication. Patients on high doses are initially seen about twice weekly until tapering begins. Once clinical improvement is noted, a general rule of thumb for tapering topical steroids is to **decrease dosage by not more than 50% at any given time.** The lower the dose, the longer it is maintained before the next step down. Once-daily drops of a weak steroid may be used for months before further taper is tried—or never stopped at all if necessary. Intraocular pressure and other evidence of drug adverse side effect should be checked at each visit. In some cases adverse side effects may be drug related, disease related, or both, making judgment calls as to whether to increase or decrease medication difficult. At doses lower than the equivalent of 1% prednisolone once or twice daily, concurrent prophylactic topical antibiotics and, in herpetic disease, prophylactic antivirals often may be discontinued unless the patient is predisposed to recurrence of infectious disease, eg, rosacea patients (staphylococcal

blepharitis). **Caution** should be exercised in young children on repeated dosing; at least one death has been reported in an infant due to long-term steroid effects from the use of steroid drops in a homograft rejection.

2. **Subconjunctival/subtenon** steroid injection for anterior segment inflammation or retrobulbar steroid injection for posterior segment inflammation are options that allow the rapid delivery of high steroid concentrations locally and often eliminate the need for systemic steroids. Unless there is a contraindication, it is common to inject a long-acting steroid preparation such as 20–40 mg/ml methylprednisolone acetate. The injection is most safely made in the temporal subtenon area over the pars plana (peripheral retina), or back near the macular region, depending on the disease target. Topical anesthetics are necessary, but mixing injectable anesthetic with steroid increases volume and initial pain. Preinjection oral analgesics should be given for the lingering discomfort. Such injections may be used at the end of an intraocular surgical procedure, in unilateral uveitis, in cystoid macular edema, and in children and may be repeated q1–2 weeks for 3–4 doses in acute disease. All are situations where systemic effects of steroids are minimized, yet good therapeutic doses are delivered to the target site. In chronic disease, injections may be given every few weeks to months several times.

3. **Systemic steroids** are to be initiated only when the physician has determined in his/her own mind that the inflammatory disease warrants this therapeutic approach and that topical and periocular routes will not suffice. Every effort must be made to avoid the systemic route in children unless concurrent systemic disease mandates their use. As with drops or injection, the patient should be fully informed as to prognosis, probable duration of treatment, and adverse side effects. For therapy projected for longer than about 10 days, signed informed consent may be advisable.

   a. **Duration of treatment and dosage** can not be set by hard or reliable guidelines because of the fickle nature of many inflammatory diseases. As a rule, 15–20 mg of prednisone (or equivalent) is a reasonable daily maintenance dose in an adult on **long-term** therapy. In some diseases such as acute herpes simplex iritis, where the corneal status precludes more intensive topical drug, **short-term** systemic steroid may be effectively given and discontinued over 10–14 days without rebound and allowing time for the corneal status to be improved such that topical steroid may be given. In other situations, such as severe autoimmune uveitis, systemic dosage of 20 mg prednisone daily or 40 mg every other day may be continued for at least 3 months after clinical quiescence has been achieved before further tapering of dosage. Sympathetic ophthalmia often is treated at this level for at least a year.

b. **A common starting dose** is 1–1.5 mg/kg prednisone in 2 divided doses daily (average total per day 50–80 mg). Some physicians prefer triamcinolone to reduce Na^+-K^+ and water imbalance (see Table 8-1). These doses are high and, barring unforeseen complications, are to be maintained until clinical improvement is noted. This must be within a reasonable period, however, as predetermined by the physician's knowledge of the disease state. Oral steroids should be taken with food, milk, or antacid to avoid gastrointestinal side effects and calcium supplements given to minimize drug calcium-leaching effects. Once improvement is noted, a slow, gradual dose reduction should be begun, dropping dosage by no more than 50% at any given level and extending duration of treatment the lower the dosage level, eg, prednisone 40 mg bid for 1 week to 30 mg bid for 1 week to 20 mg bid for 2 weeks, to 20 mg every morning and 10 mg every evening for 2 weeks, to 20 mg every morning for 3 weeks, to 10 mg every morning for 4 weeks, etc. Too rapid reduction of steroid dosing, other than short-term (14 days or less), will induce a rebound recurrence that may be more severe than the original inflammatory reaction as well as adrenal insufficiency.

c. **Morning dosing.** As noted in the sample taper schedule above, as one approaches the lower doses, all drug is given in the morning. This causes less suppression of the pituitary–adrenal axis and fewer side effects than the equivalent dose given in divided doses through the day or a single but long-acting steroid given in the morning.

d. **Alternate-day therapy** also minimizes adverse side effects while maintaining therapeutic efficacy. It should be initiated once the inflammatory reaction has come under control but long-term treatment is deemed necessary. In changing to alternate-day therapy, the total dose that would have been given over a 2-day period is given as a single dose once every other morning. One then may continue gradual taper as warranted. Alternate-day therapy does not disturb the hypothalamic pituitary-adrenal system, and there are fewer and less severe adverse side effects. With any long-term steroid therapy, adrenal suppression is a risk, however. Systemic drugs must never be abruptly discontinued, as an Addisonian crisis may be precipitated. To ascertain adrenal status, a cortisol-stimulation test is warranted if there is doubt that the patient can safely stop steroids altogether after months or even years of treatment.

e. **Combination therapy** using steroids with cytotoxic agents or cyclosporine is often more effective than either agent alone and allows use of lower drug dosage, thus minimizing side effects.

VI. **Immunosuppressive agents** are more specific in their action than are corticosteroids. The former modify the immunologic sensitization of the lymphoid cells; corticosteroids have a broader-spectrum, less specific action on the leukocyte system in general. Included in the cytotoxic drugs currently of use in ocular inflammatory disease are members of the classes of purine and pyrimidine analogs, alkylating agents, and folic acid analogs. Other members of the immunosuppressive groups are cyclosporine, an antibiotic, and the adjuvants colchicine and bromocriptine. All agents in this family of drugs interfere with the synthesis of nucleic acid or protein, or both. Table 8-4 lists the more commonly used immunosuppressive agents and their dosages in ocular disease.

A. **Indicated use** of immunosuppressive agents is in progressive, usually bilateral, vision-threatening, destructive ocular inflammatory immune disease of endogenous origin that is unresponsive to more conventional therapies. The physician must be convinced that there is no infectious component to the disease, and that there is, in fact, vision to be saved in the eye; that the treatment is not a desperation move to try everything in an eye beyond salvage.

B. **Before initiating immunosuppressive treatment,** the prognosis, risks, potential benefits, and projected duration of treatment must be explained to the patient or the person responsible for the patient. A signed consent form is advisable, and the patient should be evaluated by an internist for contraindications or potential problems with immunosuppressive therapy. An internist should also be involved in patient follow-up once therapy starts, unless the ophthalmologist has reasonably extensive experience with these agents. Unless the illness is life threatening, immunosuppressive drugs should not be used in pregnant women or children because of the potentially severe long-term effects on the fetus or child. In these cases an internist or pediatrician may be the primary physician. Most of these drugs induce azoospermia; the pretreatment banking of sperm may be advisable for male patients.

C. **The alkylating agents** of use in ophthalmic disease are the nitrogen mustard derivatives **chlorambucil** and **cyclophosphamide.**

1. **The mechanism of action** of all alkylating agents is via their ability to undergo reactions resulting in covalent linking (alkylation) of neutrophilic substances. Such cross-linking in cellular DNA results in an inability of the DNA to separate correctly during mitosis, ultimately resulting in cell death. The response is not specific and will, in theory, affect any actively dividing cell. In inflammatory disease, the immune cells are dividing more rapidly than normal tissue and are therefore more affected. Cyclophosphamide and chlorambucil are synthetic, but inactive forms of the active

Table 8-4. Nonsteroidal immunosuppressive agents[a]

Drug (commercial)	Usual dosage[b,c]
Alkylating Agents	
Cyclophosphamide (Cytoxan, Endoxan[a])	Starting: 2 mg/kg/d po (150–200 mg/d maximum). Reduce dosage by 25–50 mg/d when WBCC decreases (about 1 week). Adjust dosage to keep WBCC around 3500 mm^3, neutrophils not <1500, platelets not <75,000.
Chlorambucil (Leukeran)	Starting: 2 mg/d po. Increase every 3–4 days to total 6–12 mg/d. Monitor blood as per cyclophosphamide.
Antimetabolites	
Azathioprine (Imuran)	Starting: 1 mg/kg/d po. Increase to 2.5 mg/kg/d (50–100 mg/d maximum) over several days. Hematologic monitoring.
Methotrexate (amethopterin (Folex, Mexate)	Starting: weekly dose 7.5–25 mg po or IM. Hematologic, hepatic, and renal monitoring.
Fluorouracil (Fluorouracil)	5 mg/0.5 ml subconj. immediately postoperatively bid for 7 days, then daily for 7 days.
Antibiotics	
Cyclosporine A (Sandimmune)	Starting: 5 mg/kg/d po in 1–2 divided doses. Increase as needed to 7 mg/kg/d for uveitis and vasculitis. For corneal graft rejection start at 15 mg/kg/d for 2 days, then 7.5 mg/kg/d for 2 days, then 4.0 mg/kg/d for 4–12 mos.
Diphenylsulfone (4-4′diaminodiphenylsulfone)	25 mg po BID. Increase to 200 mg/d in 2–4 divided doses as needed over several days. Taper to maintenance over several months. Hematologic monitoring.
Immune-related Adjuvants	
Colchicine (Colbenemid, Probenecid)	0.6 mg po bid
Bromocriptine (Parlodel)	10 mg po each day with 4–5 mg/kg/d cyclosporine

[a] Not FDA approved for ocular use.
[b] See text for side effects, and text and Table 8-2 for clinical uses.
[c] Doses may frequently be lower in combination with systemic steroid.

agent, phosphoramide mustard. Th inactive drugs may be taken orally and then are metabolized to the active form by the microsomal system in the liver.

2. **Immune system effects** of alkylating agents vary with dose. Low, long-term dosing appears to affect T cells more than B-cell lymphocytes, but at higher doses B cell function is more affected. The drug exerts its effect on ocular disease by killing clone cells that damage the eye. This may be in the end organ itself or at a more peripheral location such as the marrow or lymph nodes.

3. **Clinical indications** and **contraindications** are still not fully worked out. The current most common indications for Behçet's disease, sympathetic ophthalmia, Wegener's granulomatosis, rheumatoid arthritis, polyarteritis nodosa, bullous pemphigoid, and malignancy. Relative indications are those noninfectious immune ocular diseases not responding to maximum steroid therapy. Possible efficacy has been noted in Eales' disease, retinal vasculitis (noninfectious), and serpiginous choroidopathy. Table 8-2 shows a more complete listing of ocular conditions in which these agents have been used with some success. **Contradindications** to cytotoxic therapy include focal chorioretinitis, herpes simplex, herpes zoster, cytomegalovirus, AIDS retinopathy, toxoplasmosis, and tuberculous and fungal infections.

4. **Cyclophosphamide dosage** in adult patients starts at about 2 mg/kg/d orally (150–200 mg/d maximum) taken on an empty stomach to prevent inactivation in the GI tract. A baseline white blood cell count (WBCC) and differential are taken on the day of initiating therapy and every 2–3 days until the WBCC begins to drop at about 1 week's time. When this occurs, dosage is reduced by 25–50 mg, aiming to stabilize the WBCC at no lower than 3000 cells/mm^3. A CBC and platelet count should be done every 2–3 weeks. The neutrophil count should not be allowed to fall below 1500–2000 cells/mm^3. Once stabilized, WBCC and differential are checked weekly.

5. **Chlorambucil dosage** is usually begun at 2 mg/d to ensure that there will be no idiosyncratic effect, and then increased every 3–4 days to total dosage of 6–12 mg/d. The WBCC and differential are monitored continuously as described for cyclophosphamide.

6. **Adverse side effects** of alkylating agents include leukopenia, a desired effect, but one that must not be allowed out of control, thrombocytopenia, and anemia. Other adverse effects are increased incidence of infection, especially viral, nausea, vomiting, stomatitis, alopecia, jaundice, pulmonary interstitial fibrosis, renal toxicity, and testicular atrophy. Hemorrhagic cystitis may develop with cyclophosphamide therapy and is a relative indication for discontinuing the drug, as secondary urinary bladder malignancies occur not infre-

quently in patients who have manifested this cystitis. Other adverse effects noted with cyclophosphamide are blurred vision, chromosomal damage, secretion in breast milk, and teratogenesis. Most disquieting, however, and of which patients must be warned, is the fact that these drugs are associated with the potential development of secondary malignancies, especially myeloproliferative and lymphoproliferative disorders. It cannot be ruled out, however, that the underlying diseases themselves are responsible for development of malignant disease.

D. **The oral antimetabolites** most important in ocular disease are the purine analog **azathioprine,** which interferes with purine metabolism, and the folate analog **methotrexate** (amethopterine).

1. **Mechanisms of action**

   a. **Azathioprine** is an orally administered prodrug that is metabolized to the active form, 6-mercaptopurine. The prodrug is well absorbed, causes less GI disturbance than the active drug form, and is less inactivated by liver enzymes. 6-Mercaptopurine apparently affects DNA and RNA metabolism through its conversion to T-IMP (thioinosine-5-PO_4), which then is incorporated into the nucleic acids as a base analog, thus leading to false transcription of genetic codes.

   b. **Methotrexate,** like all folic acid analogs, have profound effects on cellular metabolism by inhibiting dihydrofolate reductase, an enzyme essential for production of the coenzyme tetrahydrofolate. This coenzyme is integral to the production of thymidilate synthetase, in turn needed for production of thymidine for DNA synthesis and the mediation of purine nucleotide synthesis and RNA metabolism. Methotrexate is excreted unchanged in the urine.

2. **The immune system effects** of these antimetabolites vary with the point in time at which therapy is initiated with reference to antigenic challenge.

   a. **Azathioprine** has minimal humoral antibody effect and exerts a fairly selective effect on T-cell lymphocytes with suppression of mixed lymphocyte reaction in vitro, depression of recirculating T-lymphocytes, and development of monocyte precursor cells, inhibits killer cell activity (these cells themselves are derived from monocyte precursors) in antibody-dependent cytotoxicity reactions, suppresses delayed hypersensitivity reactions, and prolongs allograft survival (renal, skin, lung, heart).

   b. **Methotrexate** has little effect on nondividing cells but marked activity in rapidly proliferating cells. The drug affects both T and B lymphocytes and may suppress both cellular and humoral responses if given during an antigenic challenge. The metabolic block produced by methotrexate is reversed by folinic acid.

3. **Clinical indications** for **azathioprine** include autoimmune diseases such as rheumatoid arthritis as well as pemphigus vulgaris, bullous pemphigoid, and regional ileitis (Crohn's disease), and the ocular complications thereof. In one study on chronic uveitis patients, about 50% had a favorable response with combined azathioprine and low-dose systemic steroid. The remaining half did not respond or had adverse reactions. Azathioprine also has been used successfully in some cases of sympathetic ophthalmia, Vogt-Koyanagi-Harada syndrome pars planitis, and Behçet's disease. **Methotrexate** has been used successfully in certain recalcitrant cases of cyclitis and sympathetic ophthalmia; Behçet's disease and iridiocyclitis appear to be unresponsive.

4. **Dosage for azathioprine** starts at 1 mg/kg/d and works up to 2.5 mg/kg/d, with the average dose range being 50–100 mg/d as one dose or in divided doses. As noted above, the drug may be used with low-dose steroids (20–60 mg/d prednisone).

5. **Dosage for methotrexate** is variable because of the high toxic potential of the drug, which is, in part, dose related. This agent should be used only by or with physicians with considerable experience in the field. A number of dosage schedules have been recommended. Generally, a weekly oral (2.5-mg tablets) or IM (injectable preparation) dose of 7.5–25 mg is given until a therapeutic response is noted. Hematologic monitoring as described under cyclophosphamide should be carried out along with monthly (or more often as indicated) liver and renal function monitoring.

6. **Adverse side effects of azathioprine** seen most acutely are leukopenia (desirable level is not below 3000 cells/mm^3), thrombocytopenia, and GI disturbances. Chronic immunosuppression predisposes to secondary malignancies, but this risk appears lower in patients treated for autoimmune disease such as rhematoid disease than for allograft rejection. Allopurinol, an agent used for hyperuricemia, interferes with the metabolism of 6-mercaptopurine, thus necessitating lowering the azathioprine dose if allopurinol is being given concurrently.

7. **Adverse side effects of methotrexate** are common and may be severe, especially at higher doses. There may be marked leukopenia, thrombocytopenia, hepatotoxicity (atrophy, cirrhosis, necrosis), renal toxicity, ulcerative stomatitis, nausea, vomiting, diarrhea, interstitial pneumonitis, headache, blurred vision, drowsiness, and sterility.

E. **The locally delivered 5-fluorouracil (5-FU),** a pyrimidine analog, is under experimental study as both a subconjunctivally injected and a drop-delivered antimetabolite to prevent the inflammatory scarring of **glaucoma filtration blebs** postoperatively.

1. **The mechanism of action** of this antineoplastic

agent is through inhibition of fibroblast proliferation. Intravitreal and subconjunctival injections are well tolerated in animal studies.

2. **Clinical application** is currently the prevention of postoperative scarring of filtering blebs in glaucoma surgery.

3. **Dosage** used immediately at the conclusion of the surgical procedure is 5 mg of 5-FU in 0.5 ml of physiologic saline injected subconjunctivally 180 degrees away from the surgical site. The mixture is prepared by diluting 50 mg/ml 5-FU with 4 ml of saline for a final dose of 10 mg/ml. Concurrent subconjunctival injections of 20 mg triamcinolone diacetate and 2 mg dexamethasone also are injected 180 degrees away from the surgical site. Postoperatively, patients receive 5 mg of 5-FU twice daily subconjunctivally on postoperative days 1–7 and once daily on days 8–14. Maximum total dose is 125 mg during the 14-day period.

4. **Adverse side effects** have not been detected in terms of systemic toxicity. Local complications include postoperative corneal epithelial defects, which may persist up to 4 weeks, conjunctival needle tract leaks (which may be avoided by use of micropoint rather than spatula needles), and hemorrhagic choroidal detachment, which may have been more related to the surgery than to the use of 5-FU. No postoperative lacrimal system obstruction or postoperative cicatricial ectropion, which have been reported with nonocular 5-FU therapy, have yet been noted with subconjunctival 5-FU.

F. **Cyclosporine (Cyclosporine A),** an antibiotic, is one of a large family of naturally occurring and synthetic cyclic endecapeptides that has had a profound effect on current immunotherapy.

1. **The mechanism of action** is not fully understood, but it appears that the drug enters the cell and, like the corticosteroids, is bound to a specific receptor that has migrated to meet the molecule at the cell membrane. The receptor–cyclosporine complex then moves into the cell nucleus, where it affects mRNA production and ultimately protein synthesis.

2. **The immune system effect** is not fully established. The mode of action involves drug blockade of interleukin-2 (IL-2) receptors, inhibition of IL-2 release, prevention of IL-1 uptake (a step necessary for T-cell activation), or some or all of the above and more yet to be determined. Cyclosporine is, however, unique in mediating its effect via T-cell circuitry, and it is the inducer T-cell subset that is most affected. The drug greatly decreases antibody production to T-cell–dependent antigens, inhibits the cytotoxic activity of mixed leukocyte reactions, allograft survival of skin, kidney, heart, and possibly pancreas and cornea. It also may mitigate **graft-versus-host disease,** including the often devastating external ocular effects.

3. **Clinical indications.** Because of the potentially severe adverse side effects of the cytotoxic agents, cy-

closporine has become the second line of treatment after steroid failure in management of ocular immune disease. Indications for cyclosporine therapy include Behçet's disease (for which steroids may be contraindicated per some Japanese observers) and sympathetic ophthalmia. Relative indications are all noninfectious cases of uveitis unresponsive to maximum tolerated steroid therapy and repeated corneal graft rejection. Possible indications include Eales' disease, retinal vasculitis, and serpiginous choroidopathy. Contraindicated are all forms of infectious inflammatory disease. The FDA has not yet approved cyclosporine for any of the above indications.

4. **Dosage.** Cyclosporine is not absorbed well as a topical agent in the eye. It is far more effective, even for rejection of a corneal transplant, when given orally. The preparation for human use is in an olive oil solution, with 12.5% ethanol taken by mouth with milk or juice. About one third of the drug is absorbed from the GI tract, and aqueous humor concentration is about 40% that of plasma level in patients with quiescent uveitis. In therapy of uveitis, Behçet's disease, and other indicated conditions, cyclosporine dosage is 5 mg/kg/d given in 1 dose or as 2 divided doses. Maximum dosage is 7 mg/kg/d. Prednisone 10–20 mg/d may be used to augment this therapy and may be given at an even higher dose for short periods. **Corneal transplant rejection** was prevented in high-risk, vascularized eyes, with an initial cyclosporine dose of 15 mg/kg/d for 2 days, then 7.5 mg/kg/d for 2 days, and then 4–4.5 mg/kg/d to maintain therapeutic levels of 250–400 µg/liter of whole blood. Treatment was started on the day of transplant surgery and continued for 4 months, at which time the immunologic privilege of the cornea appeared to have been re-established. The overall success rate was nearly 90% in the year of follow-up in this poor-prognosis group. Topical cyclosporine is now under study to prevent rejection in high risk transplant patients.

5. **Adverse side effects.** Most adverse side effects of cyclosporine therapy reported in the literature were associated with the previously used higher doses of 10 mg/kg/d. Current doses of 5–7 mg/kg/d are associated with far fewer side effects; the two still of prime concern and occurrence are hypertension and partially reversible renal toxicity. It would appear, however, that the renal tubular atrophy and interstitial fibrosis previously reported may not occur with the lower drug doses, as the histologic changes have not been found in patients started and maintained on the lower-dose regimen. The systemic hypertension secondary to renal damage has also become less of a problem with the newer dosing. The concomitant use of steroid (prednisone 20–60 mg/d or bromocriptine 10 mg/d) with the regimen allows further lowering of the clinically effective dose of cyclosporine to 4–5 mg/kg/d. Opportunistic

infections with herpesviruses, *Candida,* and *Pneumocystis* may occur with progressive immunosuppression. Other reported side effects with cyclosporine (10 mg/kg/d) include paresthesias, epigastric burning, fatigue, gingivitis, anorexia, breast tenderness, hidradenitis, mild anemia, hyperuricemia, increased sedimentation rate, and hepatotoxicity. Cyclosporine does not appear to be associated with lymphomas or other neoplasms. B-cell lymphomas reported in transplant patients occurred in 1 of 100 patients, early in treatment course and always in association with multiple drug regimens.

G. **The antibiotic sulfone, 4-4'-diaminodiphenylsulfone (diphenylsulfone),** is used primarily in treating leprosy and dermatitis herpetiformis. A number of other ocular inflammatory/immune diseases also may respond to this drug (see Table 8-2).

1. **The mechanism of action** of this bactericidal/bacteriostatic drug in terms of anti-inflammatory effect is not established.

2. **The clinical indications** for IIS disease include dermatitis herpetiformis, bullous pemphigoid, pemphigus vulgaris, relapsing polychondritis, and ocular cicatricial pemphigoid. Of these conditions it is FDA approved only for treatment of dermatitis herpetiformis.

3. **Dosage** often must be individually designed. Diphenylsulfone is available as tablets of 25 and 100 mg. A common adult starting dose is 50 mg po daily, working up to 300 mg/d in 2–3 divided doses over several days. As soon as the disease process comes under control, slow dosage tapering to maintenance level should begin. Average dosage reduction time is 8 months, with a range of 4 months to 2½ years. If the patient is placed on a gluten-free diet, lower doses of drug may achieve the same therapeutic effect.

4. **Adverse side effects** are numerous and include agranulocytosis, aplastic anemia, and other blood dyscrasias, all of which necessitate hematologic monitoring (CBC, platelet count) weekly for the first month, monthly for the next 6 months, and semiannually thereafter. Drug should be discontinued if there is a significant drop in any blood parameter being followed. Folic acid antagonists such as pyrimethamine place patients at greater risk. The antagonist should be stopped, if possible, or closer hematologic monitoring maintained. The rare cutaneous reactions include a variety of bullous, exfoliative, and necrolytic reactions. Toxic hepatitis and cholestatic jaundice have been reported, as well as peripheral neuropathy. Other signs and symptoms occasionally associated with this drug are nausea, vomiting, abdominal pain, vertigo, blurred vision, tinnitus, insomnia, fever, headache, phototoxicity, psychosis, nephrotic syndrome, renal papillary necrosis, infertility, drug-induced lupus erythematosus, and, in overdosage, anoxic retinal and optic nerve

damage. Diphenylsulfone is mutagenic and carcinogenic in laboratory animals.

VII. **Adjuvant Therapy to Immunosuppressive Agents** (see Table 8-4).

A. **Colchicine** (acetyltrimethylcolchicinic acid) exerts antiinflammatory effects that are not well understood.

1. **Mechanism of action.** The drug suppresses lactic acid production in leukocytes, decreases phagocytosis, and inhibits PMN migration. As enhanced PMN migration is a characteristic of Behçet's disease, colchicine has been useful as a prophylactic agent in preventing recurrent attacks or in the rare patient with unilateral involvement in whom the physician is not prepared to start more powerful immunosuppressive therapy. This therapy is more popular in Japan than in other countries with a high incidence of Behçet's, such as Turkey, and it is of equivocal value in Caucasians.

2. **Dosage** is 0.6 mg orally bid.

3. **Adverse side effects** include nausea, vomiting, diarrhea, and abdominal pain. Long-term therapy may induce thrombocytopenia and aplastic anemia. The drug is contraindicated in pregnancy, as it causes fetal malformation.

B. **Bromocriptine** is a dopamine agonist that interferes with secretion of the anterior pituitary hormone, prolactin.

1. **Mechanism of action.** Prolactin competes with cyclosporine for receptor sites on the lymphocyte surface and will stimulate lymphocyte activity. Bromocriptine enhances the efficacy of lower doses of cyclosporine by interfering with prolactin secretion.

2. **Indications** for use of bromocriptine are not fully worked out. Animal models have shown efficacy in combined bromocriptine/low-dose cyclosporine therapy of graft-versus-host disease. There appears to be some efficacy in using bromocriptine alone in therapy of recurrent anterior uveitis. The use of bromocriptine as a cyclosporine dose-lowering agent would imply that the drug may be of use in the conditions in which cyclosporine is used. This is under study at the National Eye Institute.

3. **Dosage** currently used is 10 mg of bromocriptine daily by mouth, usually in combination with 4–5 mg/kg/d of cyclosporine.

4. **Adverse side effects** of bromocriptine include nausea and vomiting. Dosing should begin with 5 mg at bedtime and be worked up slowly to minimize intolerance.

VIII. **Summary of Clinical Indications and Use of Immunosuppressive Agents**

A. **Clinical conditions** for which systemic immunosuppressive agents have proven therapeutically effective after failure of conventional treatment are:

1. **Idiopathic chronic anterior uveitis or chronic cyclitis**

2. **Pars planitis (peripheral uveitis)**

3. **Behçet's syndrome** (Steroids may worsen disease according to some Japanese obervers. American observers do not necessarily agree and use steroids as initial therapy).
4. **Sympathetic ophthalmia**
5. **Peripheral ulcerative keratitis of Wegener's granulomatosis**
6. **Peripheral ulcerative keratitis** and **scleritis of rheumatoid arthritis, polyarteritis nodosa,** or **systemic lupus erythematosus**
7. **Ocular cicatricial pemphigoid**
8. **Mooren's ulcer**
9. **Thyroid exophthalmos**

B. **Current use** of the two more commonly used immunosuppressive agents, **cyclophosphamide** and **azathioprine,** at the Massachusetts Eye and Ear Infirmary Immunology and Uveitis Unit in Boston is as follows. Patients are generally maintained on either cyclophosphamide (1–2 mg/kg/d) or azathioprine (1–3 mg/kg/d) concurrently with prednisone (60–200 mg/d in 2–3 divided doses), until disease activity diminishes. Then gradual prednisone tapering begins with transition to alternate-day therapy, as described under Corticosteroids, if there is continued favorable therapeutic response. The dose of immunosuppressive drug is adjusted in response to therapeutic effect and adverse reactions. The WBCC is kept at 3000–3500/mm^3, the neutrophil count not below 1500/mm^3, and the platelet count not below 75,000/mm^3. Until the patient is stabilized on a given dose with respect to the above parameters and tolerance, a complete blood count and platelet count are obtained every 2 weeks, and monthly thereafter. Urinalyses are obtained monthly, with special attention to the presence of red blood cells indicative of occult or overt hemorrhagic cystitis (see Cyclophosphamide). Patients with idiopathic uveitis generally are maintained on immunosuppressive therapy for at least 4 months after disease has become quiescent. Ultimately, all therapy usually can be tapered slowly over several months and discontinued without flare-up of the disease. If cyclosporine is the immunosuppressive agent used, colchicine may be added in Behçet's disease as prophylaxis to deter recurrence and bromocriptine may be used concurrently as described earlier in chronic or recurrent anterior uveitis or graft-versus-host disease.

IX. **Nonsteroidal anti-inflammatory drugs (NSAIDs)** are prostaglandin inhibitors with both analgesic and anti-inflammatory activity. The orally administered drugs in this category used most commonly in ocular inflammatory disease are diflunisal, ibuprofen, indomethacin, naproxen, piroxicam, and sulindac. Topical preparations, flurbiprofen and suprofen, are used preoperatively to inhibit intraoperative miosis (Table 8-5).

A. **The mechanism of action** appears related to inhibition of cyclo-oxygenase, an enzyme involved in the conversion of arachidonic acid to inflammatory mediators, including the prostaglandins. The anti-inflammatory component

Table 8-5. Oral nonsteroidal anti-inflammatory drugs used in ophthalmic inflammatory disease*

Drug (commercial name)	Supplied (mg)	Recommended dose/day (mg)		Frequency of dosing (divided)
		Average (total mg)	Maximum (total mg)	
Diflunisal (Dolobid)	250, 500	500–1000	1500	bid
Ibuprofen (Motrin, others)	200, 300, 400, 600	1600	2400	qid
Indomethacin (Indocin)	25, 50	100–150	200	tid–qid
Indomethacin sustained-release (Indocin SR)	75	75–150	150	qd–bid
Naproxen (Naprosyn)	250, 375, 500	500	1000	bid
Piroxicam (Feldene)	10, 20	20	20	qd
Sulindac (Clinoril)	150, 200	300–400	400	bid

*Topical agents flurbiprofen and suprofen are described in the text.

does not appear to be related to release of endogenous corticosteroids.

B. **Clinical indications for oral NSAIDs** include treatment of cystoid macular edema (aphakic and pseudophakic) and possibly anterior uveitis in conjunction with topical steroids. There is no evidence that any of these agents used alone has a therapeutic effect on intraocular inflammatory disease. In terms of efficacy and safety, informal study at the Massachusetts Eye and Ear Infirmary indicates that diflunisal is the most effective and safest agent, with naproxen and indomethacin close seconds. Piroxicam, ibuprofen, and sulindac are the least effective for therapy of intraocular inflammation and associated cystoid macular edema. In one author's experience (DPL), ibuprofen has been useful in control and resolution of nodular scleritis in herpes zoster ophthalmicus. Oral NSAIDs also are particularly useful in long-term therapy of recurrent anterior uveitis, often allowing patients to discontinue steroid therapy or to maintain disease quiescence on minimal topical steroid dosing, eg, 1/8% prednisolone daily to bid. In managing noninfectious posterior uveitis and secondary vasculitis, disease must be brought under control initially with a combination of steroids and NSAIDs. Initial therapy may be retrobulbar depot methylprednisolone (40–60 mg) with concurrent diflunisal 500 mg po or naproxen 375 mg po bid. On occasion, prednisone 80–100 mg po each morning may be added for 7–14 days. Once the inflammatory disease is controlled and macular edema resolved, steroids are tapered and stopped, but the NSAID continued for 6–12 months as long as tolerated. For primary retinal vasculitis or other forms of ocular inflammatory/immune disease, NSAIDs appear ineffective. More intensive steroid or immunosuppressive therapy is required as indicated by disease.

C. **Dosage** for oral drugs is shown in Table 8-5. They are listed here in **decreasing order of apparent ocular efficacy:**
   1. diflunisal (Dolobid) 500 mg po bid
   2. indomethacin (Indocin SR) 75 mg po bid
   3. naproxen (Naprosyn) 250 or 375 mg po bid
   4. ibuprofen (Motrin, others) 300–600 mg po bid
   5. sulindac (Clinoril) 150 mg po bid
   6. piroxicam (Feldene) 20 mg po daily
   All oral NSAIDs should be taken with food, milk, or antacid.

D. **The topical preparations, 0.03% flurbiprofen and 1.0% suprofen,** are indicated for the inhibition of intraoperative miosis and are FDA approved to be used preoperatively in conjunction with mydriatic-cycloplegics. There is still considerable controversy over the efficacy of these agents in actually preventing intraoperative miosis. More recent studies indicate no significant difference between eyes dilated preoperatively with phenylephrine and cyclopentolate or scopolamine and those dilated with the same agents plus a topical NSAID as directed in the package inserts. Topical flurbiprofen is administered as 2 drops q30min for 4 doses total, starting 2 hours preoperatively, and suprofen 2 drops 3, 2, and 1 hour preoperatively. They also may be effective in therapy of cystoid macular edema at qid dosage, but oral NSAIDs are probably superior (not FDA approved for this use).

E. **Adverse side effects of oral NSAIDs** include blurred vision, dry eyes, oral ulcers, sore throat, headache, tinnitus, decreased hearing, alopecia, fever, nausea, gastritis, gastric ulcer, dysuria, frequent urination, hematuria, diarrhea, melena, constipation, chemical hepatitis, dyspnea, fatigue, weakness, dizziness, confusion, depression, insomnia, nervousness, renal failure, leukopenia, neutropenia, aplastic anemia, and Stevens-Johnson syndrome. These drugs are **contraindicated** in patients with the syndrome of nasal polyps, angioedema, and bronchospastic reaction to aspirin.

Topical flurbiprofen or suprofen may cause burning and stinging on application. In some patients this NSAID may interfere with thrombocyte aggregation and cause increased bleeding from ocular tissues at the time of surgery. The drug is contraindicated in patients with active infectious (dendritic/geographic ulcers) herpes simplex keratitis.

Information Sources and Suggested Reading
(*Corticosteroids, Immunosuppressive Agents, NSAIDs*)

1. Ehrlich, G., Behçet's disease: Current concepts. Compr. Ther. 15(1):27–30, 1989.
2. Ellis, P., *Ocular Therapeutics and Pharmacology,* 7th ed. St. Louis: C.V. Mosby, 1985, pp. 28–41, 158–161, 212–239 (principles of cortisone therapy, retina, uveitis, optic neuritis, orbit), pp. 293–295 (anti-inflammatory agents), pp. 297–301 (immunosuppressive agents).
3. Fiore, P., Jacobs, I., and Goldberg, D., Drug induced pemphigoid: a spectrum of diseases. Arch. Ophthalmol. 105: 1660–1664, 1987.
4. Flurbiprofen for inhibition of intraoperative miosis. In Ocular Therapy Report, American Health Consultants, Atlanta 1(11) 41–44 (Nov. 1988) and 2(11) 45–48 (Nov. 1989).
5. Foster, C.S., Basic ocular immunology. In Kaufman, H.E., Barron, B., McDonald, M., and Waltman, S. (Eds.), *The Cornea.* New York: Churchill Livingstone, 1988, pp. 85–124.
6. Foster, C.S., Nonsteroidal anti-inflammatory and immunosuppressive agents. In Lamberts, D.W., and Potter, D.E. (Eds.), *Clinical Ophthalmic Pharmacology.* Boston: Little, Brown, 1987, pp. 173–192.
7. Fraunfelder, F., and Roy F.H. (Eds.), *Current Ocular Therapy 3,* 3rd. Philadelphia: W.B. Saunders, 1990, multiple contributing authors, pp. 177–178, 197, 198, 201, 203–204, 206–207, 359, 372, 400, 411, 420, 689, 691 (external and endogenous immune ocular disorders).
8. Gery, I., and Nussenblatt, R., Immunosuppressive drugs. In

Sears, M.L. (Ed.), *Pharmacology of the Eye*. Vol. 69, Handbook of Experimental Pharmacology. New York: Springer-Verlag, 1984, pp. 585–602.

9. Havener, W.H., *Ocular Pharmacology*, 5th ed. St. Louis: C.V. Mosby, 1983, pp. 223–235 (nonsteroidal anti-inflammatory agents), pp. 433–500 (corticosteroids).

10. Hill, J., Use of cyclosporine in high-risk keratoplasty. Am. J. Ophthalmol. 107:506–510, 1989.

11. Hudson, N.P., and Whisler, R., Update: Treatment of rheumatoid disease. Compr. Ther. 14(10):51–56, 1988.

12. Jaffe, I., Drug therapy of rheumatoid arthritis. Compr. Ther. 15(1):20–26, 1989.

13. Kleinert, R., Corticosteroid use in ocular infectious disease, in Tabbara, K., Hyndiuk, R. (Eds.), *Infections of the Eye*. Boston: Little, Brown, 1986, pp. 293–302.

14. Leopold, I., and Gaster, R., Ocular inflammation and anti-inflammatory drugs. In Kaufman, H.E., Barrow, B., McDonald, M., and Waltman, S. (Eds.), *The Cornea*. New York: Churchill Livingstone, 1988, pp. 67–84.

15. Limaye, S., Pillai, S., and Tina, L., Relationship of steroid dose to degree of posterior subcapsular cataracts in nephrotic syndrome. Ann. Ophthalmol. 20:225–227, 1988.

16. Masuda, K., Anti-inflammatory agents: nonsteroidal anti-inflammatory drugs. In Sears, M.L. (Ed.), *Pharmacology of the Eye*. Vol. 69, Handbook of Experimental Psychology. New York: Springer-Verlag, 1984, pp. 539–552.

17. Moncada, S., Flower, R.J., and Vane, J., Prostaglandins, prostacyclin, thromboxane A_2, and leukotrienes. In Gilman, A.G., Goodman, L.L., Rall, T., and Murad, F. (Eds.), *The Pharmacological Basis of Therapeutics*, 7th ed. New York: Macmillan, 1985, pp. 660–673.

18. Mondino, B., Aizuss, D., and Farley, M., Steroids. In Lamberts, D.W., and Potter, D.E. (Eds.), *Clinical Ophthalmic Pharmacology*. Boston: Little, Brown, 1987, pp. 157–172.

19. Nussenblatt, R.B., and Palestine, A.G., *Uveitis: Fundamentals in Clinical Practice*. Chicago: Yearbook Medical Publ., 1989, pp. 1–53 (immune system), pp. 54–102 (clinical evaluation of uveitis patient), pp. 103–162 (therapeutic and diagnostic interventions), pp. 163–324 (endogenous uveitic entities).

20. Pavan-Langston, D., Uveal tract. In Pavan-Langston, D. (Ed.), *Manual of Ocular Diagnosis and Therapeutics*, 3rd ed. Boston: Little, Brown, 1990, pp. 163–200.

21. Polansky, J., and Weinreb, R., Anti-inflammatory agents: steroids as anti-inflammatory agents. In Sears, M.L. (Ed.), *Pharmacology of the Eye*. Vol. 69, Handbook of Experimental Pharmacology. New York: Springer-Verlag, 1984, pp. 459–524.

22. Sears, M.L. (Ed.), *Pharmacology of the Eye*. Vol. 69, Handbook of Experimental Pharmacology. New York: Springer-Verlag, 1984, pp. 459–524 (anti-inflammatory agents: steroids, Polansky, J., Weinreb, R.), pp. 539–552 (nonsteroidal anti-inflammatory drugs, Masuda, K.)

23. Smolin, G., and O'Connor, G.R., *Ocular Immunology*, 2nd ed. Boston: Little, Brown, 1986, pp. 1–102 (general immunol-

ogy), pp. 103–134 (immunologic testing), pp. 193–254 (immune disease of the external eye), pp. 255–272 (systemic immune disease and the external eye), pp. 273–306 (corneal graft rejection), pp. 307–346 (immune disease of the uvea and retina).

24. Smolin, G., and Thoft, R.A. (Eds.), *The Cornea.* Boston: Little, Brown, 1986, pp. 99–140 (immunology, Smolin, G.), pp. 321–326 (Mooren's ulcers, Schanzlin, G.), pp. 327–343 (rheumatoid, Smith, R., Schanzlin, D.), pp. 344–366 (nonrheumatic acquired collagen vascular disease, Foster, C.S.).

25. Stark, W., Fagadau, W., Stewart, R., et al., Reduction of pupillary constriction during cataract surgery using suprofen. Arch. Ophthalmol. 104:364–366, 1986.

9

Local Anesthetics

Local anesthetics, whether topical or injected, block both initiation and conduction of the nerve impulse. This action is transient, with ultimate full functional recovery and no permanent physiologic damage to affected neurons.

I. Pharmacology and Mechanism of Action of Topical and Injected Agents

Currently used local anesthetic agents comprise three structural parts: an aromatic acid, an alkyl alcohol, and a secondary or, more often, a tertiary amine group. The longer the alkyl chain, the greater are both the potency and the toxicity of the drug. The bonding at the alkyl site may be either an ester link, which is metabolized directly in the anesthetized tissues by plasma pseudocholinesterases, or an amide link, which makes the drug more stable in tissues because the amide link is not metabolized locally, but in the liver. Virtually all ester-linked anesthetic agents are delivered topically, and amide-linked agents are injected. **Allergic reactions** to local anesthetics seem to be confined to the ester-linked group because of the inherent metabolic instability of these topical agents.

The mechanism of action of local anesthetics is through physiologic effects on the cell membrane. Effective depolarization and conduction are dependent on a major shift to increased membrane permeability to Na^+. Local anesthetics block conduction by decreasing cell membrane permeability to Na^+. With sufficient drug concentration, not only nerve but also muscle membrane potentials may be similarly affected.

Local tissue pH also bears on anesthetic efficacy. Anesthetics exist in combined nonionized and ionized states, with the former being responsible for absorption and the latter for the actual anesthesia. At normal tissue or tear pH of 7.4, only 20% of an anesthetic agent will be in the unionized, lipid-soluble form absorbed by tissues, or, in the case of topical anesthetics, by the corneal and conjunctival epithelium. The lipid-soluble form is necessary for crossing the corneal epithelial barrier before the anesthetic deionizes in the hydrophilic stroma. The degree to which all local anesthetics enter the anesthetizing, ionized state is a function of tissue pH; the higher the pH, the greater the ionization. Unfortunately, anesthetics are often used in the presence of inflammation, which in itself lowers pH, thus making the agents more deionized and, therefore, less able to penetrate tissue, regardless of the route of administration.

II. Clinical Applications of Topical Anesthetics

As anesthetic action progressively develops, the threshold for electrical excitability increases; partial and ultimately complete blockage of conduction ensues. Onset of action of topical anesthesia is rapid, usually within 30 seconds, and the duration of action is up to 20 minutes. Successive instillation of a topical anesthetic drop 3–4 times, with a few minutes interval between drops (Table 9-1), will deepen the extent of the anesthesia such that intraocular procedures including laser therapy are much better tolerated by the patient. In general, however, topical anesthesia is used most frequently after application of a single drop to perform such ocular procedures as tonometry, superficial foreign body removal, conjunctival biopsy, and nasolacrimal canalicular irrigation and probing. Cocaine also is used in testing for Horner's pupil.

A. **Benoxinate (0.4%).** This ester of para-aminobenzoic acid (PABA) is available only as 0.4% concentration in combination with 0.25% sodium fluorescein (Fluress; see also Fluorocaine under proparacaine). As such, it is used primarily for applanation tonometry, but it also is effective in delineating corneal and conjunctival epithelial ulceration. The onset of anesthesia (10–20 seconds) and the intensity and duration of action (10–20 minutes) are similar to commercially available 0.5% tetracaine or proparacaine, but side effects are fewer. Stinging on instillation is less than that with tetracaine, and more than with proparacaine, but the tendency to corneal epithelial damage is less than that of proparacaine. Benoxinate possesses considerable antibacterial activity, thus making it highly suited for combination in solution with fluorescein, an agent that by itself supports growth of many microbes, including *Pseudomonas aeruginosa*.

Allergic reactions are rare, and there appears to be no cross-sensitivity between benoxinate and proparacaine, cocaine, or even tetracaine, another PABA derivative (see Side Effects).

B. **Cocaine (1–4%, 10%).** This narcotic agent is not used as a routine topical anesthetic. It is useful, however, for diagnosis of Horner's syndrome using 1 drop of a 10% solution. Cocaine uniquely alters uptake of norepinephrine and induces heightened sensitivity to catecholamines and thus mydriasis of the denervated pupil. Excellent anesthesia of cornea, conjunctiva, and the insertions of the rectus muscles beginning within 5–10 minutes and lasting 20 minutes is achieved with a 1–4% solution. This may be given as a total of 2 drops instilled 2–3 minutes apart or as a cocaine-soaked, wrung cotton pledget allowed to rest on the conjunctiva for 1 minute. This deep topical anesthesia allows painless full-thickness conjunctival biopsy, forced ductions of the rectus muscles when grasped with toothed forceps, and, as a function of the notable corneal epithelial toxicity, easy debridement of this structure. The vasoconstrictor action of cocaine whitens the eye and slows both bleeding and absorption of the drug. It should not be used with exogenous epinephrine, however, because of **cocaine-induced epinephrine hypersensitivity** (see Side Effects). Because of its vasoconstrictor activity and unique prolonged action on mucous membranes (1 hour or more), cocaine is also useful in nasal packing during dacryocystorhinostomy.

C. **Proparacaine (0.5%).** This commonly used topical an-

Table 9-1. Topical anesthetics*

Generic name (commercial)	Pharmacologic derivation	Drug forms	Maximum suggested dose/eye (compress nasolacrimal canal to decrease systemic absorption)
Cocaine HCl	Benzoic acid	1–4% solution	1–5 drops, 2–3 min apart
Benoxinate HCl (Fluress)	Para-aminobenzoic acid	0.4% benoxinate in solution with 0.25% Na fluorescein	1–3 drops, 1–2 min apart
Proparacaine HCl (AK-Taine, Alcaine, Fluorocaine, I-Paracaine, Kainaire, Ophthaine, Ophthetic)	Meta-aminobenzoic acid	0.5% solution	1–10 drops, 1–2 min apart
Tetracaine HCl (Pontocaine, others)	Para-aminobenzoic acid	0.5% solution	1–5 drops, 1–2 min apart
		0.5% ointment	¾-in. strip ointment

* All are ester linked and, therefore, potentially sensitizing.

esthetic causes little or no discomfort on instillation and therefore is the best accepted by patients. The time of onset is 10–20 seconds and duration of action about 20 minutes. If deeper anesthesia is desired, as for iris or even retinal laser surgery, this least toxic agent is probably the best for repeated topical application before initiating any procedure, eg, 1 drop every 1–2 minutes for 3 or 4 doses. Although it does not penetrate the cornea or conjunctiva as well as tetracaine, this agent is less irritating on instillation and will cause less corneal toxicity and epithelial clouding. Side effects are rare, usually mild, and less frequent than with tetracaine. Although both drugs are ester-linked aminobenzoic acid, no cross-sensitivity has been reported nor any cross-sensitivity with benoxinate or cocaine.

Proparacaine also comes as a 0.5% solution in combination with 0.25% fluorescein sodium (Fluorocaine). It is used primarily for applanation tonometry, but also as a disclosing agent for corneal or conjunctival epithelial disturbances. Toxicity and side effects are similar to those of proparacaine alone.

D. Tetracaine (0.5%). Tetracaine, another ester-linked PABA derivative, is a very commonly used topical anesthetic drop similar to benoxinate and proparacaine in onset of action of 10–20 seconds and duration of about 20 minutes. Despite the frequency of its use, tetracaine is not the most benign topical anesthetic. Many patients complain of burning and stinging for 20–30 seconds after instillation. Corneal toxicity is greater than that of proparacaine or benoxinate, and local allergic reaction is rare but more frequent than with the alternative anesthetics. Cross-sensitivity has not been reported with other ester-linked anesthetics; however, the drug is a highly effective topical anesthetic that penetrates cornea and conjunctiva more effectively than proparacaine, thus supporting its viability as an anesthetic agent.

III. Side Effects of Topical Anesthetics
A. Systemic reactions to local drug. Adverse side effects to topical anesthetics are quite rare; they may be manifested locally or systemically within a few minutes of instillation. Topical anesthetics are absorbed across conjunctival and nasolacrimal mucous membranes very rapidly, with the rate of rise of blood level similar to that of IV injection. Young healthy males appear the most likely to suffer vasovagal reactions, with syncope and even transient respiratory arrest. Other susceptible patients are the debilitated and those with a tendency toward allergic reactions, asthma, or chronic obstructive pulmonary disease, cardiovascular abnormalities, especially arrhythmias, and hyperthyroidism. Other than vasovagal reactions (which may have a large psychologic component), severe reactions to most topical agents given in recommended doses are essentially nonexistent.

Cocaine 4% in a dose equivalent to 10 drops (20 mg) may induce not only severe corneal epithelial sloughing, but also systemic toxicity characterized by initial hyperactivity, headache, irregular tachycardia, nausea and vomiting, pupillary dilation, and, in the extreme, delirium, seizures, and death at about 1.2-g dosage. As the mechanism of this toxicity is in part through β-adrenergic stimulation, β-blocking agents such as **propanalol** (Inderal) or **timolol** (Blocadren) 20–40 mg by mouth will **inhibit** the more **serious** sequelae of the progressive reaction.

B. **Local reactions** to topically applied anesthetics are largely restricted to the cornea at recommended doses. True allergic reactions due to hypersensitivity induced from previous exposures are very rare, self-resolving, and subsequently avoided by the use of an alternative anesthetic. Toxic adverse effects range from superficial punctate keratitis (SPK), which is almost universal, to epithelial sloughing developing 2–30 minutes after drug instillation. In about 0.001% of cases, there may be an edematous necrotizing keratitis with marked photophobia, decrease in vision, and conjunctival hyperemia. Most adverse reactions may be managed with reassurance (SPK), antibiotic ointment 3 times a day for 2–3 days until healed (some epithelial loss), or cycloplegia (1% cyclopentolate), antibiotic ointment, and pressure patch, with revisit for the most severe sloughing keratitides. As noted, there appears to be no cross-sensitivity among the various topical anesthetics. Future examinations may be done with an alternative drug with minimal risk of reaction.

IV. **Abuse of Topical Anesthetics**

Abuse of topical anesthetics results either from physicians giving patients prescriptions for these agents as treatment for painful corneal abrasions or from patients somehow obtaining the agents and self-treating for ocular discomfort. Regardless of cause, the results are the same. Tachyphylaxis develops rapidly with increased frequency of dosage, resulting in less and shorter relief from pain. Increasing dosing retards epithelial healing (neuroparalytic keratitis) and produces progressive toxicity ranging from diffuse SPK, central epithelial slough, stromal edema and infiltrates, and, in extreme cases, iritis and hypopyon. Treatment involves stopping the anesthetic, topical antibiotic, cycloplegia, pressure patching, and systemic analgesics. Occasionally patients must be admitted to the hospital for 1–2 days to bring the reaction under control.

Patients overdosed due to high levels of drug also may manifest a variety of systemic reactions similar to those described below under injectable anesthetics. The most common reasons for overdosage, other than delivery of too much drug to the eye, are excessive absorption across hyperemic conjunctival and episcleral vessels, inhibition of ester metabolism in patients receiving cholinesterase inhibitors such as phospholine iodide (glaucoma, accommodative esotropia), and, in the debilitated patient, inability to metabolize or eliminate the systemically absorbed drug from the body before toxic levels are achieved.

Table 9-2. Injected local anesthetics

Generic name (commercial)	Pharmacologic derivation	Drug concentration	Onset of action (min)	Duration without epinephrine	Duration with epinephrine
Bupivacaine HCl (Marcaine)	Benzoic acid amide linked	0.25, 0.5, and 0.75% solution	5–10	8–12 hrs	8–12 hrs
Etidocaine HCl (Duranest)	Benzoic acid amide linked	1 and 1.5%	3–5	5–10 hrs	5–10 hrs
Lidocaine HCl (Xylocaine)	Benzoic acid amide linked	0.5, 1.0, 1.5, 2.0, and 4%	4–6	40–60 min	2 hrs
Mepivacaine HCl (Carbocaine)	Benzoic acid amide linked	1, 1.5, 2, and 3%	3–5	2 hrs	2 hrs
Procaine HCl (Novocaine)	Benzoic acid amide linked	1, 2, and 10%	7–9	30–45 min	1 hr

V. Injected Local Anesthetics

The most commonly used injected anesthetics are the amide-linked esters. Table 9-2 lists these agents by name, dosage, onset, and duration of action with and without addition of the vasoconstrictor epinephrine to slow absorption. Side effects are discussed below.

VI. Side Effects of Injected Local Anesthetics

A. Systemic reactions to local drug. Injected anesthetics rarely induce true allergic or toxic systemic reactions. Allergic hypersensivity may be manifested by hives, angioneurotic edema, low blood pressure, bronchospasm, joint pain, and, very rarely, anaphylaxis. **Management** (adult doses) includes systemic **antihistamines** (Benadryl, 50 mg by mouth), **bronchodilators** (aminophylline, 3 mg/kg body weight IV no faster than 25 mg/min or 200–400 mg by mouth), and/or **Adrenalin** 1:1000, 0.2–1.0 ml subcutaneously.

B. Toxic reactions to injected anesthetics are more severe and include hyperactivity, tremulousness, and possible convulsions and unconsciousness. Cardiopulmonary effects are initially respiratory depression, hypertension, arrhythmias, and, later, hypotension secondary to peripheral vasodilation, cardiac slowing, or arrest, and ultimately respiratory arrest. Much central nervous system toxicity is reversed with administration of oxygen and cardiorespiratory effects by management appropriate to the phase of the reaction.

Injected local anesthetics also may induce morphologic changes in the extraocular and lid muscles, thus inducing the frequently noted postoperative lid ptosis and diplopia. The aminoacyl agents such as lidocaine and bupivacaine appear to be particularly prone to inducing myotoxicity. These local pathophysiologic changes are self-reparative, and the clinical symptoms are transient, usually lasting only a few days to 2–3 months.

VII. Effects of Local Anesthetics on Bacterial Cultures

See Chapter 3, Antibiotics.

Information Sources and Suggested Reading (*Local Anesthetics*)

1. Davies, P.H., *The Actions and Uses of Ophthalmic Drugs,* 2nd ed. Boston: Butterworths, 1981, pp. 191–210 (local anesthetics and decongestants).
2. Ellis, P., *Ocular Therapeutics and Pharmacology,* 7th ed. St. Louis: C.V. Mosby, 1985, pp. 80–88, 265–271 (local anesthetics).
3. Havener, W.H., Anesthesia, *Ocular Pharmacology,* 5th ed. St. Louis: C.V. Mosby, 1983, pp. 72–119.
4. Gandhi, S., Local anesthetics. In Lamberts, D.W., and Potter, D.E. (Eds.), *Clinical Ophthalmic Pharmacology.* Boston: Little, Brown, 1987, pp. 335–360.
5. Porter, J., Edney, D., McMahon, B.E., and Burns, L., Extra-

ocular myotoxicity of the retrobulbar anesthetic bupivacaine HCl. Invest. Ophthalmol. Vis. Sci. 29:163–174, 1988.

6. Ritchie, J., and Greene, N., Local anesthetics. In Gilman, A.G., Goodman, L.L., Rall, T., and Murad, F. (Eds.), *The Pharmacological Basis of Therapeutics,* 7th ed. New York: Macmillan, 1985, pp. 302–321.

10

Mydriatics and Cycloplegics

Mydriasis, iris pupillary dilation, and **cycloplegia,** paresis or paralysis of the ciliary muscle at the peripheral base of the iris, may be deliberately induced to varying degrees by several topical medications. Drug selection for clinical use is based on the degree of each effect desired. Most physicians will use a sympathomimetic such as phenylephrine with a parasympatholytic agent such as tropicamide or cyclopentolate for office examinations, as part of the treatment of mild to moderate anterior uveitis, and preoperatively. The advantage is an excellent but short-lived mydriatic/cycloplegic effect that may be reversed by parasympathomimetics such as acetylcholine and carbachol. These latter two agents become even more effective within an hour or two as the tropicamide and cyclopentolate molecules release the parasympathetic receptors, thus opening them to the action of the miotics. If longer-acting mydriatic/cycloplegic effect is desired, as in therapy of more severe intraocular inflammatory disease, long-term postoperative follow-up, and as home-administered agents for cycloplegic refraction of young children at a future office visit, a stronger and longer-acting parasympatholytic such as atropine, homatropine, or scopolamine will be selected. These, however, are not readily reversed by the parasympathomimetic miotics, and their effect will persist for several days.

I. Iris Anatomy, Innervation, and Vascular Supply

The iris is the anterior extension of the uveal tract (choroid) or vascular layer between sclera and neuroretinal structures. It is a muscular cone with the pupil at its apex and the ciliary body running 360 degrees around the base. The two iris layers are, anteriorly, the connective tissue stroma and, posteriorly, the pigmented epithelium, which is continuous posteriorly as a double layer: the inner, nonpigmented epithelium of the ciliary processes, which produces aqueous humor and extends to become the sensory retina, and the outer, pigmented layer, which becomes the retinal pigment epithelium. The sphincter muscle runs circumferentially around the pupillary margin and is parasympathetically innervated. The dilator muscle is sympathetically and, to a much lesser extent, parasympathetically innervated and runs radially from its origin in the ciliary body through the posterior iris stroma. Dilation may, therefore, be achieved by either inhibiting the sphincter muscle or stimulating the dilator muscle. The ciliary muscle also is sympathetically innervated, circular, and located in the ciliary body between iris and chorioretinal structures. Paralysis of this muscle results in loss of accommodation and relaxation of ciliary spasm. Vascular supply to the iris is via the major arterial circle originating from the anterior and a few posterior ciliary arteries. Radial arteries run from the major circle at the iris base to form the minor circle around the sphincter collarette. Venous drainage is via the vortex veins, which carry blood from the choroid to the superior ophthalmic vein. Iris blood vessels are innervated by the sympathetic nervous system.

II. Anticholinergic Drugs

These drugs block the actions of parasympathetic innervation and of cholinergic drugs on the muscles and vasculature of the iris and ciliary body. Agents included in this group, in decreasing order of potency, are **atropine, scopolamine, homatropine, cyclopentolate,** and **tropicamide.**

A. **The mechanism of action** of this drug group is through antimuscarinic activity as competitive antagonists of acetylcholine (ACh) and other muscarinic agonists. This antagonism may be reversed or inhibited by sufficient increase in ACh concentration at the receptor sites of the effector organ.

B. **Preparations for ocular use** (Table 10-1)
   1. **Atropine sulfate (dl-hyoscyamine).**
      a. **Dosage.** Solutions are available in concentrations of 0.5, 1, 2, and 4% with dosage 1–4 times daily. Ointment is available in 0.5 and 1% concentrations. The time to maximum mydriasis is 40 minutes and to maximum cycloplegia is 1–3 hours. The duration of action is 7–14 days.
      b. **Clinical indications.** Atropine sulfate differs from scopolamine in muscarinic activity, in that atropine has a more prolonged ocular effect, less potent action on the iris, ciliary body, secretory glands (salivary, sweat, bronchial), and CNS, and more potent action on the heart, intestines, and bronchial muscles. It is most useful, therefore, in situations where prolonged potent cycloplegia and mydriasis are desired while minimizing the CNS depression seen more often with scopolamine. Clinical uses include anterior uveitis to prevent or break synechiae, accommodative spasm, and cycloplegic refractions in infants and young children, where the full refractive error including latent hyperopia is necessary for treatment of heterotropias, heterophorias, and accommodative asthenopia and because getting medication in the eye at the time of the office visit often is difficult. Common **dosage for cycloplegic refraction** is ½% (blue eyes)–1% (brown eyes) solution or ointment bid for 3 days before exam. It is usual to add −1.00 sphere to the correction found under atropine cycloplegia to allow for tone of the ciliary muscle; this correction may be reduced if the child is esotropic.
      c. **Adverse side effects** from topical administration may be local or result from systemic absorption across the conjunctival and nasolacrimal mucous membranes.
         (1) **Ocular** effects include increased IOP in less than half of patients who have open-angle glaucoma (no IOP rise in normals), angle-closure glaucoma in eyes anatomically narrowed, allergic dermatitis, blurred vision due to loss of accommodation, and photophobia due to mydriasis.
         (2) **Systemic** side effects of topical drug may in-

Table 10-1. Mydriatic/cycloplegic agents in decreasing order of potency

Drug	Commercial name	Concentrations	Time to maximum mydriasis/cycloplegia	Duration of action	Drug type
Atropine SO$_4$	Many	0.5, 1, 2, 4%	40 min/1–3 hr	7–14 days	Parasympatholytic
Scopolamine	Isopto Hyoscine Mydramide AK-Homatropine	0.25%	30 min/30–45 min	5–7 days	Parasympatholytic
Homatropine HBr	Homatrocel Isopto Homatropine	2, 5%	15 min/30–90 min	3 days	Parasympatholytic
Cyclopentolate HCl	AK-Pentolate Cyclogyl	0.5, 1, 2%	15–30 min/ 15–45 min	1 day	Parasympatholytic
Tropicamide	Mydriacyl Tropicacyl Phenyltrope	0.5, 1%	20–30 min/ 20–30 min	4–6 hr	Parasympatholytic
Phenylephrine HCl	See Phenylephrine AK Dilate Efricel Mydfrin Neo-Synephrine Phenyltrope	2.5, 10% 2–5% phenylephrine 0.5–1.0% tropicamide	20–30 min/NA	4–6 hr	Sympathomimetic
Hydroxy-amphetamine	Paredrine	1%	30 min/NA	3–4 hr	Sympathomimetic
Epinephrine—see Chapter 5, Antiglaucoma Drugs					

clude tachycardia, confusion, hallucinations, drowsiness, ataxia, dermal flush, fever, dysarthria, thirst, urinary retention, convulsions, and even death. Children with Down's syndrome may be more susceptible to systemic side effects. When given systemically in conventional doses, eg, 0.6 mg IM, atropine has little ocular effect in comparison with systemically administered scopolamine, which causes definite mydriasis and loss of accommodation.

2. **Scopolamine hydrobromide (l-hyoscine)**
   a. **Dosage.** The single-agent ophthalmic solution is available as a 0.25% solution commonly used 1–4 times daily. Murocoll-2 is a 0.3% solution combined with 10% phenylephrine and should, therefore, be used with caution in patients with cardiovascular disease. The time of onset of maximal mydriasis is 15–30 minutes, and of maximal cycloplegia, 30–45 minutes. The duration of action is about 7 days.
   b. **Clinical indications** are similar to those of atropine. Because scopolamine has a greater adverse CNS effect, however, atropine may be preferable in older patients. It is not commonly used for cycloplegic refraction in children.
   c. **Adverse side effects**
      (1) **Ocular** effects of scopolamine are, as with atropine, elevated IOP in less than half of patients with open-angle glaucoma, angle-closure glaucoma in eyes so predisposed, allergic dermatoconjunctivitis, blurred vision, and photophobia.
      (2) **Systemic** side effects of topical drops are fewer, but include confusion, hallucinations, drowsiness, dermal flush, and disorientation. As noted, scopolamine has a greater adverse CNS effect than does atropine.

3. **Homatropine hydrobromide and hydrochloride**
   a. **Dosage.** This topical agent is available in 2 and 5% solutions. Onset of maximum mydriasis is 10–30 minutes, and of maximum cycloplegia, 60–90 minutes, with duration of action about 3 days. It is commonly used 1–3 times daily. This agent induces less cycloplegia than do scopolamine and atropine because of its weaker antimuscarinic activity. Its advantage is that of a moderately strong mydriatic/cycloplegic that wears off in a very few days.
   b. **Clinical indications** include anterior uveitis and postoperative dilation. This drug may be used for cycloplegic refraction, although the depth of cycloplegia in patients under 20 years is not reduced much below 2.00 diopters. Ciliary muscle tonus is not affected.
   c. **Adverse side effects**
      (1) **Ocular** effects are similar to those of atropine and scopolamine. Although homatropine rarely raises IOP in normals, it commonly causes a

pressure rise and a reduction in outflow facility in patients with open-angle glaucoma (with the angle remaining open). This phenomenon occurs far more often with homatropine than with the stronger two cycloplegic/mydriatics.

(2) **Systemic** side effects of topical drops include confusion, hallucinations, ataxia, fever, and dysarthria——all related to CNS effects.

4. **Cyclopentolate**

a. **Dosage.** This anticholinergic agent is available as a topical drop in concentrations of 0.5, 1, and 2%. Maximum mydriatic action is achieved in 15–30 minutes and maximum cycloplegia in 30–45 minutes. Duration of action is about 24 hours. The drop is commonly given 1–3 times daily, except as noted below for cycloplegic refraction.

b. **Clinical indications** are compatible with the relatively short action of the drug. It is used for mydriasis for fundus exam, in anterior uveitis of mild to moderate severity to prevent or break posterior synechiae, and to relieve ciliary spasm. Long term use in uveitis may be limited, however, as this drug is a **chemoattractant to inflammatory cells.** It is frequently used in cycloplegic refractions in children and adults, where it is desired to give the drops at the time of exam than in advance (as is done with atropine in infants and very young children). **Dosage** of cyclopentolate **for cycloplegic refraction** is usually 1% drops every 15 minutes for 1–2 doses, with brown eyes being less responsive than blue. There is almost always a residual accommodation of 1.5 D even at 40–60 minutes (maximum cycloplegia). Drug effects are normally gone in 24 hours.

c. **Adverse side effects** with topical cyclopentolate are numerous locally and systemically.

(1) **Ocular** effects include the **local** effects of a rare increase in IOP in patients with open-angle glaucoma, acute angle-closure glaucoma in eyes anatomically so predisposed, allergic reactions, blurred vision, and photophobia.

(2) **Systemic** reactions of topical drug include tachycardia, systemic hypertension, nausea, confusion, uncontrolled crying, hallucinations, drowsiness, weakness, ataxia, dermal flush, thirst, convulsions, and disorientation. Children are particularly susceptible to adverse CNS reactions, especially when 2% drops are used. Onset of side effects in adults and children may range from 30 minutes to 2 hours and pass spontaneously in 1–4 hours.

5. **Tropicamide**

a. **Dosage.** This ocular anticholinergic is available in 0.5 and 1.0% solutions for mydriatic/cycloplegic use. Dosage is commonly 1 drop 1–2 times over 10–15 minutes depending on intended use (see Clinical

Indications). Onset of maximal action is 30 minutes; drug effects last only a few hours.

b. **Clinical indications** are primarily a function of the brevity of action of this drug. It is useful diagnostically for a nonextended dilated fundus exam, usually being given as 1 drop of 0.5% solution every 5 minutes for 1–2 doses 15–20 minutes before the exam. It also is useful for **cycloplegic refraction** commonly given as 1 drop of 1% solution every 5 minutes for 3 doses and the refraction done within 30 minutes. Because of its weaker cycloplegic effect, tropicamide is not as effective for refractive purposes as cyclopentolate. Its use as a cycloplegic/mydriatic in refraction is probably best reserved for adults with reduced accommodative power. **Combined** 0.5–1.0% tropicamide and 2.5% phenylephrine are indicated in situations where greater mydriasis is desired, such as in dilated fundus exam or to break recently formed or weak posterior synechiae by the jerking action of repeated doses every 20 minutes for 3–4 doses.

c. **Adverse side effects**
(1) **Ocular** effects of topical tropicamide in the eye include extremely rare and mild elevation of IOP, angle-closure glaucoma in eyes anatomically predisposed, allergic blepharoconjunctivitis, and blurred vision.
(2) **Systemic** toxicity is rare because the drug tends to be used for single or very short-term application. Reported effects include psychotic reactions and cardiorespiratory collapse in children. Dry mouth, tachycardia, headache, and parasympathetic stimulation are all theoretically possible with this drug. One transient episode of unconsciousness and rigidity in a child has been reported.

C. **The antidote** for anticholinergic systemic poisoning sufficiently severe to warrant treatment is **1–2 mg of physostigmine salicylate parenterally,** repeated if necessary.

III. **Adrenergic Mydriatics**
These include phenylephrine, hydroxyamphetamine, and epinephrine.

A. **Phenylephrine** is a synthetic sympathomimetic (adrenergic) mydriatic and vasoconstrictor (see Chapter 2, Antiallergy Agents) with no cycloplegic properties.

1. **The mechanism of action of** phenylephrine, like all sympathomimetics, is by direct stimulation of the alpha-adrenergic receptors producing, in the eye, pupillary dilation and vasoconstriction.

2. **Dosage and clinical indications.** The ophthalmic solution for mydriasis is available in concentrations of 2.5 and 10% as a single agent and as a 2.5% solution in combination with 1% tropicamide. Onset of maximal action is within 20–30 minutes, and the effect wears off in about 4–6 hours. Dosage depends on intended

use: 1–2 drops of 2.5% phenylephrine topically once or twice for nonextended fundus exam, or, in conjunction with a cycloplegic (phenylephrine-tropicamide or with cyclopentolate), 1 drop of 2.5% phenylephrine solution every 10–15 minutes for 3 doses to break iris posterior synechiae and to dilate in anterior uveitis. Other uses include cycloplegic refraction where greater mydriasis is needed, preoperatively for wide mydriasis, and for extended fundus exam. 10% phenylephrine must be used with caution because of potential adverse cardiovascular effects and only when 2.5% phenylephrine, with or without other medication, will not achieve the desired effect.

3. **Adverse side effects**
   a. **Ocular.** This drug has little or no effect on accommodation or IOP in normal eyes, but may lower or raise the pressure in eyes with open-angle glaucoma. Some cases of transient pressure elevation may be due to the release of pigment from the posterior iris epithelium with clogging of the trabecular meshwork, a phenomenon commonly seen with topical phenylephrine. This agent also may induce acute angle-closure glaucoma (ACG) in eyes anatomically so predisposed. Doses of 0.12% may cause ACG within 30 minutes of administration, and a drop of 10% may cause such rapid wide mydriasis that the pupillary block and ACG do not develop until several hours later when the pupil is coming back down and reaches the critical mid-dilation position. Corneal endothelial cell toxicity with subsequent stromal swelling may occur if phenylephrine is given in the presence of unhealthy or ulcerated epithelium. Pseudopemphigus, epidermalization of the conjunctiva, lacrimal punctal occlusion, and allergic blepharoconjunctivitis all have been reported with chronic use of phenylephrine-containing medications for the eyes.
   b. **Systemic** side effects of topical phenylephrine, noted primarily with use of the 10% concentration, include transient systemic hypertension in both adults and infants (infants may be at greater risk than adults). Other patients at significant risk of undue rise in systemic blood pressure are those with cardiovascular disease or insulin-dependent diabetes and systemic hypertensives on reserpine or guanethidine. Patients taking monoamine oxidase inhibitors or tricyclic antidepressants should be monitored very carefully if also placed on phenylephrine-containing drops, and preferably taken off their psychiatric medication for 21 days before starting a drug with phenylephrine if the latter is deemed medically more important than the former. Other high-risk categories are patients taking systemic beta-adrenergic blockers, those with aneurysms, and those with untreated idiopathic systemic hypertension. The use of 5% or, preferably,

2.5% phenylephrine drops is far safer and has far fewer and less severe side effects in all the above groups of patients than the 10% concentration.

B. Hydroxyamphetamine is a topical sympathomimetic mydriatic with no cycloplegic properties.

    1. The mechanism of action, as with all sympathomimetics, is via direct alpha-adrenergic receptor stimulation in the pupillary dilator muscle, resulting in mydriasis and, in the conjunctiva, vasoconstriction.

    2. Dosage and clinical indications. The ophthalmic solution is 1% and given as 1–2 drops in the conjunctival sac to achieve good mydriasis of short duration, 2–3 hours. Hydroxyamphetamine is considered one of the safest mydriatics in the presence of some anterior chamber shallowing, as it is slow in onset and easily counteracted by miotics. This drug induces greater mydriasis in patients with Down's syndrome than in normal patients.

    3. Adverse side effects

        a. Ocular effects include blurred vision, "blue-tinged" vision, increased lacrimation, allergy, photophobia, ocular pain, paradoxical pressure rise in open-angle glaucoma, and minimal paralysis of accommodation. It is contraindicated in and may precipitate acute closure in narrow-angle glaucoma.

        b. Systemic adverse effects are rare, but the drug should be used with caution in patients with systemic hypertension, hyperthyroidism, and diabetes.

C. Epinephrine has been discussed in Chapter 5 on Antiglaucoma Agents. It is rarely used as a mydriatic and has no cycloplegic properties.

Information Sources and Suggested Reading (*Mydriatics/Cycloplegics*)

1. Abelson, M.B., and Alfonzo, E., *Pupillary Update.* Princeton, NJ: Excerpta Medica, 1986.
2. Davies, P.H., *The Actions and Uses of Ophthalmic Drugs,* 2nd ed. Boston: Butterworths, 1981, pp. 83–113 (atropine), pp. 114–155 (other cycloplegics——homatropine, cyclopentolate, tropicamide, mydriatics).
3. Ellis, P., *Ocular Therapeutics and Pharmacology,* 7th ed. St. Louis: C.V. Mosby, 1985, pp. 308–314 (mydriatics and cycloplegics).
4. Grant, W.M., *Toxicology of the Eye,* 3rd ed. Springfield, IL: Charles C Thomas, 1986, pp. 109–112, 126–129, 297–298, 486, 725–727, 802–803, 958–959.
5. Rosenberg, M., and Jampol, L., Drugs and pupil, in Sears, M.L. (ED.), *Pharmacology of the Eye.* Heidelberg: Springer–Verlag, 1984, pp. 715–720.
6. Weiner, N. (1) Atropine, scopolamine and related antimuscarinic drugs. (2) Norepinephrine and the sympathomimetic amines. In Goodman, L., Gilman, A., Rall, T., and Murad, F. (Eds.), *The Pharmacologic Basis of Therapeutics,* 7th ed. New York: Macmillan, 1985, pp. 130–145, 146–181.

Ocular Side Effects
of Systemic Drugs

In Part I, the systemic side effects of ocular medications were reviewed. These effects result from the absorption of eye medications into the circulation via the transconjunctival/transnasal mucous membrane route or via the nasolacrimal tract.

While the latter feeds into the gastrointestinal system, where much drug is detoxified by digestive enzymes or liver first-pass mechanisms, the transmembrane absorption into the circulation is comparable to an intravenous injection and may result in significant adverse bodily reactions. Similarly, oral, transdermal, or parenteral drugs may cause significant side effects on the eye and visual system. It is these effects that are addressed in Part II.

Intermediate or chronic administration of certain systemic drugs may produce a variety of side effects on one or more components of the eye or visual system. In some cases the mechanism is understood and in others still an enigma. Side effects caused by one member of a given chemical family are often, but not always, caused by other members of the same drug group. What is known about one drug, then, should be watched for in its relatives.

Because of their ectodermal origins, the lids and conjunctiva are frequently affected by the many drugs that may induce adverse dermatologic reactions such as erythema multiforme, Lyell's syndrome, lupus, or simply a histamine-mediated allergic response. Poliosis (whitening of the lashes or brows) has been particularly noted with use of **quinoline** derivatives such as **amodiaquine** and **chloroquine,** while alopecia (brow or lash loss) has been noted with several drugs, including the antineoplastics such as **actinomycin D** and the nutrient supplement, **vitamin A.** The orbit itself may be affected with development of exophthalmos with use of **corticosteroids, vitamin A, and lithium CO_3.** Extraocular muscle paralysis and ptosis are common side effects seen with such drug groups as antiarthritics, antibiotics, heavy metal antineoplastic agents, cardiac antiarrhythmics, systemic antihypertensives, CNS agents and alcohols, and may or may not be the result of a myasthenic neuromuscular block.

Of the global tissues, the four that stand out as most frequently affected are the cornea, lens, retina, and optic nerve. Corneal epithelial deposits may form in whorl, bow tie, or cat whisker formation (corneal verticillata or thesaurimosis). These verticillata are phospholipids in lysosomes unable to digest them due to drug toxicity. Their formation is associated with use of drugs from diverse chemical groups: **amiodarone, amodiaquine, chloroquine, hydroxychloroquine, monobenzone, perhexilene, tamoxifen,** and **tilorone.** Epithelial deposits also may appear as small vacuoles with use of **micothiazone** or **thiacetazone** or as fine grey, yellow, or brown granules scattered diffusely through the cell layers. These often are seen with **chloroquine, chlorpromazine,** and **mepacrine.** Similarly, the corneal stroma may be the site of fine granular deposits with intermediate to long-term use of **chlorpromazine, clofazimine, indomethacin,** and **methotrimeprazine.** Heavy metals such as **gold, copper, mercury,** and **silver** also may deposit out in the stroma, causing characteristic grey or brownish gold discoloration, usually at the limbus.

There is usually little disturbance of vision by any of the above deposits. They appear to cause no harm while present, are usually not an indication for stopping a drug, and often disappear if the drug is discontinued. In other instances, however, a systemic drug may induce increased lacrimation, burning, itching, or ocular discomfort without any physical evidence of keratitis or other ocular abnormality. These symptoms alone may be cause for ceasing drug use despite absence of physical change.

The crystalline lens may be the cause of acute transient myopia or become cataractous due to systemic drug toxicity, either event causing significant disruption of vision. The acute myopia may be induced by a wide variety of related and unrelated drugs, including **acetazolamide, arsphenamine, chlorothiazide, clofenamide, dichlorphenamide, hydrochlorothiazide, isotretinoin, prochlorperazine, promethazine, quinine, spironolactone, sulfonamides,** and **tetracyclines.** This myopia is of several diopters and often occurs in patients who have taken a given drug previously without any side effect. The reaction comes on within a few hours or days of starting the drug and is not caused by cholinergic or parasympathomimetic ciliary muscle contraction inducing spasm of near accommodation. The drug-induced myopia is not, therefore, reversed by anticholinergics such as atropine. This acute idiopathic myopia appears in at least some cases to be due to abnormal thickening of the lens or to ciliary body edema with shallowing of the anterior chamber and possible increased lens antero-posterior diameter. Whatever its cause, the myopia is reversible with discontinuing the inciting agent.

Cataractous changes due to systemic drug therapy are of greater concern, as not all are reversible. Radiomimetic cataracts (equatorial and ultimately posterior subcapsular cataracts) are commonly seen with antineoplastic drugs or other antimiotic agents such as **busulfan, dibromomannitol,** and **nitrogen mustards.** Drug effect is primarily on the actively mitotic lens equatorial cells, which opacify and then spread posteriorly. Like the posterior subcapsular cataracts induced by glucocorticoids, these opacities are usually nonprogressive and may even regress once the drug is discontinued.

Lens discoloration beneath the anterior capsule may be seen as blue-green **(copper),** rusty-yellow **(iron),** rosy-brown **(mercury),** and blue-grey **(silver),** all probably representing metal deposition as insoluble salts and, if not due to a primary illness, they may be due to patient ingestion of excessive **nutritional supplements.** Fine yellow-brown granules also may be deposited beneath the anterior capsule in patients on long-term **chlorpromazine** or **thiothixene** therapy. Fortunately, neither the discoloration nor the deposits appear to interfere with vision and do not seem to lead to true cataract formation.

Changes in the retina include edema, hemorrhages, vascular narrowing, maculopathy, ganglion or photoreceptor cell damage, lipidosis, and pigment epithelial (RPE) disturbance. The mechanisms of most of these side effects are unknown and may or may not disturb vision. Retinal hemorrhages are often associated with subconjunctival heme; both are usually due to drug-induced anemia. Retinal edema is visually disturbing and may be caused by such drugs as **chloramphenicol, ergotamine, griseofulvin, indomethacin (?), iodoquinol, quinine,** and **radiopaque media.** Similarly, maculopathy may cause a severe disturbance of central vision and is associated with such medications as **allopurinol (?), chloroquine, clofazimine, oral contraceptives (?), dapsone (?), flumequine, hydroxychloroquine, indiomethacin (?), niacin, phenothiazine derivates (lipofuchsin deposits), quinine (?), and the estrogen blocker, tamoxifen.** Retinal ganglion cell or photoceptor cell damage may be heralded clinically by "visual disturbance" (field changes, color disturbance, abnormal electrical recordings) in earlier stages but, unfortunately, if not anticipated by the physician, is often not detected until optic atrophy due to nerve fiber loss has occurred. Drugs associated with one or more of these or RPE changes include **chloramphenicol, cardiac glycosides, chlorpromazine, deferoxamine, ethambutol, quinine-derivatives, thioridazine,** and **vincristine.** The finding of retinal or optic nerve functional disturbances associated with any drug is usually an indication to discontinue the medication unless the consequences to the patient will be more serious than those occurring in the visual system.

Ocular electrical recordings are of immediate and prognostic value if there is any question as to drug-induced posterior segment side effects. The **ERG** (electroretinogram) is useful in identifying specific toxic sites within the retina and is of even greater value when correlated with the **EOG** (electrooculogram), which reflects the corneal–retinal potential, thus giving information as to the state of the RPE. Added to this information is the **VER** (visual evoked cortical response), which evaluates the quality of transmission from retina to visual cortex when the ERG is normal.

Optic neuropathy, neuritis, or retrobulbar neuritis (selective involvement of the papillomacular bundle in the optic nerve) all may result from direct drug neural toxicity or drug-induced interference with the blood supply to these structures. Examples that may induce these changes include **chloramphenicol, chlorpropamide, cisplatin, clomiphene, oral contraceptives, deferoxamine, disulfiram, ethambutol, isoniazid, mepacrine, penicillamine, perhexilene maleate, streptomycin, sulfonamides, tolbutamide, tryparsimide,** and **vincristine.** Involvement may occur anywhere from the head of the optic nerve back to the chiasm, with some substances focalizing, for unknown reasons, at the chiasm, e.g., **chloramphenicol, ethambutol,** and **vincristine.**

Intraocular pressure (IOP) changes up or down may occur

with a variety of drugs, the most notorious being the **glucocorticoids** for raising IOP and the **cardiac glycosides** and **cannabinols** for lowering the IOP.

Additionally, there are numerous visual effects of uncertain or central nervous system (CNS) origin, but specifically drug-induced. These include color vision disturbances, photophobia, visual hallucinations, flashing or flickering lights, and alteration of the flicker fusion threshold. Such symptoms are usually disturbing to the patient until explained by the physician as possible side effects. They do not constitute a reason for discontinuing a given medication unless they are particularly distressing to the patient or an equally effective alternative drug without such side effect is available.

The authors are indebted to several excellent texts and reports. *Drug-Induced Ocular Side Effects* and *Drug Interactions,* 3rd edition, by Felix Fraunfelder, M.D., and S. Martha Meyer is the result of the compilation of data reported by hundreds of physicians and scientists to the National Registry of Drug-Induced Ocular Side Effects in Portland, Oregon. Established 12 years ago by Dr. Fraunfelder, this registry is a center of continuous information gathering referable to probable medication-induced ocular side effects and possible interactions of other drugs with those capable of causing adverse ocular effects. *The Toxicology of the Eye,* 3rd edition, by W. Morton Grant, M.D., represents a lifetime of exhaustive literature search and personal investigation into toxicity of the visual system induced by drugs and nonmedicinal chemicals alike.

Much information in Part II was taken from the above two books as well as from other classic references, including Goodman and Gilman's *Pharmacologic Basis of Therapeutics, The Physicians Desk Reference,* 1989, and the several other sources listed at the end of this section. For rapid information access, the data here has been written in alphabetical tabular format by drug: (1) therapeutic category, (2) chemical family (when pertinent) and (3) generic name, and by anatomic location of the effect. The American commercial (proprietary) names are listed with generic names separately as an index after the tables to assist physicians and scientists in locating these drugs **when only commercial names are known.**

As noted, the occurrence of an ocular side effect does not necessarily indicate a need to discontinue the drug. In those instances where the side effect is intolerable or vision-threatening, almost all effects are reversible with stopping the medication. Because of the rapidity with which new drugs are entering clinical use and the scrutiny that older drugs are receiving in terms of potential adverse reactions, omissions and cases of "mistaken identity" are quite possible. Nonetheless, this section should provide the physician with rapid access to useful information when faced with a patient suffering visual symptoms of potential pharmacologic origin.

Information Sources and Suggested Reading
(*Ocular Toxicity of Systemic Drugs*)

1. Boerner, C., Total punctate keratopathy due to Dipivefrin [Letter]. Arch. Ophthalmol. 106:171, 1988.
2. Choe, U., Rothschild, B., and Laitman, L., Ciprofloxacin-induced vasculitis. [Letter]. N. Engl. J. Med. 320:257–258, 1989.
3. Drugs that cause psychiatric symptoms. The Medical Letter on Drugs and Therapeutics. The Medical Letter, 28(721):81–86, 1986.
4. Fiore, P., Jacobs, I., and Goldberg, D., Drug-induced pemphigoid: A spectrum of diseases. Arch. Ophthalmol. 105:1660–1663, 1987.
5. Font, R., Sobol, W., and Matoba, A., Polychromatic corneal and conjunctival crystals secondary to clofazimine therapy in a leper. Ophthalmology 96:311–315, 1989.
6. Fraunfelder, F.T., and Meyer, S.M., *Drug-induced Ocular Side Effects and Drug Interactions*, 3rd ed. Philadelphia: Lea & Febiger, 1989.
7. Grant, W.M., *Toxicology of the Eye*, 3rd ed. Springfield, IL: Charles C Thomas, 1986.
8. Hamed, L., Glaser, J., Schatz, N., and Perez, T., Pseudotumor cerebri induced by Danazol. Am. J. Ophthalmol. 107:105–110, 1989.
9. Havener, W., Chelating agents (pp. 428–432), Radioopaque contrast media (pp. 573–574), Vasodilators (pp. 600–607), Vitamins (pp. 608–621), in *Ocular Pharmacology,* St. Louis: C.V. Mosby, 1983.
10. Holland, E., Stein, C., Palestine, A. et al., Suramin keratopathy. Am. J. Ophthalmol. 106:216–220, 1988.
11. Johns, K., Head, S., and O'Day, D., Corneal toxicity of propamidine. Arch. Ophthalmol. 106:68–70, 1988.
12. Kooner, K., and Zimmerman, T., Antiglaucoma therapy during pregnancy—Part II. Ann. Ophthalmol. 20:208–211, 1988.
13. Lovastatin Study Group II, Lovastatin disputed as cataract cause. Ophthalmol. Times, pp. 1, 24, July 15, 1988.
14. Milay, R., Klein, M., and Illingworth, D.R., Niacin maculopathy. Ophthalmology 95:930–936, 1988.
15. Palmer, E., How safe are ocular drugs in pediatrics? Ophthalmology 93:1038–1040, 1986.
16. *Physicians Desk Reference for Ophthalmology.* Oradell, NJ: Medical Economics, 1989.
17. Rumelt, M., Blindness from misuse of over-the-counter medications. Ann. Ophthalmol. 20:26–30, 1988.
18. Samples, J., and Meyer, S.M., Use of ophthalmic medications in pregnant and nursing women. Am. J. Ophthalmol. 106:616–623, 1988.
19. Turgeon, P., and Salmovits, P., Scleritis as the presenting manifestation. A procainamide induced lupus. Ophthalmol. 96:68–71, 1989.
20. Vrabec, T., Sergott, R., Jaeger, E., et al., Reversible visual loss with high dose ciprofloxacin. Ophthalmology 97:707–710, 1990.

Abbreviations Used in Part II Tables

?	Not definitively documented
↓	Decreased
↑	Increased
BS	Blind spot
cj.	Conjunctiva
CNS	Central nervous system
EOG	Electrooculogram
EOM	Extraocular muscles
ERG	Electroretinogram
erythema multiforme	Stevens-Johnson syndrome
heme	Blood
Horner's syndrome	Ptosis, miosis, anhydrosis, ↑ sensitivity to sympathetic agents
IOP	Intraocular pressure
KC	Keratoconjunctivitis
lupoid syndrome	Systemic lupus erythematosus
Lyell's syndrome	Toxic epidermal necrolysis
OKN	Optokinetic nystagmus
PHPV	Persistent hyperplastic primary vitreous
POA	Paralysis of accommodation
PSC	Posterior subcapsular
RPE	Retinal pigment epithelium
SPK	Superficial punctate keratitis
subcj.	Subconjunctival
VF	Visual field
VEP (VER)	Visual evoked potential (visual evoked response)

11

Alcoholism Antagonists

Table 11-1. Alcoholism Antagonists

Generic drug name	Visual symptoms	Anterior segment	Posterior segment	Extraocular muscles, orbit	Visual fields, CNS	Other
Thiuram Derivatives						
Disulfiram	↓ Vision Visual hallucinations Color vision defect Red-green color vision defect	Lids or cj.: allergy, erythema Mydriasis Anisocoria	Retrobulbar or optic neuritis	Myesthenic neuromuscular block: EOM paralysis, ? ptosis	Toxic amblyopia Nystagmus Scotomas—central or cecocentral	? Teratogenesis Urticaria

12

Analgesics and Antiarthritics

Table 12-1. Analgesics and antiarthritics: Antigout agents

Generic drug name	Visual symptoms	Anterior segment	Posterior segment	Extraocular muscles, orbit	Visual fields, CNS	Other
Xanthine oxidase inhibitors						
Allopurinol	↓ Vision	Lids or cj.: allergy, erythema, edema, conjunctivitis, photosensitivity, ulceration, ? lash or brow loss; subcj. heme Scleritis Corneal: keratitis, ulcers, scarring ? Cataracts	Retinal hemorrhages Macular: ? edema, ? degeneration, ? exudates, ? hemorrhages	—	—	Urticaria Purpura Lupoid syndrome Erythema multiforme Exfoliative dermatitis Lyell's syndrome
Alkaloids						
Colchicine	Diplopia	? Lash or brow loss Subcj. heme Corneal: erosion, slow wound healing, dellen, keratitis ? Hypopyon ? Cataracts	Retinal hemorrhages Papilledema (toxic)	EOM paresis	—	? Teratogenesis

Table 12-2. Analgesics and antiarthritics: Gold therapy

Generic drug name	Visual symptoms	Anterior segment	Posterior segment	Extraocular muscles, orbit	Visual fields, CNS	Other
Gold salts Auranofin Aurothioglucose Aurothioglycanide Gold Au[198] Gold sodium thiomalate Gold sodium thiosulfate	Photophobia Diplopia	Gold deposits (red, brown, violet, purple): lids, cj., pan-corneal, lens surface Lids or cj.: allergy, hyperemia, ciliary flush, erythema, blepharoconjunctivitis, edema, photosensitivity, symblepharon, angioneurotic edema, ? lash or brow loss ? Corneal: ulcers, melting, keratitis Iritis	Retinal hemorrhages ? Papilledema	Myesthenic neuromuscular block: EOM paralysis, ptosis	Nystagmus	Urticaria Purpura Lupoid syndrome Erythema multiforme Exfoliative dermatitis Lyell's syndrome ? Activation of Guillain–Barre syndrome, aggravation of herpes simplex virus infections

Table 12-3. Analgesics and antiarthritics: Narcotic analgesics

Generic drug name	Visual symptoms	Anterior segment	Posterior segment	Extraocular muscles, orbit	Visual fields, CNS	Other
Methadone opioids						
Methadone	↓ Vision	Miosis or pinpoint pupils (toxic) Mydriasis (withdrawal)	Talc retinopathy	↓ Spontaneous eye movements	? Cortical blindness (hypoxic state)	Urticaria
Propoxyphene	↓ Vision Visual hallucinations	Lacrimation (withdrawal) KC sicca Miosis (acute or toxic) Pinpoint pupils (initial or coma) Mydriasis (withdrawal or hypoxia)	Optic atrophy (toxic)	—	—	Teratogenesis
Morphine opioids						
Codeine	↓ Vision Myopia Visual hallucinations	Angioneurotic edema Miosis (acute or toxic state)	—	—	—	Urticaria Erythema multiforme Exfoliative dermatitis

Diacetylmorphine (Heroin)	Pinpoint pupils (initial or coma) Mydriasis (withdrawal) Lids or cj.: ↑ Lacrimation, hyperemia, edema, ? lash or brow loss ↓IOP POA Uveitis Miosis Pinpoint pupils (toxic) Absent pupil light reflex Mydriasis (withdrawal) Anisocoria (withdrawal) Photophobia	Retinal vein thrombosis	—	Scotomas	Horner's syndrome Urticaria
Hydromorphone (Dihydromorphinone) Oxymorphone	Lids or cj.: allergy Miosis Pinpoint pupils (toxic) Mydriasis (hypoxic) ↓ Vision	—	—	—	Urticaria

Table 12-3. (continued)

Generic drug name	Visual symptoms	Anterior segment	Posterior segment	Extraocular muscles, orbit	Visual fields, CNS	Other
Morphine Opium	↓ Vision Myopia Diplopia ? Red-green color defect ? Visual hallucinations	POA ↑ Lacrimation (withdrawal) Lids or cj.: ↓ lacrimation, allergy, ptosis, ? lash or brow loss, conjunctivitis, keratoconjunctivitis POA Accommodative spasm ↓ IOP Miosis Pinpoint pupils (toxic) Mydriasis (withdrawal or extreme toxicity) Pupil irregularity (withdrawal)	—	Convergence	? VF scotomas, constriction, hemianopia	Urticaria

Other opioids

Meperidine (Pethidine)	↓Vision Visual hallucinations	Lids or cj.: allergy, erythema ? Corneal deposits ↓IOP Mydriasis Pupil light reflex	—	—	Nystagmus	Urticaria
Pentazocine	↓Vision Visual hallucinations Diplopia	Lids or cj.: erythema, conjunctivitis, edema ↑Lacrimation (abrupt withdrawal) Miosis	—	↓Spontaneous eye movements	Nystagmus	Urticaria

Table 12-4. Analgesics and antiarthritics: Narcotic antagonists

Generic drug name	Visual symptoms	Anterior segment	Posterior segment	Extraocular muscles, orbit	Visual fields, CNS	Other
Morphine opioids						
Levallorphan Nalorphine Naloxone Naltrexone	↓ Vision Visual hallucinations Photophobia (naltrexone)	Lids or cj.: allergy, pseudoptosis, photosensitivity (naltrexone) ? lash or brow loss (naltrexone), erythema Ocular pain, burning, edema (naltrexone) Mydriasis Miosis ? Cataracts (naltrexone)	—	—	—	Urticaria Erythema multiforme (naloxone) Exfoliative dermatitis (naltrexone)

Table 12-5. Analgesics and antiarthritics: Non-narcotic analgesics

Generic drug name	Visual symptoms	Anterior segment	Posterior segment	Extraocular muscles, orbit	Visual fields, CNS	Other
Anthranilic acids						
Mefenamic acid	↓ Vision Color vision defect	Ocular irritation Lids or cj.: erythema, conjunctivitis, edema, ? angioneurotic edema, subcj. heme	Retinal hemorrhages	—	—	Urticaria Pemphigoid
Para-aminophenols						
Acetaminophen Acetanilid Phenacetin	↓ Vision "Yellow" vision (acetaminophen, phenacetin toxic) Visual hallucinations	Lids or cj.: allergy, erythema, edema, conjunctivitis, angioneurotic edema, green or brown cj. vessel discoloration, subcj. heme Mydriasis ↓ Pupil light reflex	—	—	—	Erythema multiforme Lyell's syndrome Pemphigoid (phenacetin) Icterus ? Teratogenesis

Table 12-5. (continued)

Generic drug name	Visual symptoms	Anterior segment	Posterior segment	Extraocular muscles, orbit	Visual fields, CNS	Other
Pyrazolones Antipyrine	↓ Vision	Lids or cj.: allergy, conjunctivitis, edema, discoloration, subcj. heme Keratitis	Retinal hemorrhages Optic atrophy	—	Toxic amblyopia	Urticaria Erythema multiforme Lyell's syndrome
Salicylates Aspirin (acetylsalicylic acid) Sodium salicylate	↓ Vision Red-green color vision defect "Yellow" vision Diplopia Myopia Scintillating scotomas Visual hallucinations	Lids or cj.: ? lash or brow loss, allergy, conjunctivitis, edema, subcj. heme Keratitis ↓ IOP Mydriasis ↓ Pupil light reflex Hyphema	Retinal hemorrhages Retinal edema Papilledema Optic atrophy	EOM paralysis	Toxic amblyopia VF constriction Scotomas Hemianopia Nystagmus	Urticaria Purpura Erythema multiforme Lyell's syndrome Pemphigoid ? Teratogenesis (toxic): anophthalmos, microphthalmos, exophthalmos, cyclopia, retinal dysplasia

Table 12-6. Analgesics and antiarthritics: Nonsteroidal anti-inflammatory drugs

Generic drug name	Visual symptoms	Anterior segment	Posterior segment	Extraocular muscles, orbit	Visual fields, CNS	Other
Fenoprofen	↓ Vision Diplopia	Lids or cj.: erythema, conjunctivitis, angioneurotic edema, ? lash or brow loss, subcj. heme	Retinal hemorrhages ? Optic neuritis	—	—	Urticaria Erythema multiforme Exfoliative dermatitis
Flurbiprofen	↓ Vision Diplopia	Lids or cj.: erythema, conjunctivitis, subcj. heme	—	—	—	Urticaria
Ibuprofen	↓ Vision Diplopia Color vision defect, red-green defect, colors faded Visual hallucinations Myopia Moving colored lights Shooting streaks	Lids or cj.: erythema, conjunctivitis, edema, photosensitivity, angioneurotic edema, ? lash or brow loss, subcj. heme KC sicca Corneal opacities +/or vascularization	Retinal hemorrhages Optic neuritis Abnormal ERG or VEP ? Papilledema ? Macular degeneration	—	Paracentral or cecocentral scotomas VF constriction ↑ Blind spot Hemianopia Toxic amblyopia Nystagmus (toxic) ? Pseudotumor cerebri	Urticaria Purpura Lupoid syndrome Erythema multiforme Lyell's syndrome

Table 12-6. (continued)

Generic drug name	Visual symptoms	Anterior segment	Posterior segment	Extraocular muscles, orbit	Visual fields, CNS	Other
Indomethacin	↓ Vision Diplopia Blue-yellow vision defect Visual hallucinations Photophobia ? ↓ Dark adaptation	Lids or cj.: photosensitivity, conjunctivitis, subcj. heme, ? lash or brow loss Corneal: superficial whorls, SPK, epithelial erosion, crystalline deposits ? ↑ Lacrimation ? Mydriasis ? Cataracts	Retinal hemorrhages Abnormal ERG or EOG ? Retinal or macular: edema, degeneration, RPE disturbance, vascular occlusion Central serous retinopathy Papilledema ? Optic neuritis	EOM paralysis Orbit or periorbital pain	Pseudotumor cerebri ? Toxic amblyopia Scotomas VF constriction ↑ Blind spot	Urticaria Purpura Erythema multiforme Exfoliative dermatitis Lyell's syndrome Pemphigoid
Ketoprofen	↓ Vision Visual hallucinations	Lids or cj.: erythema, conjunctivitis, edema, discoloration, photosensitivity, ? angioneurotic edema, ? brow or lash loss,	Retinal hemorrhages Papilledema ? RPE changes	EOM paralysis	Pseudotumor cerebri ? VF defects	Urticaria Purpura Exfoliative dermatitis Eczema Aggravation of myasthenia gravis, ? herpes

	Subjective / Vision	Lids or Conjunctiva / Cornea	Retina / Optic Nerve	Extraocular Muscles	Visual Field	Skin
		pain, KC sicca, subcj. heme ? Uveitis ? POA				
Naproxen	↓Vision Color vision defect "Red" or "green" vision	Lids or cj.: allergy, erythema, edema, conjunctivitis, photosensitivity, angioneurotic edema, ? lash or brow loss, subcj. heme Corneal opacities or ? ulceration KC sicca POA	Retinal hemorrhages RPE changes ? Macular edema ? Papilledema Optic neuritis	EOM paralysis	? VF defects	Urticaria Purpura Erythema multiforme Lyell's syndrome ? Exfoliative dermatitis
Oxyphenbutazone Phenylbutazone	↓Vision Diplopia Red-green color defect Photophobia Visual hallucinations	Lids or cj: allergy, hyperemia, conjunctivitis, edema, photosensitivity, subcj. heme	Retinal detachment Optic neuritis Optic atrophy	EOM paralysis	Scotomas Toxic amblyopia	Urticaria Lupoid syndrome Erythema multiforme Lyell's syndrome Pemphigoid

Table 12-6. (continued)

Generic drug name	Visual symptoms	Anterior segment	Posterior segment	Extraocular muscles, orbit	Visual fields, CNS	Other
		Corneal: peripheral stromal vascularization, opacities, keratitis, ulceration, scarring				(phenylbutazone)
Piroxicam	↓ Vision Visual hallucinations ? Diplopia	Lids or cj.: erythema, conjunctivitis, photosensitivity, angioneurotic edema, lash or brow loss, lacrimation, edema, burning ? POA	? Optic neuritis	—	—	Urticaria Purpura Erythema multiforme Exfoliative dermatitis Lyell's syndrome Pemphigoid Eczema

Sulindac					
↓ Vision Diplopia ? Visual hallucinations	Lids or cj.: erythema, blepharoconjunctivitis, edema, photosensitivity, angioneurotic edema, subcj. heme Corneal: keratitis, ? ulcers, ? opacities KC sicca ? Cataracts	Retinal hemorrhages Macular RPE changes ? Optic neuritis	—	—	Urticaria Lupoid syndrome Erythema multiforme Lyell's syndrome Exfoliative dermatitis

13

Anesthetics

Table 13-1. Anesthetics: Adjunctive agents and gases

Generic drug name	Visual symptoms	Anterior segment	Posterior segment	Extraocular muscles, orbit	Visual fields, CNS	Other
Butyrophenones						
Droperidol	See Table 18-6					
Enzymes						
Hyaluronidase (subconjunctival or retrobulbar)	Myopia Astigmatism	Lids or cj.: allergy, follicular conjunctivitis, irritation	↑Cystoid macular edema	—	—	↓Duration of local anesthesia ↑Frequency of local anesthetic reactions
Neuromuscular blocking agents						
Metocurine iodide Tubocurarine	Diplopia	Lids: ptosis or retroaction, erythema ↓IOP	—	EOM paralysis Inferior rotation of eye	Nystagmus Enophthalmos	Urticaria
Succinylcholine	Diplopia	Lids: ? ptosis, allergy, erythema, edema ↑ then ↓IOP	—	Abduction on adduction attempt Altered forced duction	—	Urticaria
Quaternary ammonium compounds						
Methscopolamine* Scopolamine* (Hyoscine)	Visual hallucinations ↓Vision	↓Lacrimation ↓Tear lysosymes Mydriasis POA	—	—	—	Teratogenesis?

Table 13-1. (continued)

Generic drug name	Visual symptoms	Anterior segment	Posterior segment	Extraocular muscles, orbit	Visual fields, CNS	Other
Therapeutic gases Carbon dioxide	↓ Vision ↓ Dark adaptation Photophobia Color vision defect "Yellow" vision Visual hallucinations Diplopia	Ptosis ↓ Corneal reflex Mydriasis ↓ Pupil light reflex POA	Papilledema Retinal vascular engorgement	↓ Convergence Proptosis Abnormal conjugate deviations	VF constriction ↓ Blind spot	—
Oxygen	↓ Vision ↑ Color perception Myopia ↓ Dark adaptation	Mydriasis Cataracts	Retinal vascular: constriction, spasms, hemorrhages Retrolental fibroplasia (premature + young infants) Retinal detachment Abnormal ERG	—	Scotomas: central or paracentral	

* See chapter on Mydriatics and Cycloplegics.

Table 13-2. Anesthetics: Local anesthetics

Generic drug name	Visual symptoms	Anterior segment	Posterior segment	Extraocular muscles, orbit	Visual fields, CNS	Other
Para-aminobenzoic acid derivatives						
Bupivacaine Chloroprocaine Etidocaine Lidocaine Mepivacaine Prilocaine Procaine Propoxycaine	↓ Vision Diplopia Color vision defect (lidocaine) Visual hallucinations	Lids or cj.: allergy, hyperemia, edema, blepharoconjunctivitis Mydriasis (toxic) Anisocoria (toxic)	? Retrobulbar neuritis ? Papilledema ? Optic atrophy	EOM paresis Jerky pursuit (toxic) Abnormal doll's head movement (toxic)	Nystagmus Blepharoclonus	Horner's syndrome (extradural block) Urticaria Exfoliative dermatitis

See chapter on Local Anesthetics.

Table 13-3. Anesthetics: General anesthetics

Generic drug name	Visual symptoms	Anterior segment	Posterior segment	Extraocular muscles, orbit	Visual fields, CNS	Other
Chloroform	↓ Vision	Mydriasis (early) Miosis (deep anesthesia) Nonreactive mydriatic pupils (coma) ↓ IOP	—	Esotropia or exotropia	? Cortical blindness Nystagmus	—
Ether	↓ Vision	Lacrimation ↑ (early), ↓ (deep or coma) Cj. hyperemia, irritation → IOP Mydriasis (reactive—light, nonreactive—coma Miosis (reactive—deep anesthesia)	—	Slow oscillation +/or exotropia (early) Esotropia (coma)	? Cortical blindness	—
Ketamine	↓ Vision Diplopia Visual hallucinations	↑ Lacrimation ↓ IOP (deep anesthesia)	—	—	Nystagmus—horizontal Random ocular movement	—

Methoxyflurane	—	↓ IOP	Flecked retina syndrome	Myasthenic neuromuscular block; ptosis, EOM paralysis	Abnormal conjugate deviations ? Cortical blindness	—
Nitrous oxide	↓ Vision	↓ Lacrimation Mydriasis (reactive—light, nonreactive—coma) Miosis (deep anesthesia) ↓ or ↑ IOP	Abnormal ERG or VEP	—	? Cortical blindness	? Teratogenesis
Trichlorethylene	↓ Vision Photophobia Color vision defect Visual hallucinations	Lids or cj.: ptosis, conjunctivitis ↓ Lacrimation ↓ Corneal reflex Corneal ulcers ↓ or absent pupil light reflex Anisocoria POA ↓ IOP	Retrobulbar optic neuritis Optic atrophy Peripapillary hemorrhages Retinal edema	—	Nystagmus— horizontal Scotomas—central or paracentral VF constriction ↑ Blind spot	Exfoliative dermatitis

14

Antiallergy Drugs

Table 14-1. Antiallergy drugs: Antihistamines

Generic drug name	Visual symptoms	Anterior segment	Posterior segment	Extraocular muscles, orbit	Visual fields, CNS	Other
Alkylamines						
Brompheniramine	↓Vision	Lids or cj.: erythema, photosensitivity, ↓lacrimation, blepharospasm, subcj. heme	Retinal hemorrhages	—	VF constriction	Urticaria
Chlorpheniramine	Diplopia		Abnormal flicker fusion (triprolidine)			
Dexbrompheniramine	Visual hallucinations	SPK				
Dexchlorpheniramine		Aggravation KC sicca				
Dimethindene		↓Contact lens tolerance				
Pheniramine		Mydriasis				
Triprolidine		Anisocoria				
		↓Pupil light reflex				
Ethanolamine derivatives						
Carbinoxamine	↓Vision	Lids or cj.: ↓lacrimation, erythema, photosensitivity,	Retinal hemorrhages	—	Nystagmus	Urticaria
Clemastine	Diplopia				VF constriction (variable)	? Teratogenesis
Diphenhydramine	Visual hallucinations					

Table 14-1. (continued)

Generic drug name	Visual symptoms	Anterior segment	Posterior segment	Extraocular muscles, orbit	Visual fields, CNS	Other
Diphenylpyraline Doxylamine		blepharospasm, subcj. heme ↓ Contact lens tolerance Aggravate KC sicca Mydriasis Anisocoria ↓ Pupil light reflex POA				
Ethylenediamines Antazoline Pyrilamine (Mepyramine) Tripelennamine	↓ Vision Diplopia Visual hallucinations	Lids or cj.: erythema, photosensitivity, blepharospasm, subcj. heme, ↓ lacrimation ↓ Contact lens tolerance Aggravation KC sicca	Retinal hemorrhages	Strabismus (tripelennamine toxic)	Nystagmus (tripelennamine toxic) VF constriction	—

Phenothiazine analogs

Azatadine	↓Vision	POA			
Cyproheptadine	Diplopia	Mydriasis	Lids or cj.: erythema, edema, photosensitivity, subcj. heme, ↓ lacrimation	Retinal hemorrhages	Urticaria
	Visual hallucinations	↓Pupil light reflex	↓Contact lens tolerance		
		Anisocoria	Aggravation KC sicca		
			Mydriasis		
			—	—	

15

Anti-infectives

Table 15-1. Anti-infectives: Antibiotics*

Generic drug name	Visual symptoms	Anterior segment	Posterior segment	Extraocular muscles, orbit	Visual fields, CNS	Other
Aminoglycosides						
Gentamicin	↓ Vision Visual hallucinations	Lids or cj.: brow or lash loss, subcj. heme, photosensitivity	Retinal hemorrhage Papilledema (pseudotumor)	Myasthenic neuromuscular block: EOM paralysis, ptosis	Pseudotumor cerebri	Urticaria
Kanamycin	↓ Vision	Lid or cj.: allergy	? Optic neuritis	Myasthenic neuromuscular block: EOM paralysis, ptosis	—	Lyell's syndrome
Neomycin	Diplopia	↓ or absent pupil light response	—	Myasthenic neuromuscular block: EOM paralysis, ptosis	—	—
Streptomycin	↓ Vision Afterimaging Vision disturbance during motion Photophobia Color vision	Lids or cj.: allergy, erythema, edema, inflammation, angioneurotic edema, subcj. heme	Retinal hemorrhage Optic atrophy Retinal vasospasm Retrobulbar or optic neuritis	Myasthenic neuromuscular block EOM paresis, ptosis	Toxic amblyopia Scotomas Nystagmus	Urticaria Lupoid syndrome Exfoliative dermatitis Lyell's syndrome

Table 15-1. (continued)

Generic drug name	Visual symptoms	Anterior segment	Posterior segment	Extraocular muscles, orbit	Visual fields, CNS	Other
	blue-green defect "Yellow" vision	POA				
Tobramycin	↓ Vision Visual hallucinations Color vision defect	—	—	Myasthenic neuromuscular block: EOM paresis, ptosis	Nystagmus	—
Bacitracin	↓ Vision Diplopia	Lid or cj.: allergy, angioneurotic edema	—	Myasthenic neuromuscular block: EOM paralysis, ptosis	—	Urticaria
Cephalosporins						
Cefaclor, cefadroxil, cefonicid, cefoperazone, ceforanide, cefotaxime, cefotetan, cefoxitin, cefsulodin, ceftazidime, ceftizoxime,	Visual hallucinations Diplopia (cephaloridine) Color vision defect (cefaloridine)	Lids or cj.: allergy, erythema, edema, conjunctivitis, angioneurotic edema, subcj. heme Corneal peripheral edema	Retinal hemorrhage ? RPE disturbance or papilledema (cephaloridine)	—	? Nystagmus	Urticaria Erythema multiforme Exfoliative dermatitis

	↓ Vision / Color vision	Lids or conjunctiva	Retina / Optic nerve	Neuro-ophthalmic	Visual field	Skin / Other
ceftriaxone, cefuroxime, cephalexin, cephaloglycin, cephaloridine, cephalothin, cephamandole, cephapirin, cephazolin, cephradine, imipenem, moxalactam						
Chloramphenicol	↓ Vision Color vision defects "Yellow" vision	Lid or cj.: allergy, inflammation, angioneurotic edema POA Mydriasis ↓ Pupil reaction to light	RPE disturbance Retinal edema Retinal hemorrhages Retrobulbar or optic neuritis Optic atrophy	? Strabismus	Toxic amblyopia Scotomas VF constriction ? Nystagmus	Urticaria
Ciprofloxacin	Color vision alterations ↓ Vision	—	Optic neuropathy (toxic)	Cecocentral scotomas ↓ VEP		
Clindamycin	Color vision defects	Lids or cj.: allergy, hyperemia, photosensitivity, angioneurotic	Retinal hemorrhage	Myasthenic neuromuscular block: EOM paralysis, ptosis	—	Urticaria Erythema multiforme Exfoliative dermatitis

Table 15-1. (continued)

Generic drug name	Visual symptoms	Anterior segment	Posterior segment	Extraocular muscles, orbit	Visual fields, CNS	Other
		edema, subcj. heme				
Colistimethate Colistin	Diplopia	Mydriasis	—	Myasthenic neuromuscular block: EOM paralysis, ptosis	Nystagmus	—
Erythromycin	See Clindamycin; plus "yellow" vision defect					Lyell's syndrome
Lincomycin	See Clindamycin					
Nalidixic acid	Glare, flashing lights, scintillating scotomas Color vision defects: green, yellow, blue, or violet vision	Lid or cj.: photosensitivity, angioneurotic edema Mydriasis POA	Retinal hemorrhage Papilledema (pseudotumor)	EOM paralysis	Pseudotumor cerebri Nystagmus	Urticaria Lupoid syndrome ? Ocular teratogenesis
Nitrofurantoin	Diplopia ? Color vision defect	? Brow or lash loss Lid or cj.: tear-	Retinal hemorrhage Papilledema	EOM paralysis	Nystagmus Pseudotumor cerebri	Urticaria Lupoid syndrome

	? "Yellow" vision	ing, burning, allergy, photosensitivity, angioneurotic edema, icterus	(pseudotumor) ? Retrobulbar neuritis	—	Lyell's syndrome
Penicillins					
Benzathine pen. G, Hydrabamine pen. V, Potassium pen. G, Potassium pen. V, Potassium phenethicillin, procaine pen. G	↓ Vision Visual hallucinations Diplopia	Lids or cj.: allergy, erythema, edema, blepharoconjunctivitis, angioneurotic edema, subcj. heme POA Mydriasis	Retinal hemorrhages Papilledema (pseudotumor)	Visual agnosia Pseudotumor cerebri	Urticaria Lupoid syndrome Erythema multiforme Lyell's syndrome
Penicillins—Semisynthetic					
Amoxicillin, ampicillin, azlocillin, carbenicillin, cloxacillin, cyclacillin, dicloxacillin, hetacillin,	Diplopia	Lid or cj.: allergy, blepharoconjunctivitis, photosensitivity, edema, angioneurotic edema, subcj.	—	Myasthenic neuromuscular block: ptosis, EOM paralysis	Erythema multiforme Lyell's syndrome Exfoliative dermatitis

Table 15-1. (continued)

Generic drug name	Visual symptoms	Anterior segment	Posterior segment	Extraocular muscles, orbit	Visual fields, CNS	Other
methicillin, mezlocillin, oxacillin, piperacillin, ticarcillin		heme				—
Polymyxin B	↓ Vision Diplopia	Mydriasis	—	Myasthenic neuromuscular block: EOM paresis, ptosis	—	
Sulfonamides						
Sulfacetamide, sulfachlorpyridazine, sulfacytine, sulfadiazine, sulfadimethoxine, sulfamethazine, sulfamethizole, sulfamethoxazole, sulfa-	↓ Vision Myopia ↓ Depth perception, + adduction at near Photophobia Color vision defect "Yellow" vision Visual hallucinations "Lavender" reti-	Lid or cj.: tearing, allergy, inflammation, photosensitivity Keratitis Anterior chamber shallowing Iritis	Retinal hemorrhages, papilledema, optic neuritis ? Optic atrophy	Myasthenic neuromuscular block: EOM paralysis, ptosis Periorbital edema	Scotomas VF constriction Cortical blindness ? Toxic amblyopia	Urticaria Lupoid syndrome Erythema multiforme Lyelle's syndrome Pemphigoid Contact lenses stained yellow Purpura

Drug		Lids/Conj. & Skin	Retina	Neuromuscular	Visual Fields	Systemic/Allergic
methoxypyridazine, sulfaphenazole, sulfasalazine, sulfisoxazole	...nal vascular tree vision					

Tetracyclines

Drug	Symptoms	Lids or cj.	Retina	Neuromuscular	Visual Fields	Systemic/Allergic
Chlortetracycline, demeclocycline, doxycycline, methacycline, minocycline, oxytetracycline, tetracycline	↓ Vision Photophobia Diplopia (minocycline, tetracycline) Color vision defect +/or "yellow" vision (chlortetracycline) Myopia Visual hallucinations	Lids or cj.: edema, erythema, yellow discoloration (methacycline, tetracycline), hyperpigmentation (doxycycline, minocycline, tetracycline), photosensitivity, angioneurotic edema, subcj. heme ? Madarosis (minocycline, tetracycline)	Retinal hemorrhages	Myasthenic neuromuscular block: EOM paralysis, ptosis	VF enlarged blind spot Pseudotumor cerebri	Urticaria Lupoid syndrome Erythema multiforme Lyell's syndrome Ocular teratogenesis (? cataract)

Vancomycin: See Clindamycin

* See chapter on Antibiotics.

Table 15-2. Anti-infectives: Antifungal drugs*

Generic drug name	Visual symptoms	Anterior segment	Posterior segment	Extraocular muscles, orbit	Visual fields, CNS	Other
Penicillin derivatives						
Griseofulvin	↓ Vision	Lids or cj.: allergy, erythema, edema, conjunctivitis, photosensitivity, ulceration, ? lash or brow loss, subcj. heme Scleritis Corneal: keratitis, ulcers, scarring	Retinal hemorrhages Macular: ? edema, ? degeneration, ? exudates, ? hemorrhages	—	—	Urticaria Purpura Lupoid syndrome Erythema multiforme Exfoliative dermatitis Lyell's syndrome
Polyenes						
Amphotericin B	↓ Vision Diplopia	Subcj. heme	Retinal exudates +/or hemorrhages	EOM paresis	—	—
Nystatin	↓ Vision	—	Optic neuritis	—	—	—

*See Chapter 4 on Antifungal Drugs.

Table 15-3. Anti-infectives: Antileprosy drugs

Generic drug name	Visual symptoms	Anterior segment	Posterior segment	Extraocular muscles, orbit	Visual fields, CNS	Other
Amithiozone	See Antituberculosis Agents					
Phenazines Clofazimine	↓ Vision	Lids or cj.: red discoloration of tears, hyperpigmentation Polychromatic corneal crystals	Macular RPE mottling	—	—	—
Sulfones Dapsone	↓ Vision Visual hallucinations	Lids or cj.: edema, hyperpigmentation, subcj. heme	Optic atrophy Retinal hemorrhages	—	—	Urticaria Purpura Erythema multiforme Exfoliative dermatitis Lyell's syndrome
Ethionamide	See Antituberculosis Agents					
Rifampin	See Antituberculosis Agents					

Table 15-4. Anti-infectives: Antiparasitic drugs

Generic drug name	Visual symptoms	Anterior segment	Posterior segment	Extraocular muscles, orbit	Visual fields, CNS	Other
Amebicides						
Quinolones						
Iodochlorhydroxyquin Iodoquinol	↓Vision Diplopia	? Corneal opacities ? Madarosis	Optic atrophy/ neuritis Macular edema/ degen. RPE disturbance	—	Toxic amblyopia Nystagmus	Urticaria Purpura
Alkaloids						
Emetine	↓Vision Photophobia	Lids or cj.: hyperemia, tearing Mydriasis Nonreactive pupils POA	—	—	Central scotoma VF constriction	Urticaria
Antihelminthics						
Antimonials (trivalent)						
Antimony K⁺ or Na⁺ tartrate Antimony thioglycollate	↓ Vision	Lids or cj.: edema, yellow skin + sclera, subcj. heme	Optic atrophy, papilledema Retinal hemorrhages	—	Toxic amblyopia	Urticaria

Drug	Subjective / vision	Lids, conjunctiva, cornea, pupils	Retina / optic nerve	Motility	Visual field	Skin / other
Na⁺ antimonial gluconate, Stibocaptate, Stibogluconate, Stibophan		Nonreactive pupils, Mydriasis				
Benzimidazoles Thiabendazole	↓ Vision, Yellow vision, Visual hallucinations	Lids or cj.: allergy, hyperemia, edema, subcj. heme, KC sicca	Retinal hemorrhages	—	—	Erythema multiforme, Exfoliative dermatitis, Lyell's syndrome, Urticaria
Methoxyacridine Quinacrine (mepacrine)	↓ Vision, Photophobia, Color vision defects, Yellow, green, blue, or violet vision, Visual hallucinations	Lid or cj.: blue-black pigmentation, yellow discolor, eczema, subcj. heme; Cornea multicolor punctate deposits	Retinal hemorrhages, Optic neuritis	EOM paresis	Enlarged BS, Scotomas	—

Table 15-4. (continued)

Generic drug name	Visual symptoms	Anterior segment	Posterior segment	Extraocular muscles, orbit	Visual fields, CNS	Other
Piperazines						
Diethylcarbamazine	↓ Vision Photophobia	Lids or cj.: madarosis, edema, nodules, inflammation SPK Corneal opacities Iritis	Chorioretinitis RPE disturbance Papillitis	—	VF defects	Urticaria Purpura Erythema multiforme
Piperazine	↓ Vision Color vision defects Flashing lights Visual hallucinations	Lids or cj.: tearing, edema, photosensitivity, eczema, subcj. heme Miosis POA	Retinal hemorrhages	EOM paralysis	Nystagmus	Exfoliative dermatitis
Antimalarials **Aminoquinoline**						
Amodiaquine Chloroquine	↓ Vision Photophobia	Lids or cj.: poliosis, yellow	Retina: pigment retinopathy,	EOM paralysis, ptosis	Toxic amblyopia Scotomas: cen-	Erythema multiforme

Hydroxychlor-oquine	Night blindness Visual hallucinations Flashing lights Decreased dark adaptation Abnormal flicker fusion diplopia	discolor, photosensitivity, hyper- or depigmentation, madarosis, subcj. heme Cornea: whorl deposits, Hudson-Stähli lines, edema, decreased sensitivity, KC sicca Lens: anterior snowflake, posterior subcapsular cataracts POA	bull's eye maculopathy, doughnut retinopathy, edema, diffuse degeneration, vasoconstriction, hemorrhages Abnormal EOG and ERG Optic atrophy	Oculogyric crisis	tral, paracentral, annular, constriction, hemianopia	Exfoliative dermatitis ? Teratogenesis
Alkaloids					
Quinine	Similar to above antimalarials plus: Wavelike visual disturbance	Iris atrophy Mydriasis ↓ Pupil light response	Retinal exudates Papilledema	—	Vertical nystagmus	—

Table 15-4. (continued)

Generic drug name	Visual symptoms	Anterior segment	Posterior segment	Extraocular muscles, orbit	Visual fields, CNS	Other
Antiprotozoals **Nitroimidazoles**						
Metronidazole	↓Vision Photophobia Visual hallucinations Diplopia	Lids or cj.: erythema, inflammation, edema, photosensitivity, subcj. heme	Retinal hemorrhages	Oculogyric crisis	—	Urticaria
Pentavalent arsenicals						
Tryparsamide	Visual fogging + shimmering ↓Vision	—	Optic neuritis Optic atrophy	—	Toxic amblyopia	—
Polycyclic trypan dyes						
Suramin	Photophobia	Lids or cj.: tearing, edema, subcj. heme Corneal vortex whorl deposits Keratitis Iritis	Retinal hemorrhages Optic atrophy	—	—	Urticaria

* See chapter on Antiparasitic Drugs.

Table 15-5. Anti-infectives: Antituberculosis drugs

Generic drug name	Visual symptoms	Anterior segment	Posterior segment	Extraocular muscles, orbit	Visual fields, CNS	Other
Alcohols						
Ethambutol	↓ Vision Photophobia Red-green, blue-yellow color vision defect	—	Retinal or macular vascular hemorrhages, dilatation, spasm Retinal or macular edema, RPE changes ? Abnormal ERG or VEP	EOM paresis	Toxic amblyopia Annular, central, or cecocentral scotomas VF constriction, hemianopia, enlarged blind spot	Lyell's syndrome
Aminosalicylates						
Para-aminosalicylate Aminosalicylic acid	↓ Vision Red-green color vision defect	Lid or cj.: allergy, blepharoconjunctivitis, edema, angioneurotic edema, subcj. heme POA	Retinal hemorrhage Optic neuritis Optic atrophy	—	Scotomas	Lupoid syndrome Erythema multiforme Exfoliative dermatitis

Table 15-5. (continued)

Generic drug name	Visual symptoms	Anterior segment	Posterior segment	Extraocular muscles, orbit	Visual fields, CNS	Other
Amithiozones						
Thiacetazone	↓ Vision Photophobia	Ocular pain, burning Lids or cj.: allergy, hyperemia, blepharoconjunctivitis, ? madarosis, subcj. heme	Retinal edema +/or hemorrhages	—	—	Erythema multiforme Exfoliative dermatitis
Isoxazolidones						
Cycloserine	↓ Vision Visual hallucinations Flickering vision	Lids or cj.: allergy, inflammation, photosensitivity Subcj. heme ? POA	Retinal hemorrhages ? Optic neuritis ? Optic atrophy	—	—	—
Nicotinic acids						
Ethionamide	↓ Vision Diplopia Photophobia Color vision defect or height-	Lids or cj.: allergy, erythema, photosensitivity ? madarosis	Optic neuritis	—	—	Urticaria Exfoliative dermatitis

	Subjective symptoms	Lids, conjunctiva, cornea, pupil	Retina / optic nerve	EOM	Visual field / other	Skin / systemic
	...ened color vision Visual hallucinations					
Isoniazid	↓Vision Diplopia Photophobia Visual hallucinations Red-green color vision defect	Lids or cj.: allergy, angioneurotic edema, subcj. heme Keratitis Mydriasis Absent pupil light reflex POA	Retinal hemorrhages Retrobulbar or optic neuritis, optic atrophy Papilledema	EOM paresis	Toxic amblyopia Scotomas, VF Hemianopia Nystagmus	Urticaria Lupoid syndrome Erythema multiforme Exfoliative dermatitis Lyell's syndrome
Polypeptides						
Capreomycin	Flickering vision Flashing lights Color vision defect, white tinge ↓Vision ? Visual hallucinations	Lids or cj.: angioneurotic edema	—	—	—	Urticaria
Rifampin (Rifampicin)	↓Vision Red-green color defect	Lids or cj.: ↑lacrimation, hyperemia, erythema ble-	Retinal hemorrhages ? Retrobulbar or optic neuritis	—	—	Urticaria Purpura Lupoid syndrome

Table 15-5. (continued)

Generic drug name	Visual symptoms	Anterior segment	Posterior segment	Extraocular muscles, orbit	Visual fields, CNS	Other
		pharoconjunctivitis, edema, yellow or red discoloration, angioneurotic edema, subcj. heme Iritis				Erythema multiforme Exfoliative dermatitis Pemphigoid Contact lenses stain orange (tears)
Streptomycin	See Antibiotics table.					

Table 15-6. Anti-infectives: Systemic antiviral drugs*

Generic drug name	Visual symptoms	Anterior segment	Posterior segment	Extraocular muscles, orbit	Visual fields, CNS	Other
Antimetabolites						
Acyclovir	↓ Vision Visual hallucinations	Lids or cj.: erythema, ? lash or brow loss, subcj. heme	Retinal hemorrhages	—	—	—
Azidothymidine	↓ Vision	Subcj. heme	Retinal hemorrhages	—	—	—
Cytarabine	↓ Vision Photophobia Diplopia (intrathecal)	Lids or cj.: ↑ lacrimation, ocular pain, burning sensation, allergy, hyperemia, hemorrhagic conjunctivitis, hyperpigmentation, ? brow or lash loss Corneal opacities SPK	Retinal hemorrhages	EOM paresis (intrathecal)	Nystagmus (intrathecal)	Urticaria Purpura ? Teratogenesis

Table 15-6. (continued)

Generic drug name	Visual symptoms	Anterior segment	Posterior segment	Extraocular muscles, orbit	Visual fields, CNS	Other
Ganciclovir	? Visual hallucinations	Subjc. heme	Retinal hemorrhages ? Retinal detachment in CMV retinitis	—	—	? Teratogenesis Anophthalmia Microphthalmia
Vidarabine	Visual hallucinations	Lids or cj.: blepharospasm, subcj. heme	Retinal hemorrhages	—	—	—

* See chapter on Antivirals.

16

Antineoplastic Agents

Table 16-1. Antineoplastic Agents

Generic drug name	Visual symptoms	Anterior segment	Posterior segment	Extraocular muscles, orbit	Visual fields, CNS	Other
Alkylating agents						
Busulfan	↓ Vision	Lids or cj.: allergy, hypereremia (BCNU), erythema, blepharoconjunctivitis (cyclophosphamide, mechlorethamine, melphalan), edema (chlorambucil), hyperpigmentation (busulfan, BCNU, chlorambucil, cyclophosphamide, mechlorethamine, uracil mustard), photosensitivity (cyclo-	Retinal hemorrhages	—	Pseudotumor cerebri	Urticaria (busulfan, chorambucil, cyclophosphamide, DIC, melphalan)
Carmustine (BCNU)	Photophobia		Optic neuritis (BCNU)			Erythema multiforme (busulfan, mechlorethamine)
Chlorambucil	Visual hallucinations		Papilledema			
Cyclophosphamide			Retinal vascular disorders (BCNU): occlusion, thrombosis			Exfoliative dermatitis (chlorambucil, cyclophosphamide, mechlorethamine)
Dacarbazine (DIC)						
Lomustine (CCNU)						Aggravation of: herpes infections and Sjögren's syndrome
Mechlorethamine						
Melphalan						? Teratogenesis
Semustine						
Streptozocin						
Triethylenemelamine (Tretamine)						
Uracil mustard (Uramustine)						

(busulfan): microphthalmia, retinal degeneration

phosphamide, DIC), angioneurotic edema (melphalan), lash or brow loss, subcj. heme, ↓ lacrimation (busulfan)

Nonspecific irritation (cyclophosphamide): lacrimation, pain, burning

KC sicca (busulfan, chlorambucil, cyclophosphamide)

Corneal edema (melphalan)

↑ IOP (BCNU)

Absent pupil light reflex (BCNU)

Cataracts (busulfan)

Table 16-1. (continued)

Generic drug name	Visual symptoms	Anterior segment	Posterior segment	Extraocular muscles, orbit	Visual fields, CNS	Other
Antibiotics						
Bleomycin Cactinomycin Dactinomycin Daunorubicin Doxorubicin Mitomycin	↓ Vision (mitomycin)	Lids or cj.: loss of lashes or brows, allergy, erythema, conjunctivitis (doxorubicin), edema, hyperpigmentation, angioneurotic edema (daunorubicin), lacrimation (doxorubicin)	Retinal hemorrhages	—	? Nystagmus (bleomycin)	Urticaria Erythema multiforme Aggravation of herpes infections ? Teratogenesis
Plicamycin (Mithramycin)	—	Subcj. heme	Retinal hemorrhages	Periorbital pallor	—	? Teratogenesis Aggravation of herpes infections
Antimetabolites						
Floxuridine Fluorouracil	↓ Vision Photophobia Diplopia	Lids or cj.: ↑ lacrimation, hyperemia, er-	Retinal hemorrhages ? Optic neuritis	↓ Convergence or divergence	Nystagmus	Erythema multiforme (fluorouracil)

	ythema, pain, edema, burning sensation, cicatricial ectropion, blepharoconjunctivitis (fluorouracil), hyperpigmentation, photosensitivity, ulcers, lash or brow loss, drug in tear film, subcj. heme POA	(fluorouracil)		Aggravation of herpes infections ? Teratogenesis
Mercaptopurine Thioguanine	Color vision defects Red-green defect	Lids or cj.: icterus, hyperpigmentation, subcj. heme	—	—	—	? Teratogenesis Aggravation of herpes infections
Carbamic acid derivatives				
Urethan	↓ Vision	Subcj. heme Mydriasis Absent pupil light reflex	Retinal hemorrhages	—	Nystagmus	Aggravation of herpes infections ? Teratogenesis

Table 16-1. (continued)

Generic drug name	Visual symptoms	Anterior segment	Posterior segment	Extraocular muscles, orbit	Visual fields, CNS	Other
Chlorophenyl ethane derivatives						
Mitotane	↓ Vision Diplopia	Lids or cj.: erythema, hyperpigmentation, ? brow or lash loss Cataracts	RPE disturbance Retinal hemorrhages Papilledema	—	—	? Teratogenesis Aggravation of herpes infections
Ethylenamine derivatives						
Thiotepa	—	Lids or cj.: erythema, angioneurotic edema, lash or brow loss, subcj. heme, ? Acute fibrinous iritis	Retinal hemorrhages	—	—	Urticaria ? Teratogenesis Aggravation of herpes infections
Folic acid antagonists						
Methotrexate	↓ Vision Photophobia	Lids or cj.: ↑ or ↓ lacrimation, allergy, ery-	Retinal hemorrhages RPE distur-	EOM paralysis Periorbital edema	—	Urticaria Lyell's syndrome Aggravation of

Drug	Symptoms	Lids or conjunctiva	Retina / optic nerve	Neuromuscular / EOM	Cortical / field	Other
		thema, blepharoconjunctivitis, depigmentation, photosensitivity, lash or brow loss, nonspecific ocular pain or burning, subcj. heme in tears; Keratitis	bances; ? Optic atrophy			herpes infections; ? Teratogenesis
Heavy metals (Platinum) Cisplatin (Cisplatinum)	↓ Vision; Diplopia	Lids or cj.: erythema, conjunctivitis, edema, lash or brow loss, subj. heme	Retinal hemorrhages; RPE disturbances; Retrobulbar or optic neuritis; Papilledema; Abnormal ERG, EOG, or VEP	Myasthenic neuromuscular block: ptosis, EOM paralysis; Oculogyric crisis; Orbital pain	Cortical blindness; Hemianopia	Urticaria; Aggravation of herpes infections
Interferon	↓ Vision; Visual hallucinations	Lids or cj.: conjunctivitis, ↑ lash growth, ? brow or lash	Retinal hemorrhages; Papilledema; Abnormal VEP	—	—	Urticaria; Purpura

Table 16-1. (continued)

Generic drug name	Visual symptoms	Anterior segment	Posterior segment	Extraocular muscles, orbit	Visual fields, CNS	Other
		loss, subcj. heme				
Methylhydrazine derivatives						
Procarbazine	Photophobia Nystagmus Diplopia	Lids or cj.: erythema, hyperpigmentation, photosensitivity, ? lash or brow loss, subcj. heme POA	Retinal hemorrhages Papilledema ? Optic neuritis	—	Nystagmus	Urticaria Purpura Exfoliative dermatitis ? Teratogenesis Aggravation of herpes infections Lyell's syndrome
Nonsteroidal antiestrogens (triphenylethylene derivatives)						
Tamoxifen	↓ Vision	? Lash or brow loss Subepithelial corneal whorl opacities	Retinal or macular: hemorrhages, edema, yellow-white refractile opacities, degeneration, RPE disturbances	—	VF constriction Paracentral scotomas	? Teratogenesis ? Aggravation of herpes infections

		Papilledema ? Optic neuritis			
Urea derivatives					
Hydroxyurea	Visual hallucinations	Lids or cj.: erythema, atrophy, scaling, hyperpigmentation, ? brow or lash loss, subcj. heme	Retinal hemorrhages	—	—	? Teratogenesis Aggravation of herpes infections
Vinca alkaloids					
Vinblastine Vincristine	Visual hallucinations Photophobia Diplopia Color vision defect Red-green color vision defect ↓ Dark adaptation	Lids or cj.: photosensitivity, lash or brow loss, subcj. heme, hyperemia ↓ Corneal reflex Corneal deposits or ulcers Scleritis Iritis	Retinal hemorrhages Retrobulbar or optic neuritis Optic atrophy Abnormal ERG	Neuromuscular block: ptosis, EOM paralysis	? Nystagmus VF constriction Scotomas: central or paracentral Hemianopia Cortical blindness	? Teratogenesis Aggravation of herpes infections

17

Cardiovascular Drugs

Table 17-1. Cardiovascular drugs: Antianginal agents

Generic drug name	Visual symptoms	Anterior segment	Posterior segment	Extraocular muscles, orbit	Visual fields, CNS	Other
Benzofurans						
Amiodarone	↓ Vision Color vision defect Colored halos on lights Photophobia	Lids or cj.: ble-pharoconjunc-tivitis, photo-sensitivity, discoloration, chalazia, ? brow or lash loss KC sicca Corneal ulcers → Corneal reflex Yellow-brown deposits: cj., cornea epith. whorls, lens ? Cataracts	Papilledema ? Retinal depig-mentation ? Optic neuritis	—	Pseudotumor cerebri VF defects Nystagmus	Urticaria Erythema multiforme Lyell's syndrome
Calcium channel blockers						
Diltiazem Nifedipine Verapamil	↓ Vision Visual hallucina-tions	Lids or cj.: ery-thema, con-junctivitis, photosensitiv-ity, angioneu-rotic edema,	Retinal hemor-rhages or thrombosis (diltiazem, nifedipine)	Periorbital edema	Nystagmus ro-tary (nifedi-pine, verapa-mil) Transient blind-ness at peak	Urticaria Purpura Erythema multiforme Exfoliative dermatitis

Table 17-1. (continued)

Generic drug name	Visual symptoms	Anterior segment	Posterior segment	Extraocular muscles, orbit	Visual fields, CNS	Other
		↑ lacrimation, ocular pain, edema, subcj. heme ↓IOP ? Cataracts (nifedipine, verapamil)			plasma levels (diltiazem)	Lyell's syndrome (diltiazem)
Lidocaine analogs Flecainide Mexiletine Tocainide	↓ Vision Visual hallucinations Diplopia Photophobia	Lids or cj.: pain (flecainide), erythema, angioneurotic edema, subcj. heme, ? lash or brow loss	Retinal hemorrhages	—	Nystagmus	Urticaria (flecainide) Lupoid syndrome ? Erythema multiforme (tocainide) Exfoliative dermatitis (flecainide)
Nitrates Erythrityl tetranitrate Isosorbide dinitrate	↓ Vision Myopia (isosorbide)	? Ptosis (isosorbide) ? Miosis (isosorbide)	—	—	—	Exfoliative dermatitis

Mannitol hexanitrate Pentaerythritol tetranitrate Trolnitrate		↓ IOP ? ↑ IOP			—
Nitrites Amyl nitrite (inhalation administration)	↓ Vision "Yellow" vision Blue or yellow halos around lights Color hallucinations	Lids or cj.: allergy Mydriasis ↓ IOP (transient)	Retinal vasodilation	—	—
Perhexilene	↓ Vision Color vision defect ? Visual hallucinations	KC sicca Corneal deposits	Papilledema Retinal vascular thrombosis, hemorrhages, engorgement	—	Nystagmus Pseudotumor cerebri VF ↑ blind spot
Trinitrates Nitroglycerin	↓ Vision Colored halos around lights, yellow or blue ? Visual hallucinations	Subcj. heme ↓ IOP ? ↑ IOP	Retinal vasodilation Retinal hemorrhages Papilledema ? Optic atrophy	—	Pseudotumor cerebri Exfoliative dermatitis

Table 17-2. Cardiovascular drugs: Antiarrhythmics

Generic drug name	Visual symptoms	Anterior segment	Posterior segment	Extraocular muscles, orbit	Visual fields, CNS	Other
Anticholinergics						
Disopyramide	↓ Vision Visual hallucinations Photophobia Diplopia	Lids or cj.: ↓ lacrimation, erythema, conjunctivitis, photosensitivity Mydriasis POA	—	EOM paralysis	—	? Aggravate myasthenia gravis
β-Adrenergic blockers						
Oxyprenolol	↓ Vision Visual hallucinations Photophobia	Lids or cj.: ↓ lacrimation, allergy, hyperemia, erythema, conjunctivitis, edema, hyperpigmentation, ? lash or brow loss, ocular pain, burning ? KC sicca	—	Myasthenic neuromuscular block: ptosis, EOM paresis	—	Purpura Oculomucocutaneous syndrome

Practolol	↓Vision Visual hallucinations Photophobia	Corneal ulcers Corneal opacities ↑ or ↓ Lacrimation Ocular pain or burning ↓Tear lysozymes Lids: edema, erythema, cafe au lait pigmentation cj.: hyperemia, papillary conjunctivitis Patchy ↑ or ↓ vascularity, keratinization, scarring, edema Cornea: yellow or white stromal opacities, ulcers, perforation ↓IOP	—	Myasthenic neuromuscular block: ptosis, EOM paresis	—	Oculomucocutaneous syndrome Lupoid syndrome Urticaria Exfoliative dermatitis Eczema Pemphigoid
Propranolol	↓Vision Diplopia	Lids or cj.: allergy, erythema	—	Exophthalmos (withdrawal	—	Urticaria Lupoid

Table 17-2. (continued)

Generic drug name	Visual symptoms	Anterior segment	Posterior segment	Extraocular muscles, orbit	Visual fields, CNS	Other
	Visual hallucinations Photophobia	thema, conjunctivitis, ? lash or brow loss, ↑ or ↓ lacrimation Ocular pain ? KC sicca POA ↓ IOP		state) Myasthenic neuromuscular block: ptosis, EOM paresis Inflammatory ocular pseudotumor		syndrome Erythema multiforme Exfoliative dermatitis Pemphigoid Oculomucocutaneous syndrome
Neuromuscular blocker						
Procainamide	—	Scleritis	—	—	—	Lupoid syndrome
Quaternary ammonium parasympathomimetics						
Methacholine	—	↑ Lacrimation POA	—	—	—	—

Quinines

Quinidine					
↓ Vision Color vision defect Red-green defect Photophobia Diplopia Night blindness Visual hallucinations	Lids or cj.: allergy, hyperpigmentation, photosensitivity, angioneurotic edema, subcj. heme KC sicca Corneal deposits Iridocyclitis Mydriasis	Retinal hemorrhages Optic neuritis	Myasthenic neuromuscular block: ptosis, EOM paralysis	Toxic amblyopia	Urticaria Lupoid syndrome Exfoliative dermatitis

Table 17-3. Cardiovascular drugs: Antihypertensives

Generic drug name	Visual symptoms	Anterior segment	Posterior segment	Extraocular muscles, orbit	Visual fields, CNS	Other
Alpha-adrenergic agonists						
Clonidine	↓ Vision Visual hallucinations ? Diplopia ? Flashing lights	Lids or cj.: burning sensation, angioneurotic edema, ↓ lacrimation, ? KC sicca Miosis (toxic) Absent pupil light reflex	? Retinal or macular degeneration or RPE changes ? Abnormal EOG	—	—	Urticaria ? Pemphigoid
Adrenergic blockers						
Acebutolol Atenolol Labetalol Metoprolol Nadolol Pindolol	↓ Vision Visual hallucinations Diplopia Photophobia	Lids or cj.: hyperemia (metoprolol), → lacrimation, erythema, blepharoconjunctivitis (metoprolol), ? lash or brow loss, ocular pain, subcj. heme	Retinal hemorrhages ? Papilledema (nadolol)	Myasthenic neuromuscular block: ptosis, ? EOM paralysis	—	Oculomucocutaneous syndrome Urticaria (labetalol, metoprolol) Purpura (metoprolol) Lupoid syndrome (acebutolol, labetolol, labe-

Guanethidine	↓Vision Photophobia Diplopia Flashing lights	Corneal ulcers (metoprolol) ↓IOP Lids or cj.: hyperemia, ? lash or brow loss, edema, subcj. heme, Accommodative spasm ↓IOP	Retinal hemorrhages ? Retinal vasospasm		—	talol) Eczema (metoprolol) Horner's syndrome
Methyldopa	↓Vision Visual hallucinations Diplopia Photophobia	Lids or cj.: allergy, hyperemia, conjunctivitis, edema, subcj. heme, ↓lacrimation KC sicca ±↓IOP	Retinal hemorrhages	EOM paralysis	Hemianopia	Urticaria Lupoid syndrome Eczema
Angiotensin-converting enzyme inhibitors						
Captopril Enalapril	↓Vision Visual hallucinations ? Photophobia	Lids or cj.: erythema, blepharoconjunctivitis, edema, brown discoloration, photosensitivity, ? lash or brow	Retinal hemorrhages		—	Urticaria Lupoid syndrome Erythema multiforme Exfoliative dermatitis Pemphigoid

Table 17-3. (continued)

Generic drug name	Visual symptoms	Anterior segment	Posterior segment	Extraocular muscles, orbit	Visual fields, CNS	Other
		loss, subcj. heme, angioneurotic edema ? POA				Eczema
Benzothiadiazines						
Diazoxide	↓ Vision Diplopia	Lids or cj.: lacrimation, allergy, erythema, subcj. heme Cataracts	Retinal hemorrhages	Oculogyric crises	Ring scotomas	—
Beta-adrenergic blockers						
Timolol	↓ Vision Visual hallucinations	Lids or cj.: allergy, ↓ lacrimation, erythema, hyperpigmentation, lash or brow loss ? KC sicca ↓ IOP	—	Myasthenic neuromuscular block: ptosis, EOM paresis	—	Oculomucocutaneous syndrome

Ganglionic blockers						
Hexamethonium	↓Vision Red-green color vision defect	↓Lacrimation Cj. edema Mydriasis ↓IOP	Retinal vasodilation Macular edema Optic atrophy	? Periorbital edema	VF constriction Hemianopia Toxic amblyopia	—
Mecamylamine Tetraethylammonium Trimethaphan Trimethidinium	↓Vision Colored lights (mecamylamine)	Cj: edema POA Mydriasis ↓IOP	—	Myasthenic neuromuscular block: ptosis —	—	Urticaria (trimethaphan)
Monoamine oxidase inhibitors						
Pargyline	Visual hallucinations Color vision defects Red-green vision defect	Mydriasis (toxic) ↓Pupil light reflex (toxic) POA	—	Hyperactive eye movements (toxic)	—	—
Phthalazines						
Hydralazine	↓Vision Photophobia Colored flashing lights	Lids or cj.: pain, lacrimation, allergy, erythema, edema, conjunctivitis, subcj. heme	Retinal hemorrhages	Periorbital edema	—	Urticaria Lupoid syndrome

Table 17-3. (continued)

Generic drug name	Visual symptoms	Anterior segment	Posterior segment	Extraocular muscles, orbit	Visual fields, CNS	Other
Pyrimidinediamine						
Minoxidil	↓ Vision	Lids or cj.: erythema, hyperemia, ? brow or lash loss, conjunctivitis, hyperpigmentation, ? discoloration of lashes or brows ? ↑ IOP	? RPE disturbance ? Abnormal ERG or VEP ? Optic neuritis	—	—	—
Quinazolines						
Prazosin	↓ Vision Visual hallucinations	Lids or cj.: erythema, conjunctivitis, edema, ? lash or brow loss Aggravation of KC sicca Scleritis ? Cataracts	? RPE disturbance ? Central serous retinopathy	—	—	Urticaria

Rauwolfia alkaloids

Alseroxylon Deserpidine Rauwolfia serpentina Rescinnamine Reserpine Syrosingopine	↓ Vision Color vision defects "Yellow" vision	Lids or cj.: lacrimation, hyperemia Mydriasis ? Iritis ↓ IOP	Retinal hemorrhages ? Optic atrophy	Oculogyric crises ↓ Spontaneous movements, abnormal conjugate deviations Jerky pursuit	—	Horner's syndrome Lupoid syndrome ? Teratogenesis (reserpine)

Veratrum alkaloids

Alkavervir Cryptenamine Protoveratrines A and B Veratrum viride alkaloids	↓ Vision	Mydriasis	—	Extraocular myotonia	VF constriction	—

Table 17-4. Cardiovascular drugs: Antimigraine agents

Generic drug name	Visual symptoms	Anterior segment	Posterior segment	Extraocular muscles, orbit	Visual fields, CNS	Other
Ergot alkaloids						
Ergonovine (Ergometrine) Ergotamine Methylergonovine Methysergide	↓Vision Color vision red-green defect "Red" vision Visual hallucinations (methysergide) ↓Dark adaptation	Lids or cj.: allergy, erythema, edema, ? lash or brow loss Miosis (ergotamine) ? Cataracts ↓IOP POA	Retinal vascular: spasm, constriction, thrombosis, occlusion Abnormal ERG Optic neuritis ? Optic atrophy	—	Scotomas Hemianopias ? Cortical blindness (methylergonovine)	Lupoid syndrome

Table 17-5. Cardiovascular drugs: Cardiac glycosides

Generic drug name	Visual symptoms	Anterior segment	Posterior segment	Extraocular muscles, orbit	Visual fields, CNS	Other
Cardiac glycosides						
Acetyldigitoxin Deslanoside Digitalis Digitoxin Digoxin Gitalin Lanatoside C Ouabain	↓ Vision Blue-yellow or red-green color defect "Yellow, green, blue," or "red" vision Colored halos around lights (often blue) Flickering vision (often yellow or green) Objects have colored edges White, brown, or orange "snow glare" to objects	Lids or cj.: ptosis, allergy, angioneurotic edema Mydriasis Accommodative spasm	Abnormal ERG Retrobulbar or optic neuritis	EOM paresis	Scotomas: central or paracentral VF constriction Toxic amblyopia	Urticaria Lupoid syndrome

Table 17-5. (continued)

Generic drug name	Visual symptoms	Anterior segment	Posterior segment	Extraocular muscles, orbit	Visual fields, CNS	Other
	Scintillating scotomas Objects "frosted" Photophobia Visual hallucinations (often bright spots) Diplopia ? Myopia					

Table 17-6. Cardiovascular drugs: Peripheral vasodilators

Generic drug name	Visual symptoms	Anterior segment	Posterior segment	Extraocular muscles, orbit	Visual fields, CNS	Other
Alpha-adrenergic blockers						
Phenoxybenzamine	—	Lids or cj.: ptosis, hyperemia ? ↓ IOP Miosis	—	—	—	—
Tolazoline	—	Subcj. heme ↑ IOP → IOP (usually in hypertensive patients)	Retinal hemorrhages	—	—	—
Nicotinic acid						
Aluminum nicotinate Niacin (nicotinic acid) Niacinamide (nicotinamide) Nicotinyl alcohol	↓ Vision	Lids or cj.: allergy, hyperpigmentation, angioneurotic edema, ? brow or lash loss ? ↑ IOP ? Episcleritis	Cystoid macular edema	Proptosis	Toxic amblyopia ? Paracentral scotomas	Urticaria

Table 17-7. Cardiovascular drugs: Vasopressors and bronchodilators

Generic drug name	Visual symptoms	Anterior segment	Posterior segment	Extraocular muscles, orbit	Visual fields, CNS	Other
Sympathomimetic amines						
Albuterol	→ Vision Visual hallucinations ? Diplopia	Lids or cj.: ↑ lacrimation, erythema, blepharoconjunctivitis, edema, angioneurotic edema Mydriasis → IOP	—	—	—	Urticaria
Ephedrine	Visual hallucinations	Mydriasis ? Rebound miosis → IOP	—	—	—	—
Epinephrine	Red-green color vision defect "Green" vision	Mydriasis	—	—	Hemianopia	—

						Nystagmus—horizontal
Mephentermine Metaraminol Methoxamine Norepinephrine (Levarterenol)	Photophobia (norepinephrine) Diplopia (norepinephrine) Visual hallucinations (mephentermine)	Rebound cj.: hyperemia ↓IOP (norepinephrine) Mydriasis	—	—	—	
Phenlyephrine (nasal application)	Visual hallucinations	—	—	—	—	

Table 17-8. Cardiovascular drugs: Uterine contractants

Generic drug name	Visual symptoms	Anterior segment	Posterior segment	Extraocular muscles, orbit	Visual fields, CNS	Other
Ergot alkaloids						
Ergot	↓ Vision ? Scintillating scotomas ? Diplopia Hypermetropia	POA Mydriasis (acute) Miosis ↓ Pupil light reflex ? Cataracts	Retinal edema Retinal vasoconstriction ? Optic atrophy	—	Toxic amblyopia VF constriction Scotomas ↑ Blind spot ? Nystagmus	—

18

Central Nervous System Agents

Table 18-1. Central nervous system agents: Analeptics (mental stimulation of the elderly)

Generic drug name	Visual symptoms	Anterior segment	Posterior segment	Extraocular muscles, orbit	Visual fields, CNS	Other
Pentylenetetrazol						
(pentetrazol)	Visual hallucinations Scintillating scotomas "Yellow" vision Color vision defects	Blepharospasm Mydriasis Absent pupil light reaction Hippus	—	Strabismus Abnormal conjugate deviations	—	—

Table 18-2. Central nervous system agents: Anorexiants (therapy of exogenous obesity)

Generic drug name	Visual symptoms	Anterior segment	Posterior segment	Extraocular muscles, orbit	Visual fields, CNS	Other
Sympathomimetic amines						
Amphetamine Dextroamphetamine Methamphetamine Phenmetrazine	↓ Vision Visual hallucinations "Blue" vision (amphetamine)	Lids or cj.: ? lash loss, widened palpebral fissure, blepharospasm POA Mydriasis Decreased pupil light reaction ? PSC cataracts (phenmetrazine)	Retinal vein occlusion (phenmetrazine)	Decreased convergence	—	Teratogenesis (methamphetamine)
Benzphetamine Chlorphentermine Diethylpropion (Amfepramone) Fenfluramine	↓ Vision Photophobia Visual hallucinations Diplopia	Lids or cj.: pain, burning, allergy, erythema, ? lash loss, subcj. heme Mydriasis	Retinal hemorrhage Retinal vein occlusion ? Optic neuritis (diethylpropion)	—	Rotary nystagmus (fenfluramine)	Urticaria

Table 18-2. (continued)

Generic drug name	Visual symptoms	Anterior segment	Posterior segment	Extraocular muscles, orbit	Visual fields, CNS	Other
Phendimetrazine Phentermine		Absent pupil light reaction (fenfluramine) POA ? PSC cataracts				
Phenylpropan-olamine	↓ Vision Visual hallucina-tions	Mydriasis Anisocoria Absent pupil light reflex	Retinal vein spasm, throm-bosis, hemor-rhage Papilledema	—	Pseudotumor cerebri Nystagmus	Aggravation of hyperthyroid-ism

Table 18-3. Central nervous system agents: Antianxiety agents, muscle relaxants

Generic drug name	Visual symptoms	Anterior segment	Posterior segment	Extraocular muscles, orbit	Visual fields, CNS	Other
Benzodiazepines Alprazolam Chlordiazepoxide Clonazepam Chlorazepate Diazepam Flurazepam Halazepam Lorazepam Midazolam Oxazepam Prazepam Temazepam Triazolam	↓ Vision ↓ Depth perception Diplopia Visual hallucinations Color vision defect Photophobia	Lids or cj.: ? lash and brow loss (clonazepam), allergy, erythema, inflammation, photosensitivity, angioneurotic edema, ↑ lacrimation, subcj. heme, blepharospasm (lorazepam) ↓ Corneal reflex (chlorazepate, diazepam)	Retinal hemorrhages	Abnormal EOG Oculogyric crisis ↓ Spontaneous movements Abnormal conjugate deviations Jerky pursuit ↓ Saccadic movements EOM paralysis	Nystagmus: horizontal or gaze evoked	Urticaria Purpura Erythema multiforme

Table 18-3. (continued)

Generic drug name	Visual symptoms	Anterior segment	Posterior segment	Extraocular muscles, orbit	Visual fields, CNS	Other
		POA Mydriasis Miosis (midazolam) Decreased pupil light reflex Ocular pain or burning ? Brown lens deposits (diazepam)				

Carbamates						
Carisoprodol Meprobamate	↓ Vision Diplopia	Lids or cj.: allergy, burning, angioneurotic edema, subconj. heme, edema ↓ Corneal reflex Mydriasis Miosis Decreased pupil light reflex POA ? Hypotension	Retinal hemorrhages	EOM paralysis Random ocular movements	VF constriction Nystagmus	Urticaria Erythema multiforme Exfoliative dermatitis
Piperidines						
Pimozide	↓ Vision Visual hallucinations	Lids or cj.: ↓ lacrimation, erythema, edema POA	Retinal hemorrhages	Oculogyric crisis	—	—

Table 18-4. Central nervous system agents: Anticonvulsants

Generic drug name	Visual symptoms	Anterior segment	Posterior segment	Extraocular muscles, orbit	Visual fields, CNS	Other
Carboxylic acid derivatives						
Divalproex sodium Valproate sodium Valproic acid	Diplopia Visual hallucinations	? Lash and brow loss	—	—	Nystagmus	—
Hydantoins						
Ethotoin Mephenytoin	Diplopia Photophobia	Lids or cj.: allergy, inflammation, ? brow or lash loss, subcj. heme ? Corneal or lens opacities	Retinal hemorrhages	? Myasthenic neuromuscular block: ptosis, EOM paralysis	Nystagmus	Urticaria Lupoid syndrome Erythema multiforme Lyell's syndrome
Phenytoin	↓ Vision Glare "White snow cover" Flashing lights Oscillopsia Colors fade	Lids or cj.: allergy, ulceration, subcj. heme Mydriasis ↓ Pupil light reflex	Retinal hemorrhages Papilledema	Myasthenic neuromuscular block: EOM paralysis, ptosis ↓ Convergence Orbital or periorbital pain	Nystagmus: downbeat horizontal, or vertical Pseudotumor cerebri	Urticaria Purpura Lupoid syndrome Erythema multiforme Lyell's syndrome

	White-tinged vision Visual hallucinations Diplopia	POA Cataracts				Teratogenesis: hypertelorism, ptosis, epican- thus, strabis- mus, glau- coma, optic nerve or iris hypoplasia, retinal colo- boma or schisis, trichomegaly
Oxazolidinediones						
Paramethadione Trimethadione	Glare "White snow" vi- sion Photophobia Night blindness Red-green or yel- low-blue color vision defect White halos Color fading Diplopia	Lids or cj.: ? lash loss, allergy, photosensitiv- ity, angioneu- rotic edema, subcj. heme	Retinal hemor- rhages	Myasthenic neu- romuscular block: EOM paralysis, pto- sis	Scotomas Gaze-evoked nystagmus	Lupoid syndrome Erythema multiforme Exfoliative dermatitis Lyell's syndrome Teratogenesis ("V" eyebrows, epicanthus, myopia, stra- bismus, hyper- telorism)

Table 18-4. (continued)

Generic drug name	Visual symptoms	Anterior segment	Posterior segment	Extraocular muscles, orbit	Visual fields, CNS	Other
Succinimides						
Ethosuximide Methsuximide Phensuximide	↓Vision Diplopia Photophobia Myopia Visual hallucinations	Lids or cj.: allergy, angioneurotic edema, subcj. heme	Retinal hemorrhages	Periorbital edema or hyperemia	—	Lupoid syndrome Erythema multiforme Exfoliative dermatitis
Sulfonamides						
Sulthiame (Sultiame)	↓Vision Diplopia Color vision defect "Red" vision	Lids or cj.: edema, ptosis	Papilledema	—	—	Erythema multiforme

Table 18-5. Central nervous system agents: Antidepressants

Generic drug name	Visual symptoms	Anterior segment	Posterior segment	Extraocular muscles, orbit	Visual fields, CNS	Other
Iminostilbenes						
Carbamazepine	↓ Vision Diplopia Visual hallucinations	Lids or cj.: ? lash or brow loss, allergy, inflammation, edema, photosensitivity, subcj. heme, blepharoclonus POA Mydriasis ? Cataracts	Retinal hemorrhages Papilledema RPE changes	EOM paresis Downbeat nystagmus Oculogyric crisis ↓ Spontaneous movements	—	Urticaria Purpura Lupoid syndrome Erythema multiforme Lyell's syndrome Icterus ? Teratogenesis
Monoamine oxidase inhibitors						
Isocarboxazid Nialamide Phenelzine Tranylcypromine	↓ Vision Diplopia Photophobia Color vision defect Red-green vision defect Visual hallucinations (mialam-	Lids or cj.: photosensitivity, subcj. heme Mydriasis Miosis Anisocoria Absent pupil light reflex	? Retrobulbar neuritis ? Papilledema (isocarboxazid, phenelzine, tranylcypromine) Retinal hemorrhages	Myasthenic neuromuscular block: EOM paralysis, ptosis	VF defects (nialamide, phenelzine) Nystagmus (phenelzine, tranylcypromine)	Lupoid syndrome

Table 18-5. (continued)

Generic drug name	Visual symptoms	Anterior segment	Posterior segment	Extraocular muscles, orbit	Visual fields, CNS	Other
	ide, phenelzine)					
Oxazolidinones						
Pemoline	↓Vision Visual hallucinations Diplopia	—	—	Oculogyric crisis Strabismus	Nystagmus	Aggravation of Tourette's syndrome
Piperidines						
Methylphenidate Oral administration	Visual hallucinations	Lids or cj.: blepharoclonus, subcj. heme Mydriasis ?↑IOP	Retinal hemorrhages	—	—	Urticaria Erythema multiforme Exfoliative dermatitis
IV administration	↓Vision	—	Talc retinopathy—small yellow-white emboli, hemorrhages, late neovascularization Traction retinal detachment	—	—	—

Propylamine HCl

Drug	Subjective symptoms	Lids or cj / ocular	Retina	Neuro-ophthalmic		Dermatologic
Fluoxetine	↓ Vision Photophobia Diplopia Eye pain	Lids or cj: blepharoconjunctivitis, subcj. heme Corneal deposits Mydriasis Iritis Cataract	—	Ptosis, EOM paresis	|	Aggravation of herpes simplex virus infections Lyell's syndrome

Tetracyclics

Drug	Subjective symptoms	Lids or cj / ocular	Retina	Neuro-ophthalmic		Dermatologic
Maprotiline Mianserin	↓ Vision Visual hallucinations	Lids or cj: erythema, inflammation, edema, photosensitivity, angioneurotic edema, ? lash or brow loss, subcj. heme Mydriasis POA	Retinal hemorrhages	—	|	Erythema multiforme Urticaria

Triazolopyridines

Drug	Subjective symptoms	Lids or cj / ocular	Retina	Neuro-ophthalmic		Dermatologic
Trazodone	↓ Vision Visual hallucinations Diplopia	Ocular, pain or burning Lids or cj:: allergy, ery-	Retinal hemorrhages	—	|	Erythema multiforme

Table 18-5. (continued)

Generic drug name	Visual symptoms	Anterior segment	Posterior segment	Extraocular muscles, orbit	Visual fields, CNS	Other
	Photophobia Palinopsia (persistence of recently viewed image)	thema, blepharoconjunctivitis, photosensitivity, subcj. heme Mydriasis				
Tricyclics Amitryptiline Desipramine Imipramine Nortriptyline Protriptyline	↓ Vision Diplopia Photophobia Visual hallucinations ? Color vision defect	Lids or cj.: ↓ lacrimation, blepharospasm, erythema, edema, photosensitivity, subcj. heme, ? lash or brow loss ↓ Corneal reflex Mydriasis ↓ Pupil light reflex	Retinal hemorrhages Retrobulbar or optic neuritis	EOM paralysis (lateral rectus) Oculogyric crises Nystagmus Jerky pursuit ↓ Spontaneous movements Abnormal conjugate gaze	Toxic amblyopia	Urticaria Purpura

Amoxapine Clomipramine Doxepin Trimipramine	↓Vision Visual hallucinations Photophobia (doxepin)	Lids or cj.: ↑lacrimation (amoxapine), erythema, edema, photosensitivity, ? blepharospasm, ? lash or brow loss (amoxapine, doxepin) KC sicca (doxepin) Mydriasis ↓Pupil light reflex POA	—	EOM paresis Abnormal conjugate gaze (amoxapine)	Nystagmus—horizontal or rotary Oculogyric crisis (doxepin)	Urticaria Lyell's syndrome

Table 18-6. Central nervous system agents: Antipsychotic drugs

Generic drug name	Visual symptoms	Anterior segment	Posterior segment	Extraocular muscles, orbit	Visual fields, CNS	Other
Butyrophenones						
Droperidol Haloperidol Trifluperidol	↓ Vision Visual hallucinations Myopia	Lids or cj.: allergy, photosensitivity, angioneurotic edema, blepharospasm, ? lash or brow loss, subcj. heme Mydriasis Miosis Hypotension ? Subcapsular cataracts	Retinal hemorrhages	Oculogyric crisis	—	Exfoliative dermatitis

Dibenzoxapines

Loxapine	↓ Vision	Lids or cj.: ptosis, edema, hyperpigmentation, photosensitivity, subcj. heme Mydriasis	Retinal hemorrhages	Oculogyric crisis	—	Urticaria

Phenothiazines

Acetophenazine Butaperazine Carphenazine Chlorpromazine Ethopropazine (Profenamine) Fluphenazine Mesoridazine Methdilazine Methotrimeprazine (Levomepromazine) Perphenazine Piperacetazine Prochlorperazine Promazine Promethazine Propiomazine	↓ Vision Night blindness Color vision defect Red-green defect "Yellow" or "brown" vision Colored halos Visual hallucinations Myopia Photophobia Diplopia	Lids or cj.: ↑ lacrimation, allergy, edema, hyperpigmentation, photosensitivity, angioneurotic edema, blepharospasm, subcj. heme Corneal: pigment deposits, edema, SPK Mydriasis Miosis ↓ Pupil light reflex	Retinal hemorrhages, edema, RPE changes Optic atrophy Papilledema Abnormal ERG or EOG	Oculogyric crisis Myasthenic neuromuscular block: EOM paralysis, ptosis Jerky pursuit	Toxic amblyopia Scotomas: annular, central, paracentral VF constriction Nystagmus	Lupoid syndrome Erythema multiforme Exfoliative dermatitis Horner's syndrome ? Teratogenesis

Table 18-6. (continued)

Generic drug name	Visual symptoms	Anterior segment	Posterior segment	Extraocular muscles, orbit	Visual fields, CNS	Other
Thiethylperazine Thioridazine Trifluoperazine Trifluopromazine Trimeprazine (NB, Not all ocular side effects reported for each drug)		Nuclear stellate cataracts				
Lithium salts						
Lithium carbonate Lithium citrate	↓ Vision Photophobia Visual hallucinations Diplopia	Lids or cj.: inflammation, edema, ? lash or brow loss, subcj. heme, ↑ lacrimation, burning POA ? Cataracts	Retinal hemorrhages Abnormal EOG or VER Papilledema	Oculogyric crisis ↓ Spontaneous movements Lateral conjugate deviations Jerky pursuit Exophthalmos Myasthenic neuromuscular block: EOM paralysis	Nystagmus: horizontal or vertical Scotomas Pseudotumor cerebri	? Teratogenesis

Thioxanthenes

Chlorprothixine Thiothixine	↓ Vision Diplopia	Lids or cj.: allergy, photo-sensitivity, angioneurotic edema, subcj. heme Corneal fine particulate deposits SPK Lens fine particulate deposits Stellate cataract Miosis Mydriasis POA	Retinal hemorrhages RPE changes	Oculogyric crisis	—	Urticaria Lupoid syndrome Exfoliative dermatitis

Table 18-7. Central nervous system agents: Psychedelic drugs

Generic drug name	Visual symptoms	Anterior segment	Posterior segment	Extraocular muscles, orbit	Visual fields, CNS	Other
Cannabinols						
Dronabinol (Tetrahydrocannabinol, THC) Hashish Marihuana	↓ Vision Visual hallucinations Color vision defect or ↑ color perception "Yellow" or "violet" vision Colored flashing lights ↓ Dark adaptation Diplopia Photophobia	Lids or cj.: hyperemia, conjunctivitis, burning, blepharospasm, ↓ lacrimation ↓ IOP POA Miosis Anisocoria	—	? Abnormal conjugate deviations ↓ Oculomotor coordination	Nystagmus	? Teratogenesis
Cyclohexylamines						
Phencyclidine	↓ Vision Visual hallucinations Diplopia	Ptosis ↓ Corneal reflex ↑ IOP Miosis ↓ Pupil light reflex	—	Nystagmus: vertical, rotary, or horizontal Jerky pursuit Oculogyric crisis	—	—

Indolealkylamines

LSD Lysergide Mescaline Psilocybin	Visual hallucinations Macro- or micropsia Color vision defect ↑ Color perception Prolonged afterimages Phosphene stimulation Colored flashing lights → Vision → Dark adaptation	Mydriasis Anisocoria ↓ or absent pupil light reflex POA	Abnormal ERG or VEP	—	? Teratogenesis: cataract, iris coloboma, microphthalmos, corneal opacities, PHPV, retinal dysplasia, optic disc hypoplasia or coloboma, anophthalmia

Table 18-8. Central nervous system agents: Sedatives and hypnotics

Generic drug name	Visual symptoms	Anterior segment	Posterior segment	Extraocular muscles, orbit	Visual fields, CNS	Other
Alcohols						
Chloral hydrate	↓ Vision Visual hallucinations (often minification)	Lids or cj.: ↑ lacrimation, ptosis, allergy, hyperemia, edema, irritation Mydriasis (toxic) Miosis	? Optic neuritis	↓ Convergence EOM paralysis Jerky pursuit (toxic)	Nystagmus ? Toxic amblyopia	—
Ethanol Ethyl alcohol Acute intoxication	↓ Vision Diplopia ↓ Dark adaptation ↑ Glare recovery ↓ Depth perception Blue-yellow or red-green color defect "Blue" vision Visual hallucinations	Ptosis Mydriasis ↓ Pupil light reflex Anisocoria Miosis (coma) ↓ IOP POA	Abnormal ERG or VEP or flicker fusion	EOM paralysis Eso- or exophoria Convergent strabismus ↓ Convergence Jerky pursuit ↓ Spontaneous movements → Oculomotor coordination ↓ OKN Peripheral gaze nystagmus	Nystagmus Toxic amblyopia VF constriction	—

| Chronic intoxication | ↓Vision
Red-green color defect
Visual hallucinations
Oscillopsia | ↑Lacrimation
Corneal deposits (arcus)
Miosis
↓ or absent pupil light reflex
↓IOP | Optic neuritis | Paralysis
Jerky pursuit
Downbeat nystagmus | Central scotomas
Toxic amblyopia | Teratogenesis: narrow palpebral fissure, hypertelorism, microphthalmos hypertelorism, epicanthus, ptosis, strabismus, retinal vascular tortuosity, pseudopapilledema, myopia
May aggravate: Wernicke's encephalopathy
Cerebellar degeneration
Purtcher's retinopathy
? Retards ocular arteriosclerosis and recurrent optic neuritis |

Table 18-8. (continued)

Generic drug name	Visual symptoms	Anterior segment	Posterior segment	Extraocular muscles, orbit	Visual fields, CNS	Other
Ethchlorvynol	↓ Vision Diplopia Visual hallucinations Color vision defect "Yellow" vision	POA Anisocoria	Optic neuritis	—	Nystagmus—lateral gaze or horizontal Toxic amblyopia VF constriction Central or cecocentral scotomas	—
Mythylpentynol	Diplopia Visual hallucinations	Ptosis Cj. edema Mydriasis	—	—	Nystagmus	—
Barbiturates Allobarbital Amobarbital Aprobarbital Barbital Butabarbital Butalbital Butallylonal Cyclobarbital	↓ Vision Diplopia Oscillopsia Color vision defect "Yellow" or "green" vision Color vision	Lids or cj.: ptosis, blepharoclonus, allergy, inflammation, edema, KC sicca, photosensitivity, angioneurotic	Retinal hemorrhages Retinal vasoconstriction Retrobulbar or optic neuritis Papilledema Optic atrophy	↓ Convergence EOM paresis Jerky pursuit Random movements Vertical gaze palsy Nystagmus: jerk,	Toxic amblyopia Scotomas VF constriction ? Cortical blindness (thiopental)	Urticaria Lupoid syndrome Erythema multiforme Exfoliative dermatitis Lyell's syndrome

Generic Name	Subjective	Objective	Fundus / Electrophysiology	Ocular motility	Visual field	Other / Conditions
Hexethal Hexobarbital Mephobarbital Metharbital Methitural Methohexital Pentobarbital Phenobarbital Primidone Probarbital Secobarbital Talbutal Thiamylal Thiopental	defect Visual hallucinations	edema, subconj. heme Mydriasis Miosis (coma) ↓ Pupil light reflex Hippus ↓ IOP POA (primidone)	Abnormal ERG, VEP, or flicker fusion	gaze evoked, vertical, or horizontal ↓ OKN Nystagmus: latent, positional, voluntary, or congenital		? Teratogenesis (primidone): optic atrophy, ptosis, hypertelorism, epicanthus, strabismus
Bromides	↓ Vision Color vision defects Visual hallucinations (often minification) Diplopia Photophobia Oscillopsia	Lids or cj.: allergy, erythema, blepharoconjunctivitis ↓ Corneal reflex Mydriasis Miosis ↓ Pupil light reflex Anisocoria POA	? Papilledema ? Optic atrophy	↓ Convergence ↓ Spontaneous movements Jerky pursuit	Nystagmus Scotomas VF constriction	Erythema multiforme

Table 18-8. (continued)

Generic drug name	Visual symptoms	Anterior segment	Posterior segment	Extraocular muscles, orbit	Visual fields, CNS	Other
Brominated monouridines						
Bromisovalum (Bromisoval) Carbromal	↓ Vision Diplopia	Ptosis (carbromal) Mydriasis Miosis ↓ Pupil light reflex Anisocoria ? Cataracts (carbromal)	Retinal edema (carbromal) Optic atrophy Retrobulbar or optic neuritis	↓ Convergence (bromisovalum)	Nystagmus: horizontal or vertical Central scotomas VF constriction	Erythema multiforme
Piperidines						
Glutethimide Methyprylon	↓ Vision Diplopia Visual hallucinations	Lids or cj.: allergy, subconj. heme ↓ Corneal reflex POA Mydriasis Miosis (methylprylon) ↓ or absent pupil light reflex	Retinal hemorrhages Papilledema	—	—	Urticaria Purpura Exfoliative dermatitis

Polyethers

Paraldehyde	↓Vision Visual hallucinations	↓Corneal reflex Mydriasis (toxic) Miosis	—	—	? Hemianopia	—

Quinazolines

Methaqualone	↓Vision Diplopia Color vision defect "Yellow" vision Visual hallucinations	↑Lacrimation Subcj. heme Mydriasis (toxic) ↓Pupil light reflex ? POA	Retinal hemorrhages ? Papilledema	—	—	Urticaria Purpura Erythema multiforme

19

Dermatologic Agents

Table 19-1. Dermatologic agents: Germicides

Generic drug name	Visual symptoms	Anterior segment	Posterior segment	Extraocular muscles, orbit	Visual fields, CNS	Other
Chlorinated biphenols						
Hexachlorophene (Systemic absorption across skin)	Diplopia	Lids or cj.: erythema, photosensitivity Mydriasis	Retinal hemorrhages Papilledema	EOM paresis	Pseudotumor cerebri	—
(Accidental ingestion)	↓ Vision	Miosis Absent pupil light reflex	Optic atrophy	—	Toxic amblyopia	? Teratogenesis

Table 19-2. Dermatologic agents: Psoriasis therapy, cystic acne

Generic drug name	Visual symptoms	Anterior segment	Posterior segment	Extraocular muscles, orbit	Visual fields, CNS	Other
Chrysophanic acid derivatives						
Chrysarobin (Systemic absorption from skin)	—	Nonspecific ocular irritation Lids or cj.: hyperemia, brown-violet discoloration, keratoconjunctivitis SPK Gray corneal opacities	—	—	—	—

Retinoids

Etretinate Isotretinoin					
↓Vision Myopia ↓Dark adaptation	Lids or cj.: ↓lacrimation, erythema, blepharoconjunctivitis, edema, hyperpigmentation, photosensitivity, ? brow or lash loss ↓Contact lens tolerance Corneal: opacities, keratitis, ulcers ↓Cataracts	Papilledema Optic neuritis Abnormal ERG	—	Pseudotumor cerebri	Urticaria Teratogenesis: microphthalmia, optic nerve hypoplasia, hypertelorism, cortical blindness

Table 19-3. Dermatologic agents: Vitiligo therapy

Generic drug name	Visual symptoms	Anterior segment	Posterior segment	Extraocular muscles, orbit	Visual fields, CNS	Other
Psoralen derivatives						
Methoxsalen Trioxsalen (Systemic absorption across skin)	Photophobia	Lids or cj.: ↓ lacrimation, erythema, hyperpigmentation, photosensitivity Keratitis Pigmentary glaucoma ? Cataracts	—	—	Scotomas: central	↑ Incidence skin cancer

20

Diuretics and Osmotics

Table 20-1. Diuretics and osmotics: Diuretics

Generic drug name	Visual symptoms	Anterior segment	Posterior segment	Extraocular muscles, orbit	Visual fields, CNS	Other
Aldosterone antagonists						
Spironolactone	↓ Vision Myopia	Lids or cj.: erythema ↓ IOP	—	—	—	Lupoid syndrome
Phenoxyacetic acid derivatives						
Ethacrynic acid	↓ Vision	Subcj. heme	Retinal hemorrhages	—	Nystagmus	—
Sulfonamides						
Furosemide	↓ Vision "Yellow" vision Visual hallucinations ? Photophobia	Lids or cj.: allergy, photosensitivity, subcj. heme ? POA ↓ IOP ↓ Contact lens tolerance	Retinal hemorrhages	—	—	Urticaria Purpura Lupoid syndrome Erythema multiforme Exfoliative dermatitis Pemphigoid

Thiazides

Bendroflumethiazide Benzthiazide Chlorothiazide Chlorthalidone Cyclothiazide Hydrochlorothiazide Hydroflumethiazide Indapamide Methyclothiazide Metolazone Polythiazide Quinethazone Trichlormethiazide	↓ Vision Myopia "Yellow" vision "Yellow" spots on white background Visual hallucinations	Lids or cj.: ↓ lacrimation, allergy, conjunctivitis, photosensitivity, subcj. heme → IOP POA	Retinal hemorrhages	—	? Cortical blindness	Urticaria Purpura Lupoid syndrome Erythema multiforme Lyell's syndrome

Table 20-2. Diuretics and osmotics: Osmotic agents*

Generic drug name	Visual symptoms	Anterior segment	Posterior segment	Extraocular muscles, orbit	Visual fields, CNS	Other
Hyperosmotics						
Glycerin (Glycerol)	↓ Vision Visual hallucinations	Subcj. heme ↓ IOP	Retinal hemorrhages Retinal tear ? Expulsive hemorrhage	—	—	—
Isosorbide Mannitol	↓ Vision Visual hallucinations	Lids or cj.; edema, ? blepharitis, subcj. heme ↓ IOP	Retinal hemorrhages ? Expulsive hemorrhage	—	—	Urticaria
Urea	↓ Vision Visual hallucinations	↓ IOP Rebound glaucoma ↓ Tear lysozymes	Retinal hemorrhages Retinal tear ? Expulsive hemorrhage	—	? Nystagmus	—

* See chapter on Antiglaucoma Drugs.

21

Gastrointestinal Agents

Table 21-1. Gastrointestinal agents: Antacids

Generic drug name	Visual symptoms	Anterior segment	Posterior segment	Extraocular muscles, orbit	Visual fields, CNS	Other
Bismuth salts						
Bismuth oxychloride	? ↓ Vision (toxic) Visual hallucinations (toxic)	Lids or cj.: ? lash or brow loss, ? blue discoloration, subcj. heme Corneal deposits	—	—	—	Exfoliative dermatitis Lyell's syndrome
Bismuth sodium tartrate						
Bismuth sodium thioglycollate						
Bismuth subcarbonate						
Bismuth subsalicylate						

Histamine (H₂) blockers

Cimetidine	↓ Vision Visual hallucinations Photophobia ? "Yellow" or "pink" vision ? Myopia	Lids or cj.: ? lash or brow loss, hyperemia, erythema, conjunctivitis, subcj. heme Mydriasis (toxic) ↓ Pupil light reflex	Retinal hemorrhages	—	—	Urticaria Purpura Exfoliative dermatitis
Ranitidine	↓ Vision Visual hallucinations	Lids or cj.: ? lash or brow loss, erythema, conjunctivitis, angioneurotic edema, subcj. heme ? Mydriasis	Retinal hemorrhages	—	—	Urticaria

Table 21-2. Gastrointestinal agents: Antiemetics

Generic drug name	Visual symptoms	Anterior segment	Posterior segment	Extraocular muscles, orbit	Visual fields, CNS	Other
Butyrophenones						
Droperidol	See Antipsychotic Agents					
Orthopramides						
Metoclopramide	↓ Vision Color vision defect Photophobia Diplopia	Lids or cj.: edema, angioneurotic edema Mydriasis	—	Oculogyric crisis EOM paralysis Strabismus	Nystagmus	Urticaria
Piperazine antihistamines						
Chlorcyclizine Cyclizine Meclizine (Meclozine)	↓ Vision Diplopia Visual hallucinations	KC sicca aggravation ↓ Contact lens tolerance Mydriasis ↓ Pupil light reflex	—	—	—	? Teratogenesis: cataracts, tapetoretinal degeneration

Table 21-3. Gastrointestinal agents: Antihyperglycemics

Generic drug name	Visual symptoms	Anterior segment	Posterior segment	Extraocular muscles, orbit	Visual fields, CNS	Other
Insulin*	↓ Vision Diplopia	Lids or cj.: allergy, erythema, blepharoconjunctivitis, angioneurotic edema, ↓ tear lysozymes Mydriasis Absent pupil light reflex ↑ or ↓ IOP	? Immunogenic retinopathy	EOM paresis Strabismus	Nystagmus	Urticaria

Table 21-3. (continued)

Generic drug name	Visual symptoms	Anterior segment	Posterior segment	Extraocular muscles, orbit	Visual fields, CNS	Other
Sulfonylureas*						
Acetohexamide Chlorpropamide Glyburide Tolazamide Tolbutamide	↓ Vision Diplopia Photophobia Color vision defect Red-green defect ? Hypermetropia (tolbutamide)	Lids or cj.: ? lash or brow loss, allergy, hyperemia, conjunctivitis, edema	Retinal hemorrhages Retrobulbar or optic neuritis	EOM paresis	Scotomas—central or cecocentral (chlorpropamide, tolbutamide)	Purpura Lupoid syndrome (tolazamide) Erythema multiforme Exfoliative dermatitis May aggravate Wernicke's syndrome

* Side effect caused by antihyperglycemics are often similar to those of diabetes mellitus itself. Drug effects, however, are generally reversible and limited to the duration of drug-induced hypoglycemia.

Table 21-4. Gastrointestinal agents: Antispasmodics

Generic drug name	Visual symptoms	Anterior segment	Posterior segment	Extraocular muscles, orbit	Visual fields, CNS	Other
Anticholinergics*						
Atropine SO₄ Belladonna Homatropine	↓ Vision Photophobia Micropsia Visual hallucinations Color vision defect "Red" vision	↓ Lacrimation Absent pupil light reflex (toxic) POA Mydriasis	—	—	—	Erythema multiforme
Quaternary ammonium compounds						
Adiphenine Ambutonium Anisotropine Clidinium Diphemanil Glycopyrrolate Hexocyclium Isopropamide Mepenzolate Methantheline Methixene	↓ Vision Photophobia Diplopia Color vision defect (piperidolate) Colored flashing lights (propantheline) Flashing lights (piperidolate)	Lids or cj.: allergy, ? lash or brow loss (glycopyrrolate) POA Mydriasis	—	—	—	—

Table 21-4. (continued)

Generic drug name	Visual symptoms	Anterior segment	Posterior segment	Extraocular muscles, orbit	Visual fields, CNS	Other
Methyl atropine nitrate Oxyphenonium Pipenzolate Piperidolate Propantheline Tridihexethyl	See Quaternary ammonium compounds plus					
Tertiary amines						
Dicyclomine Oxyphency- clamine			—	—	—	? Teratogenesis (dicyclomine)

* See chapter on Mydriatics and Cycloplegics.

Table 21-5. Gastrointestinal agents: Stimulants (gastrointestinal and genitourinary)

Generic drug name	Visual symptoms	Anterior segment	Posterior segment	Extraocular muscles, orbit	Visual fields, CNS	Other
Quaternary ammonium parasympathomimetics						
Bethanechol		↓Lacrimation Cj. hyperemia Burning sensation POA Miosis	—	—	Scotomas: central	↑Incidence skin cancer
Carbachol*		POA Miosis	—	—	—	—

* See chapter on Antiglaucoma Drugs.

22

Heavy Metal Chelators

Table 22-1. Heavy metal chelators

Generic drug name	Visual symptoms	Anterior segment	Posterior segment	Extraocular muscles, orbit	Visual fields, CNS	Other
Amino acid derivatives						
Penicillamine	Myopia Hypermetropia Diplopia Photophobia Color vision defect Red-green color vision defect	Lids or cj.: ↑ lacrimation, edema, hyperemia, blepharoconjunctivitis, yellowing and wrinkling, chalazia, ? lash or brow loss ? Corneal punctate keratitis or delayed wound healing ? Cataracts	Retinal: hemorrhage, RPE disturbance, serous detachment Papilledema Retrobulbar or optic neuritis	Myasthenic neuromuscular block: ptosis, EOM paralysis ↓ Convergence	VF constriction Scotomas—cecocentral	Urticaria Lupoid syndrome Lyell's syndrome Pemphigoid
Dithiol derivatives						
Dimercaprol (BAL)	—	Lids or cj.: lacrimation, burning sensation,	—	—	—	—

Table 22-1. (continued)

Generic drug name	Visual symptoms	Anterior segment	Posterior segment	Extraocular muscles, orbit	Visual fields, CNS	Other
		edema, allergy, blepharospasm, conjunctivitis, subcj. heme				
Iron-free ligands						
Deferoxamine	↓ Vision Photophobia Color vision defect Red-green color vision defect ↓ Dark adaptation	Lids or cj.: allergy, erythema, ? subcj. heme ? Cataracts	Retinal hemorrhages Retinal or macular: degeneration, RPE disturbances, ERG, EOG, or VEP abnormalities Optic atrophy Retrobulbar or optic neuritis	—	VF constriction Scotomas: central or cecocentral	Urticaria

Hematologic Agents

Table 23-1. Hematologic agents: Anticoagulants

Generic drug name	Visual symptoms	Anterior segment	Posterior segment	Extraocular muscles, orbit	Visual fields, CNS	Other
Coumarin derivatives						
Dicumarol Ethyl biscoumacetate Phenprocouman Warfarin	↓ Vision (dicumarol, warfarin) Color vision defect	Lids or cj.: allergy, conjunctivitis, ? brow or lash loss, ↑ necrosis, ↑ lacrimation (dicumarol, warfarin), subcj. heme Hyphema	Retinal hemorrhages	—	—	Urticaria Teratogenesis: optic atrophy, cataracts, microphthalmia

Glycosaminoglycans

Heparin	↓ Vision	Lids or cj.: allergy, ↑ lacrimation, conjunctivitis, angioneurotic edema, necrosis, ? lash or brow loss, subcj. heme Hyphema	Retinal hemorrhages	—	—	Urticaria Lyell's syndrome

Indandione derivatives

Anisindione Diphenadione Phenindione	↓ Vision Color vision defect (phenindione)	Lids or cj.: ? lash or brow loss, allergy, subcj. heme, conjunctivitis, necrosis POA	Retinal hemorrhages	—	—	Urticaria Exfoliative dermatitis

Table 23-2. Hematologic agents: Plasma expanders

Generic drug name	Visual symptoms	Anterior segment	Posterior segment	Extraocular muscles, orbit	Visual fields, CNS	Other
Glucose polymers						
Dextran	Photophobia	Lids or cj.: erythema, conjunctivitis, angioneurotic edema, ↑ lacrimation, edema, burning sensation Keratitis	—	—	—	Urticaria

24

Hormonal Agents

Table 24-1. Hormonal agents: Adrenal steroids

Generic drug name	Visual symptoms	Anterior segment	Posterior segment	Extraocular muscles, orbit	Visual fields, CNS	Other
Androgens						
Danozol	↓ Vision Diplopia	Lids or cj.: erythema, edema, photosensitivity, ? lash or brow loss ? Cataracts	Papilledema	EOM paresis	Pseudotumor cerebri VF defects	Urticaria Purpura Erythema multiforme
Corticosteroids* (Glucocorticoids and Mineralocorticoids)						
Adrenal cortex injection Aldosterone Betamethasone Cortisone Desoxycorticosterone Dexamethasone	↓ Vision Myopia Diplopia Color vision defects Visual hallucinations	Lids or cj.: hyperemia, edema, angioneurotic edema, ↓ tear lysozyme, subcj. heme ↑ IOP	Retinal hemorrhages Retinal edema Abnormal ERG or VEP Retinal emboli (injection) Papilledema	Exophthalmos Myasthenic neuromuscular block: ptosis, EOM paralysis	Toxic amblyopia Pseudotumor cerebri VF: scotomas, constriction, enlarged blind spot, glaucoma field defect	Lyell's syndrome ? Teratogenesis: cataracts ↓ Resistance to infection

Fludrocortisone Fluprednisolone Hydrocortisone Meprednisone Methylprednisolone Paramethasone Prednisolone Prednisone Triamcinolone	PSC cataracts (some reversible) Delayed corneal wound healing Mydriasis Ciliary body epithelial microcysts

* See chapter on Corticosteroids for side effects of local injection or topical application.

Table 24-2. Hormonal agents: Antithyroid drugs

Generic drug name	Visual symptoms	Anterior segment	Posterior segment	Extraocular muscles, orbit	Visual fields, CNS	Other
Iodine derivatives						
Iodide or iodine solutions or compounds Radioactive iodides (Oral)	↓ Vision	Lids or cj.: allergy, ↑ lacrimation, pain, burning, hyperemia, conjunctivitis, edema, angioneurotic edema, nodules POA SPK Hypopyon Hemorrhagic iritis	Vitreous floaters	Exophthalmos	—	Urticaria Exfoliative dermatitis Teratogenesis (radioactive iodides)

(Intravenous)	As per oral administration plus: Color vision defects "Green" vision Visual hallucinations	Mydriasis	Retinal degeneration Retinal or macular edema Retinal vasoconstriction Retrobulbar neuritis Optic atrophy	—	VF: scotomas, constriction, hemianopia Toxic amblyopia	—
Thioamides						
Methimazole (thiamazole) Methylthiouracil Propylthiouracil	—	Lids or cj.: allergy, conjunctivitis, depigmentation, ? lash or brow loss, ↓ lacrimation (methylthiouracil), subcj. heme Keratitis	Retinal hemorrhages	Exophthalmos	Nystagmus (methylthiouracil)	Urticaria Lupoid syndrome Exfoliative dermatitis

Table 24-3. Hormonal agents: Oral contraceptives

Generic drug name	Visual symptoms	Anterior segment	Posterior segment	Extraocular muscles, orbit	Visual fields, CNS	Other
Ovarian steroids						
Estrogen-progesterone combinations	↓ Vision Diplopia Myopia Red-green or yellow-blue color vision defect "Blue" vision Colored halos around lights (often blue)	Lids or cj.: ptosis allergy, edema, hyperpigmentation, photosensitivity, angioneurotic edema, ? lash or brow loss ↓ Contact lens tolerance ? KC sicca Uveitis Mydriasis Anisocoria Iridocyclitis ? Cataracts	Retinal vascular: occlusion, thrombosis, hemorrhage, retinal or macular edema, vasospasm Optic or retrobulbar neuritis Papilledema	EOM paralysis	VF constriction Scotomas—central or paracentral Quadrantopia or hemianopia ↑ Blind spot Pseudotumor cerebri Nystagmus	Urticaria Lupoid syndrome Erythema multiforme ? Aggravation of retinitis pigmentosa

Table 24-4. Hormonal agents: Ovulatory drugs

Generic drug name	Visual symptoms	Anterior segment	Posterior segment	Extraocular muscles, orbit	Visual fields, CNS	Other
Nonsteroidal antiestrogens						
Clomiphene (Clomifene)	↓ Vision Flashing lights Scintillating scotomas Wave or glare distortion of images Colored lights (often silver) Phosgene stimulation Prolonged afterimage Photophobia Diplopia	Lids or cj.: allergy, ? brow or lash loss ↓ Contact lens tolerance ?PSC cataracts	? Posterior vitreous detachment ? Retinal vasospasm ? Optic neuritis	—	VF constriction Scotomas	Urticaria ? Teratogenesis: retinal aplasia
Tamoxifen	See Antineoplastic Agents					

Table 24-5. Hormonal agents: Thyroid replacement

Generic drug name	Visual symptoms	Anterior segment	Posterior segment	Extraocular muscles, orbit	Visual fields, CNS	Other
Thyroid derivatives						
Dextrothyroxine Levothyroxine Liothyronine Liotrix Thyroglobulin Thyroid	↓ Vision Photophobia Visual hallucinations	Lids or cj.: edema, hyperemia, blepharospasm, ? lash or brow loss (dextrothyroxine) ? Cataracts (dextrothyroxine)	Papilledema ? Optic neuritis ? Optic atrophy	Myasthenic neuromuscular block: ptosis, EOM paralysis; exophthalmos	Pseudotumor cerebri VF constriction Scotomas—central Hemianopia	

25

Immunosuppressants

Table 25-1. Immunosuppressants*

Generic drug name	Visual symptoms	Anterior segment	Posterior segment	Extraocular muscles, orbit	Visual fields, CNS	Other
Cyclic peptides						
Cyclosporine (Cyclopsorine A)	↓ Vision Visual hallucinations	Lids or cj.: erythema, conjunctivitis, subcj. heme, hypertrichosis	Retinal hemorrhages	—	Cortical blindness	Urticaria
Mercaptopurine derivatives						
Azathioprine	—	Lids or cj.: ? lash or brow loss, subcj. heme Delayed corneal wound healing	Retinal hemorrhages RPE disturbances	—	—	? Teratogenesis Aggravation of herpes infections ↓ Resistance to infection

* See chapter on Immunosuppressive Agents.

Neuromuscular Agents

Table 26-1. Neuromuscular agents: Muscle relaxants and antiparkinsonian drugs

Generic drug name	Visual symptoms	Anterior segment	Posterior segment	Extraocular muscles, orbit	Visual fields, CNS	Other
Aliphatic polyalcohols						
Mephenesin Methocarbamol	↓ Vision Diplopia	Lids or cj.: ptosis (mephenesin), ciliary hyperemia (mephenesin), erythema, and/or conjunctivitis (methocarbamol) ↓ IOP	—	EOM paresis (mephenesin)	Nystagmus: rotary, horizontal, or vertical	Urticaria
Anticholinergics						
Benztropine Biperiden Chlorphenoxamine Cycrimine Procyclidine Trihexyphenidyl	↓ Vision Visual hallucinations	POA Mydriasis ↓ Pupil light reflex	? RPE disturbance	—	—	? Teratogenesis
Caramiphen	—	Mydriasis POA	—	Retrobulbar neuritis	Scotomas	—

Antihistamines

Orphenadrine	↓Vision Diplopia Visual hallucinations	Subcj. heme? ↓Contact lens tolerance Aggravation KC sicca POA Mydriasis Absent pupil light reflex	Retinal hemorrhages	—	—	—
β-Adrenergic blockers						
Levodopa	↓Vision Diplopia Visual hallucinations	Lids or cj.: allergy, edema, ? lash or brow loss, subcj. heme, blepharoclonus, blepharospasm, ↑ palpebral fissure Mydriasis Miosis	Retinal hemorrhages ? Papilledema	EOM paralysis Oculogyric crisis	? Pseudotumor cerebri	Horner's syndrome Lupoid syndrome ? Malignant melanoma stimulant
Dantrolene	↓Vision Diplopia Visual hallucinations	Lids or cj.: ↑ lacrimation, photosensitivity	—	—	—	Urticaria

Table 26-1. (continued)

Generic drug name	Visual symptoms	Anterior segment	Posterior segment	Extraocular muscles, orbit	Visual fields, CNS	Other
Gamma aminobutyric acids (GABA)						
Baclofen	↓ Vision Diplopia Visual hallucinations	Mydriasis Miosis ↓ Pupil light reflex POA	—	Strabismus	Nystagmus	—
Tricyclic amines						
Amantadine	↓ Vision Diplopia Visual hallucinations	Lids or cj.: photosensitivity, ? brow or lash loss Corneal edema Punctate keratitis Mydriasis	—	Oculogyric crisis	—	Purpura Eczema

Table 26-2. Neuromuscular agents: Myasthenia gravis and antidote drugs

Generic drug name	Visual symptoms	Anterior segment	Posterior segment	Extraocular muscles, orbit	Visual fields, CNS	Other
Anticholinesterases						
Ambenonium Edrophonium Pyridostigmine	↓ Vision Diplopia	Lids or cj.: ↑ lacrimation, blepharoclonus (toxic), ? brow or lash loss (pyridostigmine) Miosis	—	Paradoxic response: ptotic eye up, nonptotic eye down	—	—
Cholinesterase reactivator*						
Pralidoxime	↓ Vision Diplopia	POA	—	—	—	—

* Also used in poisoning by organophosphate pesticides or other anticholinesterases.

27

Radiographic Contrast Agents

Table 27-1. Radiographic contrast agents

Generic drug name	Visual symptoms	Anterior segment	Posterior segment	Extraocular muscles, orbit	Visual fields, CNS	Other
Iodide derivatives						
Diatrizoate meglumine or sodium	↓ Vision Photophobia	Lids or cj.: ↑ lacrimation, pain, burning sensation, allergy, hyperemia, erythema, follicular conjunctivitis, edema, angioneurotic edema Corneal infiltrates	Retinal hemorrhages, thrombosis	—	Hemianopia Scotomas—paracentral	Urticaria
Iodipamide meglumine	—	Lids or cj.: allergy, erythema, edema, angioneurotic edema Corneal infiltrates	—	—	—	Urticaria

Table 27-1. (continued)

Generic drug name	Visual symptoms	Anterior segment	Posterior segment	Extraocular muscles, orbit	Visual fields, CNS	Other
Iophendylate	↓ Vision Abnormal visual sensations Flickering lights	Ocular pain	—	EOM paresis or paralysis	Nystagmus	Urticaria
Iothalamate meglumine or sodium Iothalamic acid	↓ Vision Photophobia Diplopia	Lids or cj.: ↑ lacrimation, allergy, erythema, edema, conjunctivitis, angioneurotic edema	Retinal or macular: edema, wedge-shaped lesions	Myasthenic neuromuscular block: ptosis, EOM paralysis Exotropia	Scotomas—paracentral	Urticaria
Metrizamide	↓ Vision Visual hallucinations Diplopia Color vision defect Red-green color vision defect Photophobia	Lids or cj.: allergy, edema, angioneurotic edema, subcj. heme	Retinal hemorrhages	EOM paresis or paralysis Strabismus	Nystagmus: horizontal, vertical, downbeat Scotomas: central Cortical blindness	Urticaria

28

Solvents

Table 28-1. Solvents

Generic drug name	Visual symptoms	Anterior segment	Posterior segment	Extraocular muscles, orbit	Visual fields, CNS	Other
Alcohols*						
Methanol (methyl alcohol) (Absorbed across skin or accidental ingestion)	↓Vision Photophobia Red-green or blue-yellow color vision defect Diplopia	—	Retinal: edema, hemorrhages, engorgement of vessels Retrobulbar neuritis Optic atrophy ? Abnormal ERG Papilledema	Ptosis EOM paresis	Nystagmus: horizontal VF constriction Scotomas: central, cecocentral, paracentral Toxic amblyopia	Urticaria
Sulfas						
Dimethylsulfoxide (DMSO) (Systemic absorption across skin)	Photophobia Color vision defect	Lids or cj.: allergy, erythema, subcj. heme	Retinal hemorrhages	—	—	Urticaria Potentiates adverse effects of agents dissolved in it

* See Ethanol in Table 18-8, Sedatives and Hypnotics.

Vaccines

Table 29-1. Vaccines

Generic drug name	Visual symptoms	Anterior segment	Posterior segment	Extraocular muscles, orbit	Visual fields, CNS	Other
BCG antitubercular vaccine						
	↓ Vision	Lids or cj.: erythema, subcj. heme Iritis ? Cataracts	Retinal hemorrhages	—	Nystagmus	Vitiligo Urticaria Purpura Lupoid syndrome Erythema multiforme Eczema Urticaria Eczema (DT)
Diphtheria (D) toxoid adsorbed **Diphtheria & tetanus (DT) toxoids adsorbed** **Diphtheria & tetanus & pertussis (DPT) toxoids adsorbed**						
	↓ Vision	Lids or cj.: allergy, erythema, conjunctivitis (DPT), angioneurotic edema, subcj. heme (DPT)	Retinal hemorrhages (DPT) Papilledema (DPT) Optic neuritis	Myasthenic neuromuscular block: EOM paresis or paralysis Ptosis (DPT)	VF defect (DT) Pseudotumor cerebri (DPT)	—

Influenza virus vaccine

↓ Vision Color vision defect Red-green color vision defect	Lids or cj.: pain, allergy, erythema, blepharoconjunctivitis, subcj. heme	Iritis Mydriasis (D) ↓ Pupil light reflex (D) POA	Retinal hemorrhages Papilledema Optic neuritis Optic atrophy Posterior multifocal placoid pigment epitheliopathy	EOM paresis or paralysis —	? Nystagmus VF constriction Scotomas: central or paracentral	Horner's syndrome Urticaria Purpura ? Erythema multiforme

Measles and/or mumps and/or rubella live vaccine

↓ Vision	Lids or cj.: pain, allergy, hyperemia, erythema, conjunctivitis, angioneurotic edema, subcj. heme Mydriasis ? Iritis (rubella) ? POA (rubella)		Retinal hemorrhages Retinitis Papilledema Optic neuritis	Myasthenic neuromuscular block: ptosis (measles) EOM paresis or paralysis Strabismus	Scotomas: ceco-central (rubella)	Urticaria Purpura Eczema ? Teratogenesis

Table 29-1. (continued)

Generic drug name	Visual symptoms	Anterior segment	Posterior segment	Extraocular muscles, orbit	Visual fields, CNS	Other
Poliovirus vaccine						
	↓ Vision	Lids or cj.: edema, erythema, angioneurotic edema, subcj. heme	? Optic neuritis	Exophthalmos	—	Urticaria Lyell's syndrome
Rabies immune globulin, rabies vaccine						
	↓ Vision Diplopia Photophobia	Lids or cj.: allergy, erythema, angioneurotic edema	Optic neuritis	—	Scotomas: cecocentral	Urticaria
Smallpox vaccine						
	↓ Vision	Lids or cj.: erythema, blepharoconjunctivitis, edema, photosensitivity	Optic neuritis	—	—	Urticaria Purpura Erythema multiforme Lyell's syndrome Eczema

Tetanus immune globulin, tetanus toxoid

Visual hallucinations ? Photophobia	Cornea: SPK, ulcers Iritis Lids or cj.: allergy, erythema, conjunctivitis, angioneurotic edema ↓ Pupil light reflex	? Optic neuritis	—	Nystagmus: horizontal	Urticaria Purpura

30

Vitamins

Table 30-1. Vitamins

Generic drug name	Visual symptoms	Anterior segment	Posterior segment	Extraocular muscles, orbit	Visual fields, CNS	Other
Vitamin A						
Retinol	Diplopia "Yellow" vision Red dyschromatopsia	Lids or cj.: yellow or orange discoloration, conjunctivitis, lash or brow loss, subcj. heme, drug in tears ? Calcium deposits in cj., cornea, sclera Miosis ↓ IOP	Retinal hemorrhages Optic atrophy Papilledema	Exophthalmos Strabismus EOM paresis	Nystagmus Scotomas ↑ Blind spot Pseudotumor cerebri	? Teratogenesis

Table 30-1. (continued)

Generic drug name	Visual symptoms	Anterior segment	Posterior segment	Extraocular muscles, orbit	Visual fields, CNS	Other
Vitamin D*						
Calcitriol Cholecalciferol (Vitamin D$_3$) Ergocalciferol (Vitamin D$_2$)	Diplopia Visual hallucinations	Lids or cj.: epicanthus, subcj. heme ? Calcium deposits in cj., cornea, sclera ↓ Pupil light reflex ? Cataracts	Retinal hemorrhages Papilledema Optic atrophy ? Optic neuritis Small optic discs	Strabismus Narrowed optic foramina ? EOM paresis	Nystagmus ? Hemianopia	? Teratogenesis

* Adverse side effects are seen primarily in infants.

Part I Index

Note: Proprietary drug names begin with a capital letter and are cross referenced to their generic drug names. *Generic drug names* appear in lower case letters in this index.

Part II Index: Proprietary and Generic Names

Note: Proprietary drug names begin with a capital letter and are cross referenced to their generic drug names. Proprietary drug names *do not* appear in the Part II tables; only generic names are listed. *Generic drug names* appear in lower case letters in this index. *Street names* appear in quotation marks, followed by their generic form.

Alysine (sodium salicylate), 252
amantadine, 384
ambenonium, 385
ambutonium, 361
Ambutonium (ambutonium), 361
Amcill (ampicillin), 273-274
Amcort (triamcinolone), 373
amebicides, 278
Amer-Tet (tetracycline), 275
A-Methapred (methylprednisolone), 373
amfepramone (diethylpropion), 321
amino acid derivatives, 365
aminoglycosides, 269-270
aminoquinolones, 280-281
aminosalicylates, 283
aminosalicylic acid, 283
amiodarone, 299
Amipaque (metrizamide), 388
Amithiazone (thiacetazone), 284
amithiozones, 284
Amitid (amitriptyline), 332
amitryptiline, 332
amobarbital, 342-343
amodiaquine, 280
Amosene (meprobamate), 325
amoxapine, 333
amoxicillin, 273-274
Amoxil (amoxicillin), 273-274
Amperil (ampicillin), 273-274
Amphedex (dextroamphetamine), 321
amphetamine, 321
Amphicol (chloramphenicol), 271
amphotericin B, 276
ampicillin, 273-274
Amtet (tetracycline), 275
amyl nitrite, 301
Amytal (amobarbital), 342-343
Anapap (acetaminophen), 251
Anaprox (naproxen), 255
Ancef (cefazolin), 271
androgens, 372
Anectine (succinylcholine), 259
Anelix (acetaminophen), 251
Anestacon (lidocaine), 261
"angel dust" (phencyclidine), 338
"angel's mist" (phencyclidine), 338
Angidil (isosorbide dinitrate), 300
Angijen (pentaerythritol tetratnitrate), 301
Anginar (erythrityl tetranitrate), 300
Angio-Conray (iothalamate meglumine or sodium), 388

angiotensin-converting enzyme inhibitors, 307-308
Ang-O-Span (nitroglycerin), 301
Anhydron (cyclothiazide), 353
"the animal" (LSD), 339
anisindione, 369
anisotropine, 361
Anorex (phendimetrazine), 322
Anspor (cephradine), 271
Antabuse (disulfiram), 242
Antagonate (chlorpheniramine), 265
antazoline, 266
Antepar (piperazine), 280
anthranilic acids, 251
antibiotics, 292
anticholinergics, 302, 361, 382
anticholinesterases, 385
antihelminthics, 278-279
antihistamines, 383
antimalarials, 280-281
Antime (pentaerythritol tetratnitrate), 301
antimetabolites, 287-288, 292-293
antimonials, trivalent, 278-279
antimony K$^+$ tartrate, 278
antimony Na$^+$ tartrate, 278
Antimony Sodium Tartrate (antimony Na$^+$ tartrate), 278
Antimony Sodium Thioglycollate (antimony thioglycollate), 278
antimony thioglycollate, 278
antiprotozoals, 282
antipyrine, 252
Antispas (dicyclomine), 362
Antitrem (trihexyphenidyl), 382
Antivert (meclizine), 358
Antora (pentaerythritol tetratnitrate), 301
Antrenyl (oxyphenonium), 362
Anucaine (procaine), 261
Anuphen (acetaminophen), 251
Anusol-HC (hydrocortisone), 373
Apamide (acetaminophen), 251
Apap (acetaminophen), 251
A.P.B. (aprobarbital), 342-343
A-Poxide (chlordiazepoxide), 323-324
Apresoline (hydralazine), 309
aprobarbital, 342-343
Aquachloral (chloral hydrate), 340
Aquapres (benzthiazide), 353
Aqua-Scrip (benzthiazide), 353
Aquasec (benzthiazide), 353
Aquasol (vitamin A), 397
Aquatensen (methyclothiazide), 353
Aquatog (benzthiazide), 353

Ro-Cillin (potassium phenethicillin), 273
Ro-Cillin VK (potassium penicillin V), 273
Rocinolone (triamcinolone), 373
"rocket fuel" (phencyclidine), 338
Roclizine (meclizine), 358
Ro-Cycline (tetracycline), 275
Rocyclo (dicyclomine), 362
Ro-Diet (diethylpropion), 321
Rodryl (diphenhydramine), 265
Roferon-A (interferon), 295-296
Rohydra (diphenhydramine), 265
Ro-Hydrazide (hydrochlorothiazide), 353
Rolabromophen (brompheniramine), 265
Rolamethazine (promethazine), 335-336
Rolaphent (phentermine), 322
Rolathimide (glutethimide), 344
Rolazid (isoniazid), 285
Romethocarb (methocarbamol), 382
Rondomycin (methacycline), 275
Roniacol (nicotinyl alcohol), 315
Ropanth (propantheline), 362
"rope" (marihuana), 338
Ropledge (phendimetrazine), 322
Ropoxy (propoxyphene), 246
Ropred (prednisone), 373
Ropredlone (prednisolone), 373
Roquine (chloroquine), 280
Rotyl (dicyclomine), 362
Roxanol (morphine), 248
RP-Mycin (erythromycin), 272
RTU (metronidazole), 282
rubbing alcohol (methanol), 390
Rufen (ibuprofen), 253
"Rx diet pills" (amphetamine, dextroamphetamine, methamphetamine), 321

St. Joseph Aspirin (aspirin), 252
Salazopyrin (sulfasalazine), 275
salbutamol (albuterol), 316
salicylates, 252
Salicylazosulfapyridine (sulfasalazine), 275
Saluron (hydroflumethiazide), 353
Sandimmune (cyclosporine), 380
Sandoptal (butalbital), 342-343
Sandril (reserpine), 311
Sansert (methysergide), 312
S-Aqua (benzthiazide), 353
Sarocycline (tetracycline), 275
Sarodant (nitrofurantoin), 272-273
Sarogesic (prednisone), 373

Saropen-VK (potassium penicillin V), 273
S.A.S-50 (sulfasalazine), 275
S.A.S.P. (sulfasalazine), 275
Satric (metronidazole), 282
Savacort 50/100 (prednisolone), 373
Savacort D (dexamethasone), 372
"scag" (diacetylmorphine), 247
"schmeck" (diacetylmorphine), 247
"schoolboy" (codeine), 246
scopolamine, 259
Scotrex (tetracycline), 275
Screen (chlordiazepoxide), 323-324
Scrip-Dyne (propoxyphene), 246
S.D.M. 23/35 (pentaerythritol tetratnitrate), 301
S.D.M.N. 50 (mannitol hexanitrate), 301
Sebizon (sulfacetamide), 274-275
Seco-8 (secobarbital), 343
secobarbital, 343
Seconal (secobarbital), 343
Sectral (acebutolol), 306-307
Sedadrops -Square (phenobarbital), 343
Sed-Tens SE (homatropine), 361
Seffin (cephalothin), 271
Semitard (insulin), 359
semustine, 290-291
Serax (oxazepam), 323-324
Serensil (ethchlorvynol), 342
Serentil (mesoridazine), 335-336
Serfia (rauwolfia serpentina), 311
Serfin (reserpine), 311
Serfolia (rauwolfia serpentina), 311
Seromycin (cycloserine), 284
Serp (reserpine), 311
Serpalan (reserpine), 311
Serpaloid (reserpine), 311
Serpanray (reserpine), 311
Serpasil (reserpine), 311
Serpate (reserpine), 311
Serpena (reserpine), 311
Sertabs (reserpine), 311
Sertina (reserpine), 311
Servisone (prednisone), 373
"714s" (methaqualone), 345
"sheets" (phencyclidine), 338
"shit" (diacetylmorphine), 247
"shrooms" (psilocybin), 339
Sigazine (promethazine), 335-336
Sigpred (prednisolone), 373
Sinequan (doxepin), 333
SK-65 (propoxyphene), 246